Applied Principles of Biomaterials in Nanomedicine

Applied Principles of Biomaterials in Nanomedicine

Edited by **Ralph Seguin**

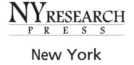

New York

Published by NY Research Press,
23 West, 55th Street, Suite 816,
New York, NY 10019, USA
www.nyresearchpress.com

Applied Principles of Biomaterials in Nanomedicine
Edited by Ralph Seguin

Printed in the United States of America.

Contents

Preface

This book is a collection of reviews and original researches by experts and scientists working in the field of biomaterials, its development and applications. It offers readers the potentials of distinct synthetic and engineered biomaterials. This book gives a comprehensive summary of the applications of various biomaterials, along with the techniques required for designing, developing and classifying these biomaterials without any intervention by any industrial source. Biomaterial structures and supramolecules are examined as protein carriers, tissue scaffolds etc. The researches and reviews focus on the functions of novel and familiar macromolecular compounds in nanotechnology and nanomedicine. The book also elucidates the chemical and mechanical modeling of these compounds so as to serve biomedical needs.

This book unites the global concepts and researches in an organized manner for a comprehensive understanding of the subject. It is a ripe text for all researchers, students, scientists or anyone else who is interested in acquiring a better knowledge of this dynamic field.

I extend my sincere thanks to the contributors for such eloquent research chapters. Finally, I thank my family for being a source of support and help.

Editor

Part 1

Biomaterials Processing and Engineering

Collagen- vs. Gelatine-Based Biomaterials and Their Biocompatibility: Review and Perspectives

Selestina Gorgieva[1] and Vanja Kokol[1,2]
[1]University of Maribor, Institute for Engineering Materials and Design, Maribor
[2]Center of Excellence NAMASTE, Ljubljana,
Slovenia

1. Introduction

Selection of a starting material, which will somehow mimic a naturally-existing one, is one of the most important points and crucial elements in biomaterials development. **Material biomimetism** is one of those approaches, where restoration of an organ's function is assumed to be obtained if the tissues themselves are imitated (Barrere et al., 2008). However, some of the biopolymers as e.g collagen can be selected from within a group of biomimetic materials, since they already exist, and have particular functions in the human body.

Collagen is one of the key structural proteins found in the extracellular matrices of many connective tissues in mammals, making up about 25% to 35% of the whole-body protein content (Friess, 2000; Muyonga et al., 2004). Collagen is mostly found in fibrous tissues such as tendons, ligaments and skin (about one half of total body collagen), and is also abundant in corneas, cartilages, bones, blood vessels, the gut, and intervertebral discs (Brinckmann et al., 2005). It constitutes 1% to 2% of muscle tissue, and accounts for 6% of strong, tendinous muscle-weight. Collagen is synthesized by fibroblasts, which originate from pluripotential adventitial cells or reticulum cells. Up to date 29 collagen types have been identified and described. Over 90% of the collagen in the body is of type I and is found in bones, skins, tendons, vascular, ligatures, and organs. However, in the human formation of scar tissue, as a result of age or injury, there is an alteration in the abundance of types I and III collagen, as well as their proportion to one another (Cheng et al., 2011).

Collagen is readily isolated and purified in large quantities, it has well-documented structural, physical, chemical and immunological properties, is biodegradable, biocompatible, non-cytotoxic, with an ability to support cellular growth, and can be processed into a variety of forms including cross-linked films, steps, sheets, beads, meshes, fibres, and sponges (Sinha & Trehan, 2003). Hence, collagen has already found considerable usage in clinical medicine over the past few years, such as injectable collagen for the augmentation of tissue defects, haemostasis, burn and wound dressings, hernia repair, bioprostetic heart valves, vascular grafts, a drug –delivery system, ocular surfaces, and nerve regeneration (Lee et al., 2001). However, certain properties of collagen have adversely influenced some of its usage: poor dimensional stability due to swelling in vivo; poor in vivo mechanical strength and low elasticity, the possibility of an antigenic response (Lynn et al., 2004) causing tissue irritation due to residual aldehyde cross-linking agents, poor patient tolerance of inserts, variability in releasing kinetics, and ineffectiveness in the management of infected sites (Friess, 1998). In addition, there is the high-cost of pure type I collagen, variability in the enzymatic degradation rate when compared with hydrolytic degradation, variability of isolated collagen in cross-link density, fibre size, trace impurities, and side-effects, such as bovine spongeform encephalopathy (BSF) and mineralization. The above-mentioned disadvantages must be considered during collagen use in medical applications (Pannone, 2007).

In this review collagen will be presented and compared to its degradation product, gelatine, taking into account their molecular and submolecular structural properties, possibilities to overcome common problems related to their usage as biomaterial, i.e. the solubility and degradation rate mechanisms, as well as their applications in combination with other types of (bio)polymers.

2. Molecular and submolecular structure of collagen vs. gelatine

2.1 Collagen

The **collagen** rod-shape molecule (or *tropocollagen*) is a subunit of larger collagen fibril aggregates. The lengths of each subunit are approximately 300 nm and the diameter of the triple helix is ~1.5 nm. It is made up of three polypeptide α-chains, each possessing the conformation of a left-handed, polyproline II-type (PPII) helix (Fig. 1). These three left-handed helices are twisted together into a right-handed coiled coil, a triple-helix which represent a **quaternary structure** of collagen, being stabilized by numerous hydrogen bonds and intra-molecular van de Waals interactions (Brinckmann et al., 2005) as well as some covalent bonds (Harkness, 1966), and further associated into right-handed microfibrils (~40 nm in diameter) and fibrils (100-200 nm in diameter), being further assembled into collagen fibres (He et al., 2011) with unusual strength and stability.

The **primary structure** of collagen shows a strong sequence homology across genus and adjacent family line (Muyonga et a., 2004), thus a distinctive feature of collagen is the regular arrangement of amino acids in each of the three chains of collagen subunits. The sequence of amino acids is characterized by a repetitive unit of glycine (Gly)-proline (Pro)-X or Gly-X- hydroxyproline (Hyp), where Gly accounting for the 1/3 of the sequence, whilst X and Y may be any of various other amino acid residues. However, the X-position is occupied almost exclusively by Pro, whereas Hyp is found predominantly in the Y-position (Gorham, 1991), both constitute of about 1/6 of the total sequence. This kind of regular repetition and high Gly content is found in only a few other fibrous proteins, such as silk fibroin and elastin, but never in globular proteins. Thus the super-coil of collagen is stabilized by hydrogen bonds between Gly and Pro located in neighbouring chains and by an extensive water-network which can form hydrogen bonds between several carbonyl and hydroxyl peptide residues (Brinckmann et al., 2005). Furthermore, amino acids in the X- and Y-positions are able to participate in intermolecular stabilization, e.g. by hydrophobic interactions or interactions between charged residues, mostly coming from Pro and Hyp residues steric repulsion (Brinckmann et al., 2005). This helical part is further flanked by short non-helical domains (9-26 amino acids), the so called telopeptides, which play an important role in fibril formation and natural cross-linking. After spontaneous helix formation, cross-links between chains are formed within the region of the N-terminal telopeptides (globular tail portion of the chains), and then the telopeptides (containing the

Collagen- vs. Gelatine-Based Biomaterials and Their Biocompatibility: Review and Perspectives

5

cysteine (Cys) and tyrosine (Tyr) of pro-collagen) are shed leaving the rod-like ca. 3150 amino acid containing triple helix. These collagen rods assemble together with a quarter-stagger to form the collagen fibre and the fibres are stabilised by further cross-links.

Type I (Fig. 2) collagen, the predominant genetic type in the collagen family being the major component of tendons, bones and ligaments, is a heterotrimeric copolymer composed of two α1 (I) and one α2 (I) chains, containing approximately 1050 amino acids each. This collagen type contains one-third of Gly, contains no tryptophan (Trp) or Cys, and is very low in Tyr and histidine (His) (Muyonga et al., 2004). Its molecule consist of three domains: amino-terminal nontriple helical (N-telopeptide), central triple helical consisting of more than 300 repeat units and represent more than 95% of polypeptide, and carboxy-terminal nontriple helical (C-telopeptide) (Yamauchi & Shiiba, 2008). New data show that besides the telopeptides, tropocollagens still contain the N- and C-terminal propeptide sequences, called non-collagenous domains (Brinckmann et al., 2005), which are responsible for correct chain alignment and triple helix formation. The propeptides are removed before fibril formation and regulate the fibril formation process. Tropocollagens are staggered longitudinally and bilaterally by inter- and intra-molecular cross-links into microfibrils (4 to 8 tropocollagens) and further into fibrils. This periodic arrangement is characterized by a gap of 40 nm between succeeding collagen molecules and by a displacement of 67 nm. The fibrils organize into fibres which, in turn, can form large fibre bundles, being both stabilized by intermolecular cross-links (Friess, 1998).

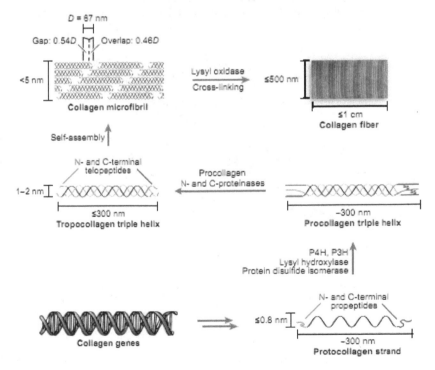

Fig. 1. Biosynthetic route of collagen fibers (Shoulders & Raines, 2009)

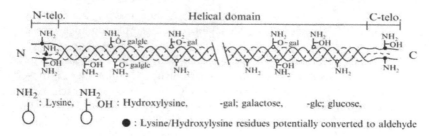

Fig. 2. Structure of type I collagen molecule. (Yamauchi & Shiiba, 2008) and (http://www.kokenmpc.co.jp/english/support/tecnical/collagen/index.html).

Collagen **types I, II, III, and V** (Fig. 3) are called fibril- forming collagens and have large sections of homologous sequences independent of species, among which first three types are known to be chemotactic (Chevallay & Herbage, 2000). Type II collagen, the main component of a nose cartilage , the outside of the ears, the knees and parts of larynx and trachea, is a homotrimer composed of three α1 (II) chain (Shoulders and Rains, 2009), whilst **type III** collagen, present in skin and blood vessels is homotrimer, composed of three α1 (III) chains (Gelse et al., 2003). In **type IV** collagen, being present in basement membrane, the regions with the triple-helical conformation are interrupted with large non-helical domains, as well as with the short non-helical peptide interruption. **Types IX, XI, XII and XIV** are fibril associated collagens with small chains, which contain some non-helical domains. **Type VI** is microfibrillar collagen and **type VII** is anchoring fibril collagen (Samuel et al., 1998).

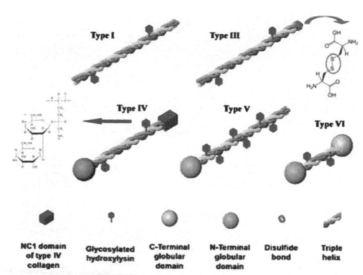

Fig. 3. Schematic presentation of main structural differences between the most abundant collagen types of extracellular matrix in human tissues (Belbachir et al., 2009).

From among all the known collagen types, three-dimensional (3D) model of fibril-forming **type II** collagen was proposed for the development of synthetic collagen tissues and the study of the structural and functional aspects of collagen (Chen et al., 1995) due its orderly arrangement of triple helix tropocollagen molecules, results in a formation of fibrils having a distinct periodicity. Thus this system also allows the studies of the stereochemistry of all the side-chain groups and specific atomic interactions, and further evaluation of its therapeutic effects on collagen related diseases.

2.1.1 Antigenicity of collagen

A chemical compound that stimulates an immune response is called an antigen, or an immunogen. A host's immune response is not directed toward the entire antigen molecule, but rather to specific chemical groups called epitopes, or antigenic determinants on the molecule, which are responsible for the immunogenic properties of the antigen. Two important characteristic of antigens are **immunogenicity** (specific immune response) and **reactivity** (ability to react with specific antigen) where "complete antigen" possess both characteristics, whilst, "incomplete antigen" do not show immunogenicity, but is able to bind with antibodies (Kokare, 2008). The status of **collagen** as an **animal-derived biomaterial** raise concerns regarding its potential to evoke immune response. Its ability to interact with secreted antibodies (**antigenicity**) and to induce an immune response–process that includes synthesis of the same antibodies (**immunogenicity**), are connected with macromolecular features of a protein, uncommon to the host species, such as collagen with animal origin. When compared with other proteins, collagens are weakly immunogenic, due to evidences of its ability to interact with antibodies (Gorham, 1991). Clinical observations indicate that 2-4 % of the total population posses an inherent immunity (allergy) to bovine type collagen (Cooperman & Michaeli, 1984).

According to Lynn (Lynn et al., 2004), antigenic determinants (epitopes, macromolecular features on an antigen molecule that interact with antibodies) of collagen can be classified into following categories (Fig. 4):
1. Helical- recognition by antibodies is dependent on 3D conformation (i.e., the presence of an intact triple helix).
2. Central- recognitions are located within the triple helical portion of native collagen, but recognition based solely on amino acid sequence and not on 3D conformation. They are often hidden, only interacting with antibodies when the triple helix has unwound, e.g. in denatured state.
3. Terminal- recognitions are major antigenic determinants (Lee et al., 2001), located in the non-helical terminal regions (telopeptides), but can be eliminated by pepsine treatment leading to atelocollagen (Fig. 5) (Chevallay & Herbage, 2000; Hsu et al., 1999; Kikuchi et al., 2004). Telopeptide cleavage results in collagen whose triple-helical conformation is intact, yet as both the amino and carboxyl telopeptides play important roles in cross-linking and fibril formation, their complete removal results in an amorphous arrangement of collagen molecules and a consequent loss of the banded-fibril pattern in the reconstituted product, and significant increase in solubility (Lynn, 2004).

The possible use of recombinant human collagen (although more expensive) could be a way of removing concerns of species-to-species transmissible diseases (Olsen et al., 2003). However, complete **immunogenic purification** of non-human proteins is difficult, which may result in immune rejection if used in implants. Impure collagen has the potential for xenozoonoses, a microbial transmission from the animal tissue to the human recipient (Canceda et al., 2003). Anyhow, although collagen extracted from animal sources may present a small degree of antigenicity, it is widely considered acceptable for tissue engineering on humans (Friess, 1998). Furthermore, the literature has yet to find any significant evidence on human immunological benefits of deficient-telopeptide collagens (Wahl & Czernuszka, 2006).

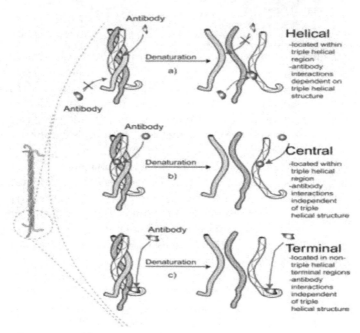

Fig. 4. Classes of antigenic determinants of collagen (Lynn et al., 2004).

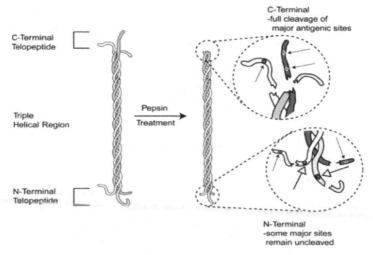

Fig. 5. Telopeptide removal via pepsin treatment (Lynn et al., 2004).

So, atelocollagen produced from type II collagen has demonstrated its potential as a drug carrier, especially for gene delivery (Lee et al., 2001). However, collagen type IV possesses a strong immunogenic character, even after pepsin treatment (Chevallay & Herbage, 2000). **Another approach** for rendering the reduction of collagen antigenicity and the immune reaction, has been presented, where the amino and carboxyl side groups are blocked by glutarladehyde cross-linking (Hardin-Young et al., 2000). However, data from studies using glutaraldehyde as the cross-linking agent are hard to interpret because glutaraldehyde treatment is also known to leave behind cytotoxic residues. It is, therefore, possible that the reduced antigenicity associated with glutaraldehyde cross-linking is due to nonspecific cytotoxicity rather than a specific effect on antigenic determinants.

2.2 Gelatine

Gelatine is the product of thermal denaturation or disintegration of insoluble collagen (Gomez-Gullien et al., 2009) with various molecular weights (MWs) and isoionic points (IEPs) depending on the source of collagen and the method of its manufacturing process of recovery from collagen. Collagen exists in many different forms, but gelatine is only derived from sources rich in **Type I collagen** thet generally contains no Cys. Collagen used for gelatine manufacturing can be from different sources, among which anyhow bovine and porcine gelatines are more-widely used. Alternative sources of collagen for gelatine production have been studied in last decade, such as fish skins, bones and fins (Nagai & Suzuki , 2000), sea urchin (Robinson, 1997), jellyfish (Nagai et al., 2000) and bird feet from Encephalopat (Herpandi et al., 2011). However, the amino acid compositions are slightly different among all types of gelatine from different sources. Amino acids from pigskin gelatine and bone gelatines do not contain Cys, but fish scale and bone gelatine instead, which has less content of Gly in comparison with mammalian sources (Zhang et al., 2010). With the exception of gelatine from pigskin origin, all other gelatines do not contain aspartic acid (Asp) and glutamic acid (Glu).

During the **denaturation-hydrolysis process** (Fig. 6), collagen triple-helix organization is hydrolyzed at those sites where covalent cross-links join the three peptides, which in case of type B gelatine produced by partial alkaline hydrolysis of collagen, leads to polydisperse polypeptide mixture with average MW of 40-90 kDa, instead of MW ~ 100 kDa as related to collagen α-chains; the collagen denaturation in its passage to gelatine can be followed polarimetrically by reduction of specific optical rotation $[\alpha]_D$ of collagen (Cataldo et al., 2008).

As the collagen matures, the cross-links become stabilised, because ε-amino groups of lysine (Lys) become linked to arginine (Arg) by glucose molecules (Mailard reaction), forming extremely stable **pentosidine type cross-links**. During the **alkaline processing**, the alkali breaks one of the initial (pyridinoline) cross-links and as a result, on heating the collagen releases, mainly, denatured α-chains into solution. Once the pentosidine cross-links of the mature animal have formed in the collagen, the main process of denaturation has to be thermal hydrolysis of peptide bonds, resulting in protein fragments being from below 100 kDa to more than 700 kDa, and with IEP between 4,6 and 9. During the **acid process**, the collagen denaturation is limited to the thermal hydrolysis of peptide bonds, with a small amount of α-chain material from acid soluble collagen in evidence. Based on this, gelatine is divided into two main types: **Type A,** which is derived from collagen of pig skin by acid pre-treatment with IEP of 7 - 9, and **Type B,** which is derived from collagen of beef hides or bones by liming (alkaline process) with IEP of 4.6 - 5.4.

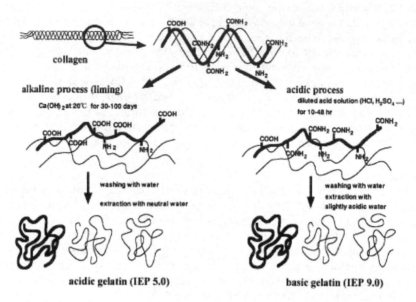

Fig. 6. Two methods for gelatine extraction from tissues containing collagen (Ikada, 2002).

Type A gelatine (dry and ash free) contains 18.5 % nitrogen, but due to the loss of amide groups, **Type B gelatine** contains only about 18% nitrogen. Amino acid analysis of gelatine is variable, particularly for the minor constituents, depending on the raw material and process used, but proximate values by weight are: Gly 21 %, Pro 12 %, Hyp 12 %, Glu 10 %, alanine (Ala) 9 %, Arg 8 %, Asp 6 %, Lys 4 %, serine (Ser) 4 %, leucine (Leu) 3 %, valine (Val) 2 %, phenylalanine (Phe) 2 %, threonine (Thr) 2 %, isoleucine (Ile) 1 %, hydroxylysine (Hyl) 1 %, methionine (Met), His < 1 % and Tyr < 0.5 %. It should be remembered that the peptide bond has considerable aromatic character; hence gelatine shows an absorption maximum at ca. 230 nm.

Collagen is resistant to most proteases and requires special collagenases for its enzyme hydrolysis. Gelatine, however, is susceptible to most proteases, but they do not break gelatine down into peptides containing much less than 20 amino acids (Cole, 2000).

Gelatine forms physical gels in hydrogen-bond friendly solvents above a concentration larger than the chain overlap concentration (~ 2 % w/v). The gelatine sol undergoes a first order thermo-reversible gelation transition at temperatures lower then Tg with is ~30°C, during which gelatine molecules undergo an association-mediated conformational transition from random coil to triple helix. The sol has polydisperse random coils of gelatine molecules and aggregates, whereas in gel state there is propensity of triple helices stabilized through intermolecular hydrogen bonding, during which, three dimensional (3D) interconnected network connecting large fractions of the gelatine chains is formed (Mohanty & Bohidar, 2003, 2005).

On cooling, gelatine chains can rewind, but not within the correct register, and small triple-helical segments formed may further aggregate during gel formation. The lateral aggregation of gelatin triple helix that give rise to collagen fibrils in vivo, does not occur in gelatine gels (Chavez et al., 2006). Hydrogel formation, accompanied by a disorder-order rearrangement in which gelatine chains partially recover the triple helix collagen structure, leads to forming of renaturated gelatine with amorphous main regions of randomly-coiled gelatine chains interconnected with domains of spatially-ordered microcrystallites, stabilized by hydrogen bonds between N-H of Gly and C=O from Pro. Stabilization of molecular conformation and inter-helix interactions are a consequence of the existence of a highly-ordered hydration shell with water bridges linking two groups within the same or different gelatine chains. Hydrogen bond formation is responsible for the increase in denaturation temperature of the fixed tissue; when compared to the pig-skin and bovine gelatines, which have ~30% Pro and Hyp, fish gelatines possess a lesser percentage of Pro and Hyp (~20 %), the impact of which is thermal stability and shifting by 5-10°C to lower gelling and melting temperatures (Farris et al., 2009) and gel strength (Herpandy et al., 2011).

Despite gelatine being one of the polymers recognized for millennia, questions about its structure and functionality are still being discussed today. The 3D network of gelatine has been defined by several authors using "fringed micelle" model in which there are micro-crystallites interconnected with amorphous regions of randomly-coiled segments, whilst other authors propose the existence of local regions of protein quaternary structure, self-limiting in size, which can be triple-helical, only partially triple-helical or also include β-turn and β-sheet motifs (Pena et al., 2010).

2.2.1 Antigenicity of gelatine

Due to modern manufacturing sites and the use of highly advanced, controlled manufacturing processes with numerous purification steps (washing, filtration), heat-treatments including a final ultra-heat treatment (UHT) sterilization step followed by a drying of the gelatine solution, gelatine with highest quality can be prepared in regard to physical, chemical, bacteriological and virological safety.

During Bovine Spongiform Encephalopathy (BSE), all products of bovine origin were under suspicion as being possible transmitters of disease to humans. Thus several studies have been done to demonstrate the capability of certain steps during gelatine production to inactivate BSE infectivity, showing a reduction of SE infectivity for acid demineralization and lime-treatment of 10 and 100 times, respectively. The combined reduction has been found to be 1000 times.

The classical UHT sterilization used in gelatin manufacture should also reduce any residual infectivity 100 times, or more probably 1000 times (Taylor et al., 1994). Washing, filtration, ion exchange and other chemicals or treatments used in the manufacture of gelatine would reduce the SE activity even further (by an assumed ratio of 100 times).

However, it is also a known fact that gelatine is a non-immunogenic material, yet very little research has been done on this theme, thus most knowledge is based on early experiments (Hopkins & Wormall, 1933), where this gelatine property was described to be connected with the absence of aromatic ring. Gelatine non-antigenicity has attracted attention by (Starin, 1918) who, in particular, carried out an extensive investigation, using the precipitin, anaphylactic, complement fixation and meiostagmin reactions, and decided that the injection of gelatine into rabbits, guinea-pigs and dogs failed to produce antibodies by gelatine. This failure of gelatine to incite antibody production has been interpreted in several ways, but the view most commonly held suggests that the non-antigenicity, in this instance, is due to the absence of aromatic groupings, as gelatine is deficient in Tyr and Trp, and contains only a very small amount of Phe. A similar explanation for gelatin´s non-immunogenic property was given by (Kokare, 2008), where is stated that gelatine is non-antigenic because of the absence of aromatic radicals.

3. Cross-linking of collagen vs. gelatine and their immuno response effect

Collagen isolation by pepsin digestion involves de-polymerization of collagen by removing amino and carboxyl- terminal telopeptides containing the intermolecular cross-links. The isolated collagen thus exhibits poor thermal stability, mechanical strength and water resistance, due to the destruction of natural cross-links and assembly structure by neutral salt, acid, alkali, or proteases during the extraction process (Sisson et al., 2009). In order to increase their strength and enzyme resistance, and to maintain their stability during implantation, especially for long term application, collagenous matrices are usually stabilized by cross-linking (Yannas, 1992; Tefft et al., 1997). In addition, cross-linking permits a reduction in the antigenicity of collagen and, in some forms, decreases its calcification (Damnik, 1996).

Method	Collagen	Gelatine
Chemical cross-linking		
Aldehydes e.g. glutaraldehyde (GTA)	Charulatha et al., 2003; Kikuchi et al., 2004; Mu et al., 2010, Ma et al., 2003	Sisson et al.; 2009, Farrist et al.; 2009
Dialdehide starch (DAS)	Mu et al., 2010	Martucci & Ruseckaite, 2009
Acyl azide	Charulatha et al.; 2003, Friess; 1999,	
Diphenylphosphorylazide (DPPA)	Khor, 1997, Roche et al.; 2001	
Carbodiimides, e.g.1-ethyl-3- (3 dimethylamino-propyl)(EDC)	Park et al.; 2002, Pieper et al.; 1999, Kim et al., 2001, Song et al., 2006	Barbetta et al.; 2010, Natu et al.; 2007, Chang et al.; 2007, Kuijpers et al.; 2000
Hexamethylene diisocyanate	Friess, 1999	
Ethylene glycol diglycidyl ether		Vargas et al.; 2008
Polyepoxy compounds	Friess, 1999; Khor, 1997, Zeeman et al., 1999	
Phenolic compounds	Han et al.; 2003; Jackson et al., 2010	Kim et al.; 2005; Zhang et al.; 2010; Pena et al.;2010
Genipin	Ko et al.; 2007; Yan et al., 2010	Yao et al.; 2005, Lien et al.; 2010, Bigi et al., 2002; Chiono et al., 2008; Mi et al., 2005
Citric acid derivative (CAD)		Saito et al., 2004
Enzymatic crosslinking		
Transglutaminase	Jus et al.; 2011	Bertoni et al., 2006; Fuchs et al., 2010, Sztuka & Kolodziejska, 2008
Tyrosinase	Jus et al.; 2011	Chen et al., 2003
Laccasse	Jus et al.; 2011	
Physical crosslinking		
Dehydrothermal treatment (DHT)	Pieper et al., 1999; Tangsadthakun, et al., 2006	Dubruel et. al.; 2007
UV irradiation	Torikai & Shibata, 1999	Bhat & Karim, 2009
γ-radiation	Labout , 1972	Cataldo et al.; 2008

Table 1. Overview over cross-linking methods for collagen vs. gelatine materials

Different ways of collagen (as well as gelatine) cross-linking, **either chemical, enzymatic or physical**, have been carried out and often the method is prescribed by the target application (see Table 1).

Aldehydes have a long tradition as cross-linking reagents. Treatment with **glutaraldehide (GTA)**, in particular, is intensively used. Besides its good efficiency, this cross-linking method is fast, inexpensive and mechanical properties are enhanced (Friess, 1999). Cross-linking reaction occurs between carboxyl groups on the Glu and amine groups of Lys, or Arg forming a Shiff-base as presented on Fig. 7. However, due to the polymerization of GTA, cross-linking is sometimes restricted to the surface of the device and a heterogeneous cross-linking structure can then occur (Cheung et al., 1984). Additionally, GTA is incorporated into the new linkage and unreacted GTA can cause local incompatibility, inflammation or calcification (Luyn et al., 1995), along with limited cell ingrowth (Jayakrishnan et al.; 1996) and cytotoxicity (Sisson et al., 2009) even at concentrations of 3.0 ppm after being released into the host as a result of collagen biodegradation. From other side, glutaraldehide-based cross-linking is the current standard procedure for the production of heart valves, providing the prosthesis with low incidences of thrombo-embolism and satisfactory haemodynamic performance (Everaerts et al., 2007).

Reconstituted collagen membranes cross-linked with **3,3'-dithiobispropionimidate (DTBP)** and **diimidoesters-dimethyl suberimidate (DMS)** (Fig. 8) are shown to be more biocompatible than those treated with GTA (Charulatha & Rajaram, 2001).

Non-toxic, water soluble substances which only facilitate the reaction, without becoming part of the new linkage, are **acyl azides** and carbodiimides. **Carbodiimides, e.g. EDC**, couple carboxyl groups of Glu or Asp with amino groups of Lys or Hyl residues, thus forming stable amide bonds (Fig. 9). Reaction efficacy is increased by addition of **N-hydroxysuccinimde (NHS)** which prevents hydrolysis and rearrangement of the intermediate (Friess, 1999; Gorham, 1991; Olde Damink et al., 1996), thus causing the formation of a coarse structure instead of tougher microstructure, in its absence (Chang & Douglas, 2007). Because EDC can only couple groups within a distance of 1 nm, this treatment enhances intra- and interhelical linkages within or between tropocollagen molecules (Sung et al., 2003), without an inter-microfibrillar cross-links (Zeeman et al., 1999). EDC cross-linked collagens show reduced calcification, with no cytotoxicity and slow enzymatic degradation (Khor, 1997; Pieper et al., 1999).

Some natural non-toxic and biodegradable molecules with favourable biocompatibility have been exploited as protein cross-linkers, such as **D,L-glycceraldehyde** (Sisson et al., 2009), **oxidized alginate** (Balakrishnan & Jayakrishnan, 2005**), dialdehyde starch (DAS** (Mu et al., 2010), Fig. 10) **and genipin**.

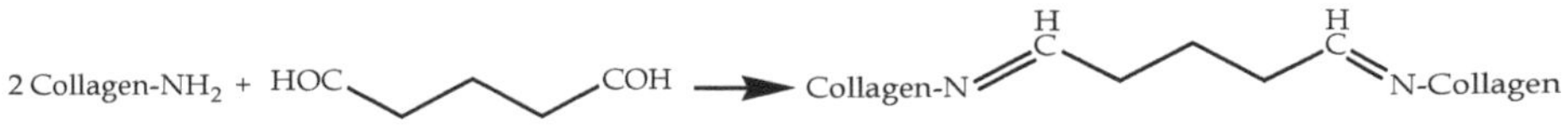

$$2\,\text{Collagen-NH}_2 + \text{HOC} \diagup\diagdown\diagup\diagdown \text{COH} \longrightarrow \text{Collagen-N} = \overset{H}{\underset{}{C}} \diagup\diagdown\diagup\diagdown \overset{H}{\underset{}{C}} = \text{N-Collagen}$$

Fig. 7. Crosllinking of collagen with glutaraldehyde (GTA)

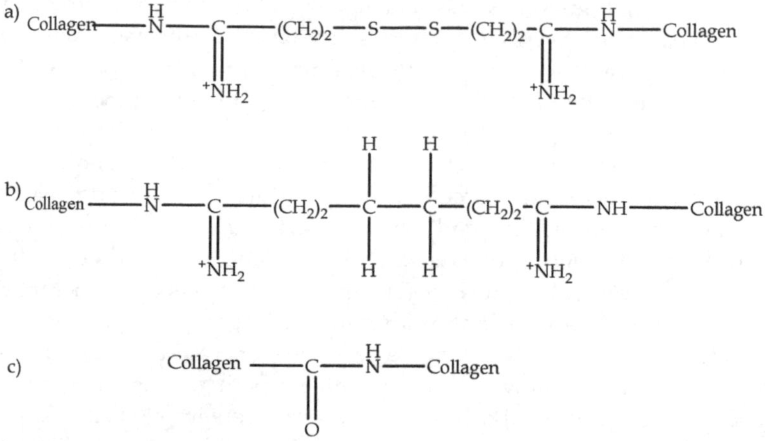

Fig. 8. Structure of cross-links obtained by (a) DTBP, (b) DMS and (c) acyl azide treatments (Charulatha & Rajaram, 2003).

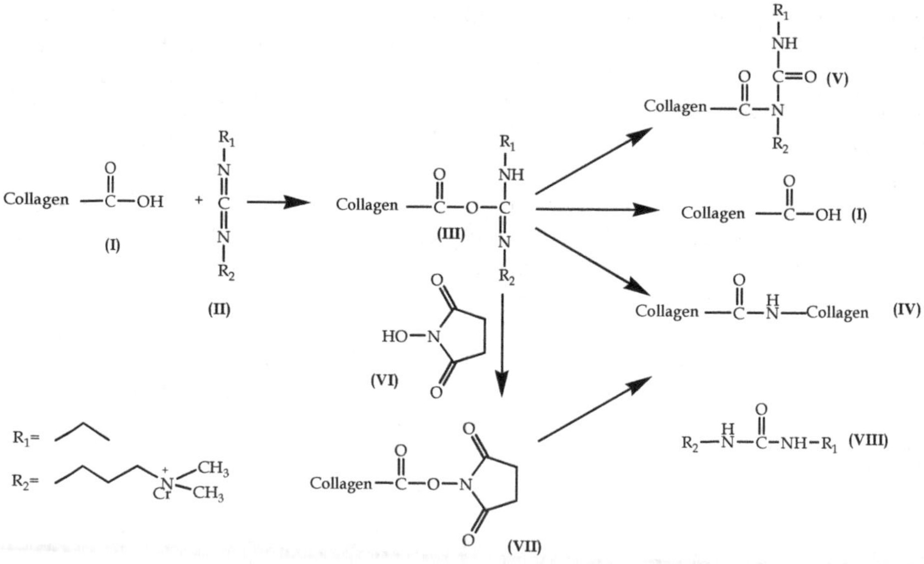

Fig. 9. Crosllinking of collagen with EDC and NHS: (I) collagen, (II) EDC, (III) O-acylurea intermediate, (IV.) CO-NH bond formation, (V) N-acylurea intermediate (VI) NHS, (VII) NHS-activated carboxylic group in collagen and (VIII) substituted urea (Damnik et al., 1996).

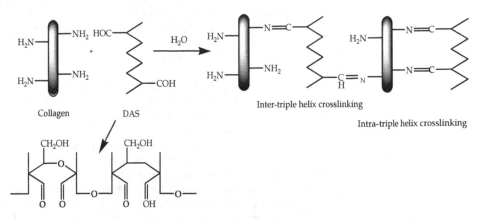

Fig. 10. Cross-linking of collagen with DAS involving Schiff's base formation between ε-amino groups from Lys or Hyl side-groups of collagen and aldehyde groups in DAS (Sission et al., 2009)

Recently, **polyphenols,** such as procyanidin (He, 2011), proanthocyanidin (Kim et al., 2005; Han et al., 2003), caffeic and tannic acids (Zhang et al., 2010), epigallocatehin and epicatehin gallates (Jackson et al., 2010), and other tannins (Pena et al., 2010) have also been used for this purpose, additionally bringing antioxidant activity, pharmacological activity, and therapeutic potential to the biomaterial due their free-radical scavenging capacities. Not only the antioxidant activity of polyphenols, but also their other physiological properties, such as anti-allergenic, anti-inflammatory, antimicrobial, cardioprotective, and anti-thrombotic make these compounds very interesting raw materials for medical applications (Pena et al., 2010). It has been shown that some of them are able to stabilize collagen and protect the chains from collagenase degradation more effectively than glutaraldehyde and carbodiimides, thus extend the implanted material over a longer period, using very low concentration (Jackson et al., 2010). The interactions between protein and polyphenol can involve hydrogen bond, covalent linkage, ionic and hydrophobic bonding. The reaction mechanism involves an initial oxidization of phenolic structures to quinones, which can readily react with nucleophiles from reactive amino acid groups in protein: sulfuhydryl group in Cys, amino group of Lys and Arg, amide group from Asp and Glu, indole ring of Trp and imidazole ring from His (Zhang et al., 2010). Nevertheless, the effect of polyphenol on the microstructure of collagen, i.e. from triple-helixes to fibrils, remains largely unknown. In reaction mechanism between gelatin and tannin are involved hydrogen bonds between hydroxyl groups of tannin and polar groups of gelatin, and hydrophobic interactions between pyrrolidine ring of Pro and pentagalloyl glucose from tannin (Obreque-Slier et al., 2010; Pena et al., 2010).

Anti-inflammatory properties are added values during **genipin**-induced cross-linking, showing to be 10, 000 times less cytotoxic then glutaraldehide which may produce weakly clastogenic responces in CHO-K1 cells (Tsai et al., 2000; Sisson et al., 2009). Moreover, the minimal calcium content of genipin–fixed tissue was detected (Chang, 2001). Genipin is a natural product, being obtained from an iridoid glucoside, geniposide abundantly present in *Genipa Americana* and *Gardenia jasminoides Ellis.* Although the cross-linking mechanism of genipin with gelatine (or collagen) is insufficiently understood, it is known that genipin reacts with free amino groups of proteins (Fig. 11), such as Lys, Hyl and Arg, forming dark blue colour, thus acting as monomeric or oligomeric bridge which results in a comparable mechanical strength and resistence against enzymatic degradation as the glutaraldehyde-fixed tissues (Mi et al., 2005; Bigi, et al., 2002); the maximum cross-linking percentage when using genipin as a cross-linker enriched in gelatin films, is about 85% (Bigi et al., 2002). Touyama group (Touyama et al., 1994) proposed a mechanism for the reaction of genipin with a methylamine, were, reaction occurred through a nucleophilic attack of the primary amine on the C3 carbon of genipin, causing an opening of the dihydropiran ring. An attack then followed on the resulting aldehyde group by the secondary amine group. The final step in formation of the cross-linking material is believed to be dimerization produced by radical reactions, which indicate that genipin form intra- and intermolecular cross-links that have heterocyclic structure with primary amino group-containing proteins. During cross-linking reaction, genipin introduce intermicrofibrilar cross-links between adjacent collagen microfibrils, which affect the mechanical properties (Sung et al., 2003). The sizes of the interfibrilar cross-links can vary by pH variation, during cross-linking reaction, which is pH dependent: under basic conditions, genipin undergoes ring-opening polymerization, thus enlarging the spaces between fibrils, whilst under basic and neutral conditions, reaction with primary amines occur (Mi et al., 2005). Studies have been also have been conducted using material composed of genipin cross-linked gelatine and tricalcium phosphate, showing no inflammation and biocompatibility of such a composite (Yao et al., 2005). In addition, genipin cross-linking in certain polyelectrolyte multy-layer systems is shown to increase cell-adhesion and the spreading on polymeric films, thus improving tissue-implant interfaces (Hillberg et al., 2009).

Citric acid derivative (CAD) prepared by modification of citric acid carboxylic groups with NHS was introduced for cross-linking of gelatine through its amino groups leading to amide bonds formation (Saitoa et al., 2004).

Several components of **polyepoxy** family have been reported, between which **ethylene glycol diglycidyl ether**, with two epoxide functional groups located on both molecule's ends, most reactive due to the high energy is associated to the considerable strains that exist within the three-membered ring. For these type of cross-linking agent, the opening of the epoxide ring happen simultaneously to the occurrence of the cross-linking reaction, which can occur within acidic and basic media (Vargas et al., 2008).

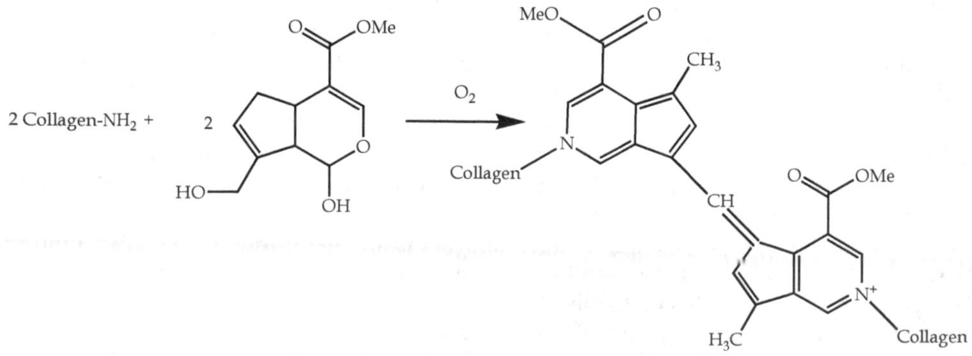

Fig. 11. Reaction between collagen and genipin proposed by (Mi, 2005).

Collagen- vs. Gelatine-Based Biomaterials and Their Biocompatibility: Review and Perspectives

17

Enzymatic cross-linking was introduced in an attempt to overcome some problems with traditional chemical approaches. The oxidative enzymes tyrosinase and laccase (Jus et al., 2011), as well as acyltransferase-transglutaminase, are capable of creating covalent cross-links in proteinaceous substrates (Fig. 12). Tyrosinases and laccases are capable of converting low-molecular weight phenols or accessible Tyr residues of proteins into quinones-reacitve species capable for non-enzymatic reactions with nucleophiles, such as reactive amino groups of other amino acid residues, without disruption of gelatines coil to helix transitions because of only 0,3% of Tyr residues in gelatine and their location outside of the Gly-X-Y tripeptide repeat region being responsible for gelatine's helix formation (Chen et al., 2003), and thus forming quiet weak gels because of the same reasons. Transglutaminase catalyses the cross-linking of gelatine by formation of isopeptide bonds between the γ-carbonyl group of a Glu residue and ε-amino group of Lys residue, and one molecule of ammonia per cross-link as by-product (Chen et al., 2003; Bertoni et al., 2006; Crescenzi et al., 2002). Presumably transglutaminase-catalyzed cross-linking occurs in the tripeptide repeat region that is responsive for gelatine's helix forming ability (Chen et al., 2003). The acyl-transfer enzyme catalyzes transamidation reactions that lead to the formation of N-ε-(γ-glutamyl)lysine cross-links in proteins (Crescenzi et al., 2002).

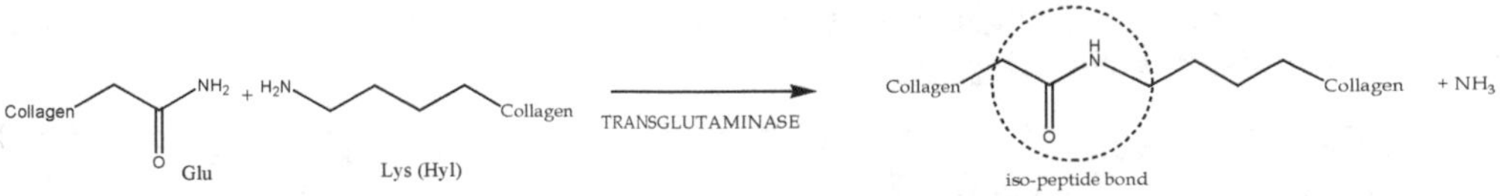

Fig. 12. Chemical cross-linking of Glu-carboxyl and Lys (Hyl)-amino groups in collagen and formation of iso-peptide bond, promote by transglutaminase (Crescenzi et al., 2002).

The treatment by **UV irradiation** only modifies the surface rather than the bulk of the collagen (Mu et al., 2010). Cross-linking of gelatine by UV–irradiation method involve pre-modification of gelatine amino groups (from Lys and Hyl side chains) (Dubruel et al., 2007), commonly by metacrilyc-anhydride (Fig. 13) (Vlierberhe et al., 2009). In subsequent step, water-soluble gelatine-methacrylamide can be cross-linked not only by UV treatment, but, also by a number of suitable polymerization processes, such as redox, thermal, γ-irradiation or e-beam curing (Van Den Bulcke et al., 2000). Prolonged exposure to UV-rays can cause also the denaturation of molecule, which can be minimized by performing the irradiation in deaerated (oxygen-poor) solutions of the gelatine derivatives (Schacht, 2004). Cross-linkage by **electron beam and x-ray** irradiation additional perform sterilization of the substrate.

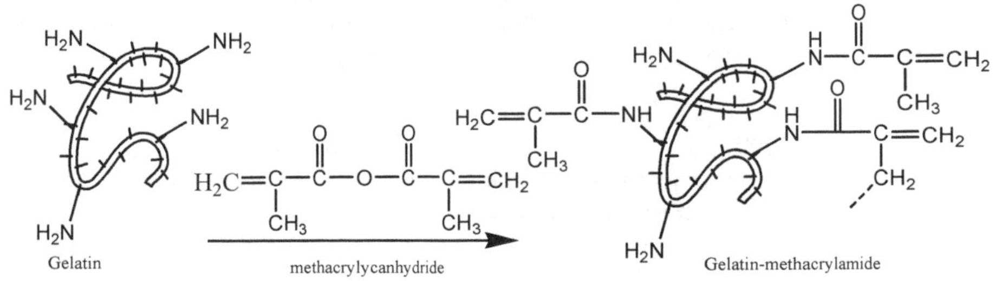

Fig. 13. Derivatization of gelatine amino groups with metacrilycanhydride (Schacht, 2004).

4. Collagen vs. gelatine as biomaterials

Collagen was first employed as a biomaterial in medical surgery in the late 19th century (Burke et al., 1983; Silver et al., 1997). Subsequently, it was used in many other medical applications, e.g. as wound dressings, hemostats or in cardiovascular, plastic or neurosurgery. Most commonly, collagen type I is used in medical devices (Silver et al.; 1997). Device production is uncomplicated and is performed in water without applying high temperatures, resulting in a variety of matrix forms, such as coatings, fibres, films, fleeces, implants, injectable solutions and dispersions, membranes, meshes, powders, sheets, sponges, tapes and tubes. Additionally, its properties can be adapted to desired requirements by additional cross-linking, although shape-instability due to swelling, poor mechanical strength, and low elasticity in vivo, may limit its unrestricted usage. Further limitations are possible antigenic responses, tissue irritations and variations in release kinetics (Sinha & Trehan, 2003). On the other hand, **gelatine** was employed as biomaterials more recently, i.e. tissue engineering from ~ 1970s and in recent years as a cell-interactive coating or micro-carrier embedded in other biomaterials (Dubruel et al., 2007). A non-exhaustive overview of the most recent publications, subdivided by application, for either collagen or gelatine alone or in a combination of other biopolymers is summarized in Table 2 which clearly indicates that gelatine has a wider- application range within the field of both soft and hard-tissue engineering.

Speciality	Collagen application	Gelatine application
Cardiology	heart valves (Everaerts et al., 2007; Taylor et al., 2006; Cox et al., 2010; Tedder et al., 2010)	heart valves– electrospun gelatine-chitosan- polyurethane (Wong et al., 2010) aortic valve –gelatine impregnated polyester graft (Langley et al., 1999) cardiac tissue engineering (Alperin et al., 2005)
Dermatology	soft tissue augmentation (Spira et al., 2004) skin replacement (Lee et al., 2001) artificial skin dermis (Harriger et al., 1998) skin tissue engineering (Ma et al., 2003; Tangsadthakun et al., 2006)	artificial skin (Choi et al., 1999; Lee et al., 2003) soft tissue adhesives (McDermott et al., 2004)
Surgery	hemostatic agent (Cameron, 1978; Browder & Litwin, 1986) plasma expander suture wound dressing and repair (Rao, 1995) skin replacement (artificial skin) nerve repair and conduits blood vessel prostheses (Auger et al., 1998; McGuigan et al., 2006, Amiel et al., 2006)	small intestine (Chiu et al., 2009) liver – chitosan/gelatine scaffold (Jiankang et al., 2007) wound dressing (Tucci & Ricotti, 2001) nerve regeneration - chitosan/gelatin scaffolds (Chiono et al., 2008) blod vesels(Mironov et al., 2005)

Orthopaedic	born, tendon and ligament repair cartilage reconstruction – collagen (Stone, 1997), composite of collagen type II/chondroitin/hyaluronan (Jančar et al., 2007) articular cartilage – collagen/chitosan (Yan et al., 2010)	bone substitute - gelatine/hydroxyapatite (Chang et al., 2007) hard tissue regeneration – gelatine/hydroxyapatite (Kim et al., 2005) cartilage (Lien et al., 2010) cartilage defects regeneration – chitosan/ gelatine (Guo et al., 2006), ceramic/ gelatine (Lien et al.; 2009) bone substitute – gelatine/tricalcium phosphate (Yao et al., 2005)
Ophthalmology	corneal graft (Lass et al., 1986) vitreous implants artificial tears (Kaufman et al., 1994) tape and retinal reattachment contact lenses eye disease treatment (http.....)	ocular inserts (Natu et al., 2007) carriers for intraocular delivery of cell/tissue sheets (Lai et al., 2010) contact lens - chitosan/gelatine (Yuan & Wei, 2004) eye disease treatment (Lai, 2010)
Urology	dialysis membrane hemodialysis (Kon et al., 2004) sphincter repair (Westney et al., 2005)	
Vascular	vascular graft (Yoshida et al., 1996) Vessel replacement, electrospin collagen (Li, 2005) angioplasty	
Others	biocoatings cell culture organ replacement skin test protein , drug and gene delivery (Mahoney & Anseth , 2007) vocal cord regeneration (Hahn et al., 2006) treatment of faecal incontinence (Kumar et al., 1998)	plasma substitutes (Kaur et al., 2002) drug delivery - gelatine/chrodroitin sulphate (Kuijpers et al., 2000) adipose tissue engineering for soft tissue remodelling (Hong et al., 2005)

Table 2. Medical applications of collagen and gelatine

Different research groups have separately evaluated collagen/gelatine-based biomaterials that differ in the applied collagen/gelatine type, cross-linking agents, additives (in the case of composites), pore size, pore geometry, and pore distribution. Beside, only a limited number of cell types have been included in most studies, which makes a meaningful understanding of how one type of (collagen/gelatine) scaffold, with its specific properties, can be applied as a suitable substrate for a variety of cell types, rather difficult. In addition, since the collagen/gelatine-based biomaterial used as scaffolds for in vivo tissue engineering in the form of gels, sponges and woven meshes are required disappear by resorption into the body after accomplishment of tissue regeneration, different tissues needs may demand biodegradable scaffolds with different physical and chemical characteristics.

4.1 Combination with other biopolymers

Fabrication of scaffolds from single-phase biomaterial with homogeneous and reproducible structures presents a challenge, due their generally-poor mechanical properties, which limit their use. Combination with different natural or synthetic polymers in composites or by introducing of e.g. ceramics is one of today´s approaches for overcoming above mentioned limitations.

Along with **hydroxyapatite (HA), collagen** is one of two major components of the bone, making up 89% of the organic matrix and 32% of the volumetric composition of bone (O´Brien, 2011). HA, being similar to bone mineral in physicochemical properties, is well known for its bioactivity and osteoconductivity in vitro and in vivo. Thus, gelatine/HA composite is a potential temporary biomaterial for hard tissue regeneratation, in view of combining the bioactivity and osteoconductivity of HA with the flexibility and hydrogel characteristics of gelatine (Chang & Douglas, 2007; Kim et al., 2004; Narbat et al., 2006; Wahl & Czernuszka, 2006). Both, collagen and HA devices significantly inhibited the growth of bacterial pathogens, being the most frequent cause of prosthesis-related infection (Carlson et al., 2004).

Modification of the collagen/gelatine scaffold materials by **glycosaminoglycans (hyaluronan and chondroitin sulphate)** was introduced in order to enhance cells migration, adhesion, proliferation and differentiation, and to promote preservation of the differentiated states of the cells, as compared to collagen/gelatine alone (Jancar et al., 2007), as well as for control release of antibacterial agents (van Wachem et al., 2000). Hyaluronic acid is a component of the extracellular matrix of some tissue (cockscomb and vitreous humour) and possesses high capacity lubrication, water-sorption and water retention, whilst chondroitin sulphate is sulfated glycosaminoglycan and is important structural component of cartilage, which provides its resistance to compression (Baeurle et al., 2009).

The better collagen delivery systems, having an accurate release control, can be achieved by adjusting the structure of the collagen matrix or adding **other proteins, such as elastin or fibronectin** (Doillon & Silver, 1986). Thus, a combination of collagen with other polymers, such as collagen/liposome (Kaufman et al., 1994) and collagen/silicone (Suzuki et al., 2000), has been proposed in order to achieve the stability of a system, and the controlled release profiles of incorporated compounds.

The addition of collagen to a **ceramic** structure can provide many additional advantages to surgical applications: shape-control, spatial adaptation, increased particle and defect wall-adhesion, and the capability to favour clot-formation and stabilisation (Scabbia and Trombelli, 2004).

cross-linked **collagen/chitosan** (Kim et al., 2001; Ma et al., 2003; Wang et al., 2003; Chalonglarp et al., 2006) as well as **gelatine/chitosan** (Kim et al., 2005; Chiono et al., 2008) matrices were presented as a promising biomaterial for tissue engineering, to be used in several specific areas, such as drug delivery, wound dressings, sutures, nerve conduit, and matrix templates for tissue engineering. Human connective tissues do not contain chitosan, but it has structural similarity to glucosaminoglycan (GAG), mostly components of ECM. GAG attached to the core protein of proteoglycan consist of repeating disaccharide unit, usually includes an uronic acid component (e.g., D and L-gluconic acid) and a hexoamine component (e.g., N-acetyl-D-glucosamine, which, together with glucosamine build the copolymer structure of chitosan and N-acetyl-D-galactosamine). Chitosan, because of it cationic nature, can promote cell adhesion, can act as modulator of cell morphology, differentiation, movements, synthesis and function. It is reported that chitosan induces fibroblasts to release interleukin-8, which is involved in migration and proliferation of fibroblasts and vascular endothelial cells, but, also promotes surface-induced thrombosis and embolization, which limits its application in blood-containing biomaterials (Wang et al., 2003). Chitosan addition enhances poor mechanical properties of gelatine and influence on more controllable biodegradation rate. Chitosan, with higher Degree of deacetilation (DD), modified with gelatine, possess more intensive cytocooplatibility, enhance cell proliferation and decline cell apoptosis. From the other hand, a flexible gelatine complex with a rigid chitosan weakens the adhesion via neutralizing cationic sites of chitosan, with suitable negative-charges borne by the gelatine, and as a consequence, a gelatine/chitosan product shows improved cell mobility, migration and multiplication (Mao et al., 2004; Yuan et al., 2004). Thus, networks composed of gelatine and chitosan have been studied extensively due its excellent ability to be processed into porous scaffolds with good cytocompatibility and desirable cellular response (Mao et al., 2004; Wang et al., 2003).

The advantageous properties of collagen for supporting tissue growth have been used in conjunction with the superior mechanical properties of **synthetic biodegradable polymers** to make hybrid tissue scaffolds for bone and cartilage. Collagen has also been used to improve cells´ interactions with electrospun nanofibers of poly (hydroxyl acids), such as poly(lactic acid), poly(glycolic acid), poly(ε-caprolactone), and their copolymers (Pachence et al., 2007).

Novel **gelatine/alginate** sponge serving as an drug carrier for silver sulfadiazine and gentamicin sulphate, used for wound healing (Choi et al., 1999). Alginate is known as a hydrophilic and biocompatible polysaccharide, and is commonly used in medical applications, such as wound dressing, scaffolds for hepatocyte culture, and surgical and dental materials. It's content in the above-mentioned sponge cause increasing in porosity, resulting in enhanced water uptake ability.

4.2 Mechanism of collagen degradation
4.2.1 In vitro degradation

Degradation of collagen requires water and enzyme penetration, and the digestion of linkages. Collagen swells to a certain extent by exposure to water, but due to its special sterical arrangement (triple helical conformation), native collagen can only be digested completely by specific collagenases and pepsin-cleaving enzymes being able to cleave collagen in its undenatured helical regions at physiological pH and temperature (Harrington, 1996; Sternlicht & Werb, 2001). Included are collagenases which cleave once across all three chains, such as tissue collagenases, as well as collagenases making multiple scissions per chain, such as collagenase from Clostridium histolyticum (CHC) (Seifter et al., 1971) whilst non-specific proteinases, such as pepsin, which can only attack the telopeptides or denatured helical regions of collagen (Weiss, 1976) are responsible for further degradation down to amino acids.

CHC types of collagenase are only present in tissue at very low- levels and tightly- bound to collagen (Woessner, 1991), while tissue collagenases cleavie to all types of collagen, with no preference for a special collagen substrate (Welgus et al.,; 1983). Depending on the collagen type, about 150-200 cleaves per chain can be made (Seifter et al., 1971).

To date, seven forms of CHC are known (Mookhtiar et al., 1992). All seven enzymes contain zinc and calcium and consist of one polypeptide chain with one active site. The zinc (II) atom is located in the active site and is therefore essential for catalysis, whereas the calcium (II) atoms are required to stabilize the enzyme conformation and, consequently, the enzymatic activity (Bond et al., 1984). On the basis of their primary and secondary structures, their substrate specifities and their method of attack, CHCs can be divided into two classes. Class I contains α-, β-, γ-, and η-collagenase, and firstly attacks the collagen triple-helix near the ends. After cleavage at the C-terminal end, a cut near the N-terminus follows, before collagen is successively degraded into smaller fragments. Class II consists of δ-, ε- and ζ- collagenase and cleaves the tropocollagen in its centre, to producing two fragments. Further digestion of the bigger fragment follows (Mookhtiar et al., 1992). Consequently, class II CHC better resembles tissue collagenases, which cleaves collagen into TCA and a TCB fragment (Seifter et al., 1971; Welgus et al., 1980).

Collagen fibrils are degraded in a non-specific manner, with no preferential cleavage site in the interior or at the ends of fibrils (Paige et al.; 2002). It was concluded that collagenase is too large to penetrate into the fibrils, so digestion can only occur at the fibrils` surface (Okada et al., 1992; Paige et al., 2002). Hence, the degradation rate is directly correlated to those substrate molecules available on the surface. If collagen forms fibres and fibre-bundles, and the tropocollagens within becomes inaccessible, the degradation rate is reduced even more (Steven, 1976).

4.2.2 In vivo degradation

In vivo, degradation of collagen is more complex than in vitro. Collagen implants are infiltrated by various inflammatory cells, e.g. fibroblasts, macrophages or neutrophils, which cause contraction of the implant and secret collagen-degrading enzymes, activators, inhibitors, and regulatory molecules. Infiltration depends on properties of the implant, such as collagen nature, shape, porosity and degree of cross-linking, implantation site and individual enzyme levels (Gorham, 1991). Collagen is degraded by endopeptidases from the four major classes (Table 3): metalloproteinases, serine proteases, cysteine proteases and aspartic proteases, although, non-enzymatic degradation mechanisms, e.g. hydrolysis, participate in collagen breakdown (Okada et al., 1992). Connective tissue, for example, is digested by the interplay between four different classes of proteinases, which are either stored within cells or released when required, while for degradation of the extracellular matrix, MMPs are mainly responsible. Cystein and aspartic proteinases (cathepsins) degrade connective tissue intracellularly at acidic pH (3-5) values, whereas serine and matrix metalloproteinases (MMP) act extracellularly at neutral pH values (Shingleton et al., 1996). Anyhow, cathepsins also play a major role in intracellular digestion of phagocytosed material, by cleaving telopeptide containing cross-links, and under certain conditions they can also act extracellularly by cleaving triple-helical regions, which is followed by denaturation of solubilised triple-helix and further degradation by proteases (such as gelatinases type MMP-2 and 9), due to susceptibility of individual α-chains (Baley, 2000).

MMP enzymes represent a family of structurally and functionally related zinc- and calcium-containing endopeptidases which degrade almost all extracellular matrix and basement membrane proteins (Wall et al., 2002; Bailey, 2000). To date, 24 different MMPs and 4 tissue inhibitors of metalloproteinases (TIMP) are characterized (Yoshizaki et al., 2002). According to their primary structure and substrate specify, MMPs are divided into five sub-classes.

Five major MMPs have been identified in humans, namely fibroblast collagenase (MMP1), gelatinase A (MMP-2), gelatinase B (MMP-9), neutrophil collagenase (MMP-8) and stromelysine (MMP-3) (Netzel-Arnett et al., 1991). Besides collagenase 4MMP-8, which is stored in specific granules of neutrophils, and membrane-type MMPs (MT-MMP), which are integral membrane cell glycoproteins, all other MMPs are synthesized if required (Imai et al., 1998) and able to cleave native triple-helical fibrilar collagens.

Enzyme class	Cellular source	Substrate	Activator
Matrix metalloproteinases			
Collagenases			
• MMP-1	Connective tissue cells Monocytes/macrophages	Native triple helix	MMP-3 Plasmin
• MMP-8	Neutrophilis	Native triple helix	MMP-3/NE
• MMP-13 (Rodent MMP-1)	as MMP-1	as MMP-q plus telopeptides	Plasmin MMP-2/3 MT-MMP
Gelatinases	Most cell types	Native type IV gelatin	
• MMP-2			MMP-1/2 MT-MMP
	Connective tissue cells		
• MMP-9	Neutriphilis/monocytes	as MMP-2	Plasmin MMP-2/3
Stromelysins	Connective tissue cells		
• MMP-3	Macrophages	Collagen types III,IV and IX	Plasmin Cathepsin G
	Macrophages	Aggrecan	
• MMP-10		as MMP-3	as MMP-3
Cystine proteinases	Lysosomal		
• Cathepsins			
• B,L,C,H,N and S			
• K		Telopeptide Bone/triple helix plus telopeptides	Cathepsin D Low pH
Serine proteinases	Granulocytes		
• Neutrophil elastase			
• Cathepsin G		Telopeptides/triple helix	
Aspartic proteases			
• Cathepsin D		Telopeptide	
		Telopeptide	

Table 3. Major collagen degrading enzymes (Bailey, 2001).

The mechanism of collagen degradation by MMPs is not totally resolved. One of hypothesis is that collagen is actually unwound by MMPs (Chung et al., 2004). Collagenases bind and locally unwind the triple-helical structure before hydrolysing the peptide bonds. According to these, MMP-1 preferentially interact with the Gly-Leu on α2 (I) chain residues and with Gly-Ileu on α1 chain and cleaves the three α chains in succession, generating two triple-helical fragments of ¾ and ¼ the molecule length, which show lower denaturation temperature then physiological one, and they both denaturate, producing random polypeptide gelatine chains (Baley, 2000), which are further degraded by gelatinases (MMP-2 and MMP-9) and other nonspecific enzymes as schematically presented on Fig. 14.

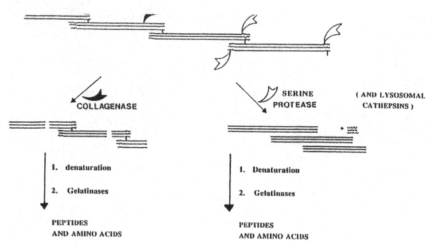

Fig. 14. Dual degradation mechanism of cross-linked fibers in the collagen implant. These mechanism include (left) neutral collagenase cleaving the three chains of the triple-helix and (right) the acid cathepsins and neutral serine proteases cleaving the nonhelical terminal regions (telopeptides) containing the intermolecular cross-links (Bailey, 2001).

Existence of locally unfolded states in collagen molecule has been also suggested (Escat, 2010), according to which, folded structure of collagen cannot fit into the catalytic site, since collagen triple-helix has a diameter of approximately 15 Å, whiles catalytic domain of MMPs has a catalytic site of only 5 Å wide. Beside, scissile bond, cleaved by collagenases is buried in collagen structure when collagen is exposed to solvent, which make it inaccessible for scission. Local unfolding is collagen triple-helix property, which occur without presence of collagenases, but necessary for collagen degradation in collagenase presence. In addition, immino-poor regions in collagen are thought to carry biological information, such as cell recognition or protein binding sites (Brodsky & Persikov, 2005), but may play also an important role in collagen degradation (Fields, 1991).

MMP expression is induced by various cytokines, e.g. interleukin-1, and growth factors (Shingleton et al., 1996). MMPs are secreted as latent inactive pro-enzymes (zymogens) which have to be activated before they have complete proteolytic activity (Overall, 1991). Four amino acids (three His and one Cys) are coordinated to the zinc atom in the active centre of zymogens (Birkedal-Hansen et al., 1993), being proposed by a "cysteine switch model". The linkage to the Cys residue is thought to be cleaved and a water molecule, which must be the fourth substituent in the active enzyme can bind (Nagase et al., 1999). In vivo, zymogens are activated by removal of a pro-peptide by proteinases, like plasmin or stromelysin, followed by a second activation step provoked by proteinases or autocatalysis

(Shingleton et al., 1996). Additionally, activation is controlled by TIMPs, which can prevent activation of zymogens and/or action of activated MMPs. In vitro, trypsin and organomercurials can be used for activation as well (Overall, 1991). Physical agents unfold the structure, the zinc-cysteine contact breaks and the propeptide is cleaved auto-catalytically (Woessner, 1991).

Tissue collagenases cleave tropocollagen at one single site, producing TCA and TCB fragments about three-quarters and one-quarter of the original molecule size. After this initial cleavage, the helical fragments spontaneously denature at body temperature and are subsequently further digested by other proteinases (Mallya et al., 1992). This secondary degradation can take place extracellularly or intracellularly after phagocytosis (Harris, et al., 1974). Apart from collagenases, gelatinases play an important role in collagen degradation. Besides, with any further degradation of initially-cleaved collagen, gelatinases can degrade native collagen type I, IV, V and VII (Overall, 1991). Furthermore, levels of gelatinases are considered to be a good index whether inflammation is present or not, because high concentrations are only available when a normal remodeling process is disrupted (Trengove et al., 1999).

4.2.3 Immunological response of collagen-based biomaterials

As already mentioned, the implantation of biomaterials often initiates acute inflammatory responses, which sometimes can cause chronic inflammatory response. Measuring the intensities and duration of the immune responses against implanted biomaterials is important for biocompatibility evaluation. The tissue response towards implanted biomaterials (also called the foreign body reaction) is influenced by morphology and composition of the biomaterial and the place where biomaterial is implanted (Ye et al., 2010; Jansen et al., 2008; Wang et al., 2008). Inflammation reaction is manifested by secretion of large amount of antibodies (secreting B cells and T cells with cytotoxic activity) and cytokines, in presence of foreign materials (as scaffolds) or pathogens. The microenvironment of the implant further changes, so, determination of immunological response after in vivo implantation is based of measuring the level of pro-inflammatory cytokine secretions and antibody secretions, and monitoring the population changes of immune cells (Song et al., 2006; Hardin-Young et al., 2000).

According to (Luttikhuizen et al., 2007), collagen-based scaffolds are mainly infiltrated by Giant cells that phagocytose and degrade the collagen bundles, until the material is completely disposed of. This is a chronic inflammatory reaction, which last until the material is completely degraded, after which the cells that are involved disappear.

As an alternative for collagens isolated from calf skin and bond, as a risk-carry materials of bovine spongiform encephalophaty and transmissible spongiform encephalopathy, novel **forms of acid-soluble collagen**, extracted from jellyfish was proposed (Song et al., 2006), because of their differences in amino acid composition: jellyfish collagen had higher content of Gln (glutamine) and Glu, lower Pro content, small Tyr content, comparing with bovine and also contains Cys, which is not common for bovine collagen.

4.2.4 New sources of gelatine

Currently gelatine for food and used by the pharmaceutical industry is derived almost exclusively from **animal products**. About 55,000 tons of animal-sourced gelatine is used each year. Recently, an advance toward turning corn plants into natural factories producing high-grade gelatine in a safe and inexpensive manner has been introduced as an alternative, enabling the development of a variety of gelatines with specific MWs and properties tailored to suit various needs. Beside, **plant-derived recombinant gelatine** would address concerns about the possible presence of infectious agents in animal by-products and the lack of traceability of the source of the raw materials currently used to make gelatine. Resourcing plant materials to recover and purify recombinant gelatine has remained a challenge because only very low levels accumulate at the early stages of the development process. Furthermore, since recently, gelatines are also produced biotechnologically by the use of recombinant DNA technology, which opens the possibility to manipulate the amino acid sequence of gelatines, and thereby to functionalize them for specific purposes. The biotechnological production of recombinant gelatine also eliminates the risk of prion contaminations, which are possible, present in non-recombinant animal source gelatines (Sutter et al., 2007). Thus, many commercial recombinant collagens already exist on the market and are becoming commonly used in the development of medical soft and hard tissue repair applications (Pannone, 2007).

5. Conclusion

This review presents the characteristic properties of both fibrous proteins including biocompatibility, non-immunogenicity, their capacities for modification at the molecular level, thus rendering or tuning their functional (surface/interfacial, mechanical, topological and morphological) properties, characteristic gelation (sol-gel transition) and gel-forming abilities and, finally, their bio-absorbability and biodegradability. In addition, their expanding applications for biomaterials are compared, with emphasis on the importance of understanding their suitability, as defined biomaterials with specific properties, for certain cell types. Finally, new perspectives for further study and development indicated, providing satisfactory interaction and imitation of biological functions.

6. References

Alperin, C., Zandstra, P.W. & Woodhouse, K.A. (2005). Polyurethane films seeded with embryonic stem cell derived cardiomycytes for use in cardiac tissue engineering applications. *Biomaterials*, Vol. 26, No. 35, pp. (7377-7386)

Amiel, G.E., Komura, M., Shapira, O., Yoo, J.J., Yazdani, S., Berry, J., Kaushai, S., Bischoff, J., Atala, A. & Soker, S. (2006). Engineering of blood vessels from acellular collagen matrices coated with human endothelial cells. *Tissue Engineering*, Vol. 12, No. 8, pp. (2355-2365)

Auger, F.A., Rouabhia, M. Goulet, F., Berthod, F., Moulin, V. & Germain, L. (1998). Tissue-engineered human skin substitutes developed from collagen-populated hydrated gels: clinical and fundamental applications. *Medical and Biologycal Engineering & Computing*, Vol. 36, No. 6, pp. (801-812)

Baeurle, S.A., Kiselev, M.G., Makarova, E.S. & Nogovitsin, E.A. (2009). Effect of the counterion behaviour on the frictional-compressive properties of chondroitin sulphate solutions. *Polymer*, Vol 50, No. 7, pp. (1805-1813)

Balakrishnan,B. & Jayakrishnan, A. (2005). Self-cross-linking biopolymers as injectable in situ forming biodegradable scaffolds. *Biomaterials*, Vol. 26, No.18, pp. (3941-3951)

Bailey, A.J.(2001).The fate of collagen implants in tissue defects. *Wound Repair and Regenration,* Vol. 8, pp. (5-12)

Barrere, F., Mahmood, T.A., de Groot, K., van Blitterswijak, C.A. (2008). Advanced biomaterials for skeletal tissue regeneration: Instructive and smart functions. *Material science and Engineering,* Vol. 59, No. 1-6, pp. (38-71)

Barbetta, A., Rizzitelli, G., Bedini, R., Pecci, R. & Dentini, M.(2010). Porous gelatin hydrogels by gas-in-liquid foam templating. *Soft Matter,* Vol. 6, pp. (1785-1792)

Belbachir, K., Noreen, R., Gouspillou, G. & Petibois, C. (2009). Collagen types analysis and differentiation by FTIR spectroscopy. *Analytical and Bioanalytical Chemistry,* Vol.395, No. 3, pp. (829-837)

Bertoni, F., Barbani,N., Giusti, P & Giardelli, G. (2006). Transglutaminase reactivity with gelatine: perspective applications in tissue engineering. *Biotechnology Letters,* Vol.28, pp. (697-702)

Bigi,A., Cojazzi,G., Panzavolta, S., Roveri,N. & Rubini, K. (2002). Stabilization of gelatin films by crosslinking with genipin. *Biomaterials,* Vol.23, pp. (4827-4832)

Birkedal-Hansen,H., Moore,W.G., Bodden,M.K., Windsor,L.J., BirkedalHansen,B., DeCarlo,A. & Engler, J.A. (1993). Matrix Metalloproteinases: a Review. *Critical Reviews in Oral Biology and Medicine : an Official Publication of the American Association of Oral Biologists,* Vol. 4, pp.(197 – 250)

Bhat, R. & Karim, A.A. (2009). Ultraviolet irradiation improves gel strength of fish gelatin. *Food Chemistry,* Vol. 113, No. 4, pp. (1160-1164)

Bond, M.D. & Van Wart, H.E. (1984). Relationship Between the Individual Collagenases of Clostridium Histolyticum: Evidence for Evolution by Gene Duplication. *Biochemistry,* Vol.23, pp. (3092 – 3099)

Brinckmann, J., Notbohm, H., Mueller,P.K. & Editors. (2005). *Collagen: Primer in Structure, Processing and Assembly,* Springer-Verlag Heidelberg, ISBN-10 3-540-23272-9, The Netherlands

Browder, I.W., & M.S. Litwin. (1986). Use of absorbable collagen for hemostasis in general surgical patients. The American Surgeon, Vol. 52, No. 9, pp. (492-494)

Brodsky, B. & Persikov, A.V. (2005). Molecular structure of the collagen triple helix. *Advances in Protein Chemistry,* Vol. 70, pp. (301-309)

Browder, I.W. & Litwin, M.S. (1986). Use of absorbable collagen for hemostasis in general patients. *Americal Surgeon,* Vol. 52, No. 9, pp. (492-494)

Burke, K.E., Naughton, G., Waldo, E. & Cassai, N. (1983). Bovine Collagen Implant: Histologic Chronology in Pig Dermis. *Journal of Dermatologic Surgery and Oncology,* Vol. 9, pp. (889 – 895)

Cameron, W.J. (1978). A new topical hemostatic agent in gynecologic surgery. *Obstet Gynecology,* Vol. 51, No. 1, pp. (118-122)

Cancedda, R., Dozin, B., Giannoni, P. & Quarto, R. (2003). Tissue engineering and cell therapy of cartilage and bone. *Matrix Biology,* Vol. 22, No.1, pp. (81-91)

Carlson, G.A., Dragoo, J.L., Samimi, B., Bruckner, D.A, Bernard, G.W., Hedrick, M. & Benhaim, P. (2004) Bacteriostatic properties of biomatrices against common orthopaedic pathogens. *Biochemical and Biophysical Research Communications,* Vol. 321, No. 2, pp. (472-478)

Cataldo, F., Ursini, O., Lilla, E. & Angelini, G. (2008). Radiation-induced crosslinking of collagen gelatin into a stable hydrogel. *Journal of Radioanalytical and Nuclear Chemistry,* Vol. 275, No. 1, pp. (125-131)

Chalonglarp, T., Sorada, K., Neeracha, S., Tanom, B. & Siriporn, D.(2006). Properties of Collagen/Chitosan Scaffolds for Skin Tissue Engineering. *Journal of Metals, Materials and Minerals,* Vol. 16, pp. (37-44)

Chang, M.C. & Douglas, W.H. (2007). Cross-linking of hydroxyapatite/gelatin nanocomposite using imide-based zero-length cross-linker. *Journal of Materials Science: Materials for Medicine,* Vol.18, pp. (2045-2051)

Charulatha, V. &. Rajaram , A. (1997). Crosslinking density and resorption of dimethyl suberimidate treated collagen. *Journal of Biomedical Materials Research,* Vol.36, pp. (478–486)

Chang, Y. Tsai CC, Liang HC, Sung HW. (2001). Reconstruction of the RVOT with a bovine jugular vein graft fixed with a naturally occurring crosslinking agent (genipin) in a canine model. *Journal of Thoracic and Cardiovascular Surgery,* Vol.122, No. 6, pp. (1208–1218)

Charulatha, V. &. Rajaram, A. (2001). Dimethyl 3,3'-dithiobispropionimidate: a novel crosslinking reagent for collagen. *Journal of Biomedical Materials Research,* Vol. 54, pp. (122–128)

Charulatha, V. &. Rajaram, A. (2003). Influence of different crosslinking treatments on the physical properties of collagen membranes. *Biomaterials,* Vol. 24, No. 5, pp. (759-767)

Chavez, F.V., Hellstrand, E. & Halle, B. (2006). Hydrogen Exchange and Hydration Dynamics in Gelatin Gels. *Journal of Physical Chemistry B,* Vol. 110, No. 43, pp. (21551-21559)

Chen,T., Embree, H.D., Brown,E.M., Taylor, M.M. & Payne, G.F. (2003). Enzyme-catalyzed gel formation of gelatin and chitosan: potential for in situ appplications. *Biomaterials,* Vol. 24, pp. (2831-2841)

Chen, J.M., Sheldon, A., & Pincus, M.R. (1995). Three dimensional energy-minimized model of human type II smith collagen microfibrill. *Journal of Biomolecular Structure & Dinamics,* Vol. 12, pp. (1129 –1156)

Cheng,W.,Yan-hua,R., Fang-gang,N. & Guo-an,Z. (2011). The content and ration of type I and type III collagen in skin differ with age and injury. *African Journal of Biotechnology,* Vol. 10, No. 13, pp. (2524-2529)

Cheung, D.T., Perelman,N., Ko, E.C. & Nimni,M.E.(1984). Mechanism of Crosslinking of Proteins by Glutaraldehyde III. Reaction With Collagen in Tissues. *Connective Tissue Research,* Vol.13, No. 2, pp. (109 – 115)

Chevallay, B. & Herbage, D. (2000). Collagen-based biomaterials as 3D scaffold for cell cultures: applications for tissue engineering and gene therapy, *Medical & Biological Engineering & Computing,* Vol. 38, No.2, pp. (211-218)

Chiono, V., Pulieri, E., Vozzi, G., Ciardelli, G., Ahluwalia, A. & Paolo Giusti, P.(2008). Genipin-crosslinked chitosan/gelatin blends for biomedical applications. *Journal of Material Science: Materials in Medicine,* Vol. 19, No. 2, pp. (889-898)

Chiu, C.H., Shin, H.C., Jwo, S.C. & Hsieh, M.F. (2010). Effect of Crosslinkers on Physical Properties of Gelatin Hollow Tubes for Tissue Engineering Application. *World Congress on Medical Physics and Biomedical Engineering,* Vol. 25, No. 10, pp.(293-296)

Choi, Y.S., Hong, S.R., Lee, Y.M., Song, K.W., Park,M.H. & Young Soo Nam, Y.S. (1999). Study of gelatin-containing artificial skin: I. Preparation and characteristics of novel gelatin-alginate sponge. *Biomaterials*, Vol. 20, pp. (409-417)

Chung, L., Dinakarpandian, D., Yoshida, N., Fields, J.L.L., Fields, G. B., Visse, R. & Nagase, H.(2004). Collagenase unwinds triple-helical collagen prior to peptide bond hydrolysis. *The European Molecular Biology Organization Journal*, Vol. 23, pp. (3020-3020)

Collagen Corneal Shields, Available online:
    http://www.uic.edu/com/eye/LearningAboutVision/EyeFacts/CollagenCorneal Shields.shtml

Collagen: The Body´s Cellular Fabric, Available online:
    http://www.kokenmpc.co.jp/english/support/tecnical/collagen/index.html)

Cole, B. (1999). Gelatin, In: *Wiley Encyclopedia of Food Science and Technology (second edition)*, Francis,F.J, John Wiley & Sons, ISBN: 0-471-19285-6, New York

Cooperman, L. & Michaeli, D. (1984). The immunogenicity of injectable collagen. 1. 1-year prospective study, Journal of the American Academy of Dermatology, Vol.10, No. 4, pp. (647-651)

Cox, M.A.J., Kortsmit, J., Driessen, N., Bouten, C.V.C. & Baaijens, F.P.T. (2010). Tissue-Engineered Heart Valves Develop Native-like Collagen Fiber Architecture, *Tissue Engineering Part A*, Vol. 16, No. 5, pp. (1527-1537)

Crescenzi V, Francescangeli A, Taglienti A. (2002). A new gelatine-based hydrogels via enzymatic networking. *Biomacromolecules*, Vol. 3, pp. (1384–1391)

Damnik, O., L.H.H., Dijkstra, P.J., van Luyn, M.J.A, van Wachem, P.B, Nieuwenhuis, P. & Feijen, J. (1996). Cross-linking of dermal sheep collagen using a water-soluble carbodiimide, *Biomaterials*, Vol. 17, No. 8, pp. (765-773)

Doillon, C.J. & Silver, F.H. (1986). Collagen — based wound dressing effects of hyaluronic acid and fibronectin on wound healing. *Biomaterials*, Vol. 7, pp. (3 –8)

Dubruel, P., Unger, R., Van Vlierberghe, S., Cnudde, V., Jacobs, P.J.S, Schacht, E. & Kirkpatrick, C.J. (2007). Porous Gelatin Hydrogels: 2. In Vitro Cell Interaction Study. *Biomacromolecules*, Vol. 8, pp. (338-344)

Escat, R.S. (2010). The role of Unfolded States in Collagen Degradation, PhD thesis Massachusetts Institute of Technology

Everaerts, F., Torrianni, M., Hendriks, M., Feijen, J. (2007). Quantification of carboxyl groups in carbodiimide cross-linked collagen sponges. *Journal of Biomedical Materials Research, Part A*, Vol. 83A, No. 4, pp. (1176-1183)

Farris,S., Schaich,K.M., Liu,L.S., Piergiovanni, L. & Yam, K.L. (2009). Development of polyon-complex hydrogels as an alternative approach for the production of bio-based polymers for food packaging applications. A review. *Trends in Food Science Technology*, Vol. 20, pp. (316-332)

Farrist, S., Song, J. & Huang, Q. (2009). Alternative Reaction mechanism for the Cross-Linking of Gelatin with Glutaraldehyde. *Journal of Agricultural & Food Chemistry*, Vol. 58, No. 2, pp. (998-1003)

Fields, G.B. (1991). A model for interstitial collagen catabolism by mammalian collagenase. *Journal of Theoretical Biology*, Vol. 153, No. 4, pp. (585-602)

Fuchs, S., Kutscher, M., Hertel, T., Winter, G., Pietzsch, M. & Coester, C. (2010). Transglutaminase: new isights into gelatin nanoparticle cross-linking. *Journal of Microencapsulation*, Vol. 27, No. 8, pp. (747-754)

Friess, W. (1998). Collagen-biomaterial for drug delivery. *European Journal of Pharmaceutics and Biopharmaceutics*, Vol.45, No. 2, pp. (113 – 136)

Friess, W. (1999). *Drug Delivery Systems Based on Collagen*, Shaker Verlag, ISBN, 3-8265-6994-6, Aachen

Gelse, K., Poschl, E., Aigner, T. (2003). Collagens-structure, function, and biosynthesis. *Advanced Drug Delivery Reviews*, Vol. 55, No.12, pp. (1531-1546)

Gomez-Guillen, M. C., Perez-Mateos, M., Gomez-Estaca, J., Lopez-Caballero, E., Gimenez, B., & Montero, P. (2009). Fish gelatin: a renewable material for developing active biodegradable films. *Trends in Food Science & Technology*, Vol. 20, No. 1, pp. (3-16)

Gorham, S.D. (1991). Collagen as a biomaterial. In: *Biomaterials*, Byron D, Stockton Press, New York, 55-122

Guo, T., Zhao, J., Chang, J., Ding, Z., Hong, H., Chen, J. & Zhang, J. (2006). Porous chitosan-gelatin scaffold containing plasmid DNA encoding transforming growth factor-β1 for chrondrocytes proliferation. *Biomaterials*, Vol. 27, No. 7, pp. (1095-1103)

Hahn, M.S., Kobler, J.B., Zeitels, S.M . & Langer, R. (2006). Quantitative and comparative studies of the vocal fold extracellular matrix II: collagen. *The Annals of Otology, Rhinology & Laringhology*, Vol. 115, No. 3, pp. (225-232)

Han, B., Jaurequi, J., Tang, B.W. & Marcel E. Nimni (2003). Proanthocyanidin: A natural crosslinking reagent for stabilizing collagen matrices, *Journal of Biomedical Materials Research Part A*, Vol 65A, No. 1, pp. (118-124)

Hardin, J.Y., Carr, R.M., Dowing, G.J., Condon, K.D. & Termin,P.L. (2000). Modification of Native Collagen Reduces Antigenicity but Preserves Cell Compatibility, *Biotechnology and Bioingeneering*, Vol. 49, No. 6, pp. (675-682)

Harriger, M.D., Supp, A.P., Warden , G.D. & Boyce, S.T. (1998). Glutaraldehyde crosslinking of collagen substrates inhibits degradation in skin substitutes grafted to athymic mice. *Journal of Biomedical research* ,Vol.5 pp. (137-145)

Harrington,D.J. (1996). Bacterial Collagenases and Collagen-Degrading Enzymes and Their Potential Role in Human Disease. *Infection and Immunity*, Vol.64, pp. (1885-1891)

Harris,E.D., Jr. & Krane,S.M.(1974). Collagenases(Second of Three Parts). *The New England Journal of Medicine*, Vol. 291, pp. (605 – 609)

Harkness, R.D. (1966). Collagen. *Science Progress*, Vol. 54, pp. (257-274)

He, L., Mu, C., Ski, J., Zhang, Q., Shi, B & Lin, Q. (2011). Modification of collagen with a natural cross-linker, procyanidin. *International Journal of Biological Macromolecules*, Vol. 48, No. 2, pp. (354-359)

Herpandi, Huda, N. & Adzitey,F. (2011). Fish Bone and Scale as a Potential Source of Halal Gelatin. *Journal of Fisheries and Aquatic Science*, Vol. 6, No. 4, pp. (379-389)

Hillberg, A.L., Christina A. Holmes, C.A. & Maryam Tabrizian, M.(2009). Effect of genipin cross-linking on the cellular adhesion properties of lyer-by –lyer assembled plyelectrolyte films. *Biomaterials* , Vol. 30, No. 27, pp. (4463-4470)

Hopkins, S.J. & Wormall, A. (1933). Phenyl isocyanate protein compounds and their immunological properties. *Biochemical Journal*, Vol. 27, pp. (740-753)

Hsu, F.Y., Chueh, S.C. & Wang, J.Y. (1999). Microspheres of hydroxyapatite/reconstituted collagen as supports for osteoblast cell growth. *Biomaterials*, Vol.20, No. 20, pp. (1931-1936)

Ikada, Y. (2002). Biological Materials, In: *Integrated Biomaterials Science*, Barbucci,R. Kluwer Academic /Plenium Publishers, ISBN: 978-0-306-46678-6, New York, USA

Imai,S., Konttinen,Y.T., Jumppanen,M., Lindy,O., Ceponis,A., Kemppinen,P., Sorsa,T., Santavirta,S., Xu,J.W. & Lopez-Otin,C. (1998). High Levels of Expression of Collagenase-3 (MMP-13) in Pathological Conditions Associated With a Foreign-Body Reaction. *Journal of Bone and Joint Surgery*, Vol. 80, pp. (701 – 710)

Jackson, J.K., Zhao, J., Wong, W. & Burt, H.B. (2010). The inhibition of collagenase induced degradation of collagen by the galloyl-containing polyphenols tannic acid, epigallocatechin gallate and epicatechin gallate. *Journal of Materials Science: Materials for Medicine*, Vol.2, pp. (1435-1443)

Yan, L.P., Wang, Y.J., Ren, L., Wu, G., Caridade, S.G., Fan,J.B., Wang, L.Y., Ji, P.H., Oliveira, J.M., Oliveira, J.T., Mano, J.F. & Reis, R.L. (2010). Genipin-cross-linked collagen/chitosan miomimetic scaffolds for articular cartilage tissue engineering applications. *Journal of Biomedical Materials Research Part A*, 95A, No. 2, pp. (465-475)

Jancar, J., Slovnikova, A., .Amler,E., Krupa, P., Kecova,H., Planka, L., Gal,P. & Necas, A. (2007). Mechanical Response of Porous Scaffolds for Cartilage Engineering. *Physiologycal Research*, Vol. 56, No. 1, pp. (17-25)

Jansen, R.G., van Kuppevelt, T.H., Daamen,W.F., Kuijpers-Jagtman, A.M. & Von den Hoff, J.W. (2008). Tissue reactions to collagen scaffolds in the oral mucosa and skin of rats: Environmental and mechanical factors. *Archives of Oral Biology*, Vol. 53, pp. (376-387)

Jayakrishnan, A. & Jameela,S.R. (1996). Glutaraldehyde as a Fixative in Bioprostheses and Drug Delivery Matrices. *Biomaterials*, Vol. 17, No. 5, pp. (471 – 484)

Jiankang, H., Dichen, L., Yaxiong, L., Bo, Y., Hanxiang, Z., Qin, L., Bingegg, L. & Yi, L. (2009). Preparation of chitosan-gelatin hybrid scaffolds with well-organized microstructures for hepatic tissue engineering. *Acta Biomaterialia*, Vol. 5, No. 1, pp. (453-461)

Jus, S., Stachel, I., Schloegl,W., Pretzler,M., Friess,W., Meyer,M., Birner-Gruenberg, R., & Guebitz,G.M. (2011). Cross-linking of collagen with laccases and tyrosinases. *Materials Science and Engineering C*, Vol. 31, No. 5, pp. (1068-1077)

Kaufman, H.E., Steinemann, T.L., Lehman, E., Thompson, H.W., Varnell, E.D., Jacob-La Barre, J.T. & Gerhardt, B.M. (1994). Collagen based drug delivery and artificial tears. *Journal of Ocular Pharmacology*, Vol.10, No.1, pp. (17 –27)

Kaur, M., Jumel, K., Hardie, K.R., Hardman, A., Meadows, J. & Melia, C.D. (2002). Determining the molar mass of a plasma substitute succinylated gelatin by size exclusion chromatography –multi- angle laser light scattering , sedimentation equilibrium and conventional size exclusion chromatography. *Journal of Chromatography A*, Vol. 957, No. 2, pp. (139-148)

Khor, E. (1997). Methods for the Treatment of Collagenous Tissues for Bioprostheses. *Biomaterials*, Vol. 18, No. 2, pp. (95 – 105)

Kikuchi, M., Matsumoto, H.N., Yamada, T., Koyama, Y., Takakuda, K. & Tanaka, J. (2004). Glutaraldehyde crosslinked hydroxyapatite/collagen self-organized nanocomposites. *Biomaterials*, Vol. 25, No. 1, pp. (63-69)

Kim, H.W., Knowles, J.C. & Kim, H.E. (2004). Hydroxyapatite and gelatin composite foams processed via novel freeze-drying and crosslinking for use as temporary hard tissue scaffolds. *Journal of Biomedical Materials Research Part A*, Vol. 72, No. 2, pp. (136-145)

Kim, S.E., Cho, Y.W., Kang, E.J., Kwon, I.C., Lee, E.B., Kim, J.H., Chung, H & Jeong, S.Y. (2001). Three-Dimensional Porous Collagen/Chitosan Complex Sponge for Tissue Engineering. *Fibers and Polymers*, Vol. 2, No. 2, pp. (64-70)

Kim, S., Nimni, M.E., Yang, Z. and Han, B. (2005). *Chitosan/gelatin-based films crosslinked by proanthocyanidin.* Journal of Biomedical Materials Research Part B: Applied Biomaterials, *Vol. 75B*, No. 2, pp. (442-450)

Ko, C.S., Wu, C.H., Huang, H.H. & Chu, I.M. (2007). Genipin Cross-linking of Type II Collagen-chondroitin Sulfate-hyaluronan Scaffold for Articular Cartilage Therapy. *Journal of Medical and Biological Engineering,*Vol. 27, No. 1, pp. (7-14)

Kokare, C.R. (2008). *Pharmaceutical Microbiology-Principles and Applications,* Nirali Prakashan, ISBN NO.978-81-85790-61-2, Pune, India

Kon, T., Mrava, G.L, Weber, D.C. & Nose, Y. (2004). Collagen membrane for hemodialysis. *Journal of Biomedical Materials Research Part A*, Vol. 4, No. 1, pp. (13-23)

Kuijpers, A.J., Engbers, G.H., Krijqsveld, J., Zaat, S.A., Dankert, J. & Feijen, J. (2000). Cross-linking and characterization of gelatin matrices for biomedical applications. *Journal of Biomaterials scince. Polymer Edition*, Vol. 11, No. 3, pp. (225-243)

Kumar, D., Benson, M.J. & Bland, J.E. (1998). Glutaraldehyde cross-linked collagen in the treatment of faecal incontinence. *British Journal of Surgery*, Vol. 85, No. 7, pp. (978-979)

Labout, J.J.M. (1972). Gamma-radiation in Collagen Solutions Influence of Solutes on the Gelatin Dose. *International Journal of Radiation Biology*, Vo. 21, No. 5, pp. (483-492)

Lai, J.Y. & Li,Y.T. (2010). Functional Assesment of Cross-Linked Porous Gelatin Hydrogels for Bioingeneered Cell Sheet Carriers, *Biomacromolecules*, Vol. 11, No. 5, pp. (1387-1397)

Lass, J.H., Ellison, R.R., Wong, K.M. & Klein, L. (1986). Collagen degradation and synthesis in experimental corneal crafts. *Experimental Eye Research*, Vol. 42, No. 3, pp. (201-210)

Langley, S.M., Rooney,S.J., Hay, M.J.R.D., Spencer,J.M.F., Lewis,M.E., Pagano, D., M Asif, M., Goddard, J.R., Tsang,V.T., Lamb, R.K., Monro, J.L., Livesey, S.A. & Bonser, R. S. (1999). Replacement of the proximal aorta and aortic valve using a composite bileaflet prosthesis and gelatin-impregnated polyester graft (Carbo-seal): early results in 143 patients. *The Journal of Thoracic and Cardiovascular Surgery*, Vol. 118, pp. (1014-1020)

Lee, C.H., Singla, A. & Lee, Y. (2001). Biomedical applications od collagen. *International Journal of Pharmaceuticals*, Vol. 221, No. 1-2, pp. (1-22)

Lee, S.B., Jeon, H.W., Lee, Y.W., Lee, Y.M., Song, K.W., Park, M.H., Nam, Y.S. & Ahn, H.C. (2003.)*Bio-artificial skin composed of gelatin and (1-->3), (1-->6)-betaglucan.* Biomaterials , Vol. 24, No. 14, pp. (2503-2511)

Li, M., Mondrinos, M.J., Gandhi, M.R., Ko, F.K., Weiss, A.S. & Lelkes, P.I. (2005). Electrospun protein fibers as matrices for tissue engineering. *Biomaterials*, Vol. 26, No. 30, pp. (5999-6008)

Lien, S. M., Chien, C. H. & Huang, T. J. (2009). A novel osteochondral scaffold of ceramic – gelatin assembly for articular cartilage repair. *Materials Science & Engineering: C*, Vol. 29, No. 1, pp. (315-321)

Lien, S., Li, W. & Huang, T. (2010). Genipin-crosslinked gelatin scaffolds for articular cartilage with a novel crosslinking method. *Materials Science & Engineering C*, Vol. 28, No. 1, pp. (36-43)

Liu, H., Peptan, I., Clark, P. & Mao, J. (2005). Ex Vivo Adipose Tissue Engineering by Human Marrow Stomal Cell Seeded Gelatin Sponge. *Annals of Biomedical Engineering*, Vol. 33, No. 4, pp. (511-517)

Luttikhuizen,D.T., Dankers, P.Y., Harmsen, M.C., van Luyn, M.J.A. (2007). Material dependent differences in inflammatory gene expression by giant cells during the foreign body reaction. *Journal of Biomedical Materials Research Part A*, Vol. 83 , pp. (879-886)

Lynn, A. K., Yannas, L.V. & Bonfield, W. (2004). Antigenicity and Immunogenicity of Collagen. *Journal of Biomadical Materials Research Part B: Applied Biomaterials B*, Vol.71B, No.2, pp. (343-354)

Ma, L., Gao, C., Mao, Z., Zhou, J., Shen, J., Hu, X. & Han,C. (2003). Collagen/chitosan porous scaffolds with improved biostability for skin tissue engineering. *Biomaterials*, Vol. 24, pp. (4833-4841)

Mahoney, M.J. & Anseth, K.S. (2007). Contrasting effects of collagen and bFGF-2 on neural cell function in degradable synthetic PEG hydrogels. *Journal of Biomedical Materials Research Part A*, Vol. 81A, No. 2, pp. (269-278)

Mallya,S.K., Mookhtiar,K.A. & Van Wart,H.E. (1992). Kinetics of Hydrolysis of Type I, II, and III Collagens by the Class I and II Clostridium Histolyticum Collagenases. *Journal of Protein Chemistry*, Vol. 11, pp. (99 – 107)

Mao, J.S., Cui,Y.L., Wang, X.H., Sun, Y., Yin, Y.Y, Zhao, H.M. & Yao, K.D.(2004). A preliminary study on chitosan and gelatin polyelectrolyte complex cytocompatibility by cell cycle and apoptosis analysis. *Biomaterials*, Vol. 25, pp. (3973-3981)

McDermott, M.K., Chen, T., Williams, C.M., Markley, K.M. & Payne, G.F. (2004). Mechanical properties of biomimetic tissue adhesive based on the microbial transglutaminase-catalysed crosslinking of gelatin. *Biomacromolecules*, Vol. 5, No. 4, pp. (1270-1279)

McGuigan, A.P. & Sefton, M.V. (2006). Vascularized organoid engineered by modular assembly enables blood perusion. *Proceedings of the National Academy of Sciences of the Unated States of America*, Vol. 103, No. 31, pp. (11461-11466)

Mi, F.L., Shyu,S.S & Peng C.K. (2005). Caracterization of ring-opening polymerization of genipin and pH dependent cross-linking reactions between chitosan and genipin. *Journal of Polymer Science Part A: Polymer Chemistry*, Vol.43, No.10, pp. (1985-2000)

Mironov, V., Kasyanov, V. & Markwald, R.R. 8Nanotechnology in vascular tissue engineering: from nanoscaffolding towards rapid vessel biofabrication. *Trends in Biotechnology*, Vol. 26, No. 6, pp. (338-344)

Martucci, J.F. & Ruseckaite, R.A. (2009). Biodegradation of three.layer films based on gelatin under indoor soil condiions. *Polymer Degradation & Stability*, Vol. 94, No. 8, pp. (1307-1313)

Mohanty, B & Bohidar, H.B. (2003). Systematic of Alcohol-Induced Simple Coacervation in Aqueous Gelatin Solutions. *Biomacromolecules*, Vol. 4, No. 4 , pp. (1080-1086)

Mohanty, B., & Bohidar, H.B. (2005). Microscopic structure of gelatin coacervates. *International Journal of Biological Macromolecules*, Vol. 36, No. 1-2, pp. (39-46)

Mohanty, B., & Bohidar, H.B. (2005). Microscopic structure of gelatin coacervates. *International Journal of Biological Macromolecules*, Vol. 36, No. 1-2, pp. (39-46)

Mookhtiar, K.A. & Van Wart,H.E. (1992).Clostridium Histolyticum Collagenases: a New Look at Some Old Enzymes. *Matrix (Stuttgart)*, Vol. 1, pp. (116 – 126)

Muyonga, J.H., Cole, C.G.B. & Duodu, K.G.(2004). Characterization of acid soluble collagen from skins of young and adult Nile perch (Lates niloticus). *Food Chemistry*, Vol. 85, No. 1, pp. (81-89)

Mu, C., Liu,F., Cheng,Q., Li,H., Wu, B., Zhang, G. & Lin, W. (2010). Collagen Cryogel Cross-Linked by Dialdehyde Starch, *Macromolecular Materials and Engineering*, Vol. 295, No. 2, pp. (100-107)

Nagai, T., & Suzuki, N. (2000). Isolation of collagen from fish waste material-skin, bone and fins. *Food Chemistry*, Vol. 68, No. 3, pp. (277-281)

Nagai, T., Worawattanamateekul, W., Suzuki, N., Nakamura, T., Ito, T., Fujiki, K., Nakao, M. & Yano, T. (2000). Isolation and characterization of collagen from rhizostomous jellyfish (*Rhopilema asamushi*). *Food chemistry*, Vol. 70, No. 2, pp. (205-208)

Nagase,H. & Woessner,J.F., Jr. (1999). Matrix Metalloproteinases. *Journal of Biological Chemistry*, Vol. 274, pp. (21491 – 21494)

Narbat, M.K., Orang, F., Hashtjin, M.S. & Goudarzi, A. (2006). Fabrication of Porous Hydroxyapatite-Gelatin Composite Scaffolds for Bone Tissue Engineering. *Iranian Biomedical Journal*, Vol. 10, No. 4, pp. (215-223)

Natu, M.V., Sadinha, J.P., Correia, I.J. & Gil, M.H. (2007). Controlled release gelatin hydrogels and liophilisates with potential application as ocular inserts. *Biomedical Materials*, Vol. 2, pp. (241-249)

Netzel-Arnett,S., Mallya,S.K., Nagase,H., Birkedal-Hansen,H. & Van Wart,H.E. (1991). Continuously Recording Fluorescent Assays Optimized for Five Human Matrix Metalloproteinases. *Analytical Biochemistry*, Vol.195, pp. (86 – 92)

Obregue-Slier, E., Solis, R.L., Neira, A.P. & Marin, F.Z. (2010). Tannin-protein interaction is more closely associated with astringency than tannin-protein precipitation: experience with two oenological tannins and a gelatin. *International Journal of Food Science & Technology*, Vol. 45, No. 12, pp. (2629-2636)

Okada,T., Hayashi,T. & Ikada,Y. (1992). Degradation of Collagen Suture in Vitro and in Vivo. *Biomaterials*, Vol. 13, pp. (448 – 454)

Olsen, D., Yang, C., Bodo, M., Chang, R., Leigh, S., Baez, J., Carmichael, D., Perala, M., Hamalainen, E.R., Jarvinen, M. & Polarek, J. (2003). Recombinant collagen and gelatin for drug delivery. *Advanced Drug Delivery Reviews*, Vol. 55, No. 12, pp. (1547-1567)

Overall, C.M. (1991). Recent Advances in Matrix Metalloproteinase Research. *Trends in Glycoscience and Glycotechnology*, Vol. 3, pp. (384 – 400)

Pachence, J.M., Bohrer, M.P. & Kohn, J. (2007). Biodegradable Polymers, In: *Principles of Tissue Engineering*, Lanza, R., Langer, R. &Vacanti, J., pp. (323-358), Elsevier Academic Press, ISBN-13:978-0-12-370615-7, Burlington, USA

Paige, M.F., Lin, A.C. & Goh, M.C. (2002). Real-Time Enzymatic Biodegradation of Collagen Fibrils Monitored by Atomic Force Microscopy. *International Biodeterioration & Biodegradation*, Vol. 50, pp. (1 – 10)

Pannone, P.J. (2007).*Trends in biomaterials research (first edition),* Nova Science Publishers, ISBN-13: 978-1600213618, New York

Park, S.N., Lee, H.J., Lee, K.H. & Suh, H. (2003). Biological characterization of EDC-crosslinked collagen-hyaluronic acid matrix in dermal tissue restoration. *Biomaterials,* Vol. 24, No. 9, pp. (1631-1641)

Pena, C., Caba, K., Eceiza, A., Ruseckaite, R. & Mondragon, I. (2010). Enhancing water repellence and mechanical properties of gelatin films by tannin addition. *Bioresourse Technology,* Vol. 101, pp. (6836-6842)

Pieper,J.S., Oosterhof,A., Dijkstra,P.J., Veerkamp,J.H. & Van Kuppevelt,T.H. (1999). Preparation and Characterization of Porous Crosslinked Collagenous Matrixes Containing Bioavailable Chondroitin Sulfate. *Biomaterials,* Vol. 20, pp. (847 – 858)

Rao, K.P. (1995). Recent developments of collagen-based materials for medical applications and drug delivery systems. *Journal of biomaterials sicence. Polymer edition,* Vol. 7, No. 7, pp. (623-645)

Roche, S., Ronziere, M.C., Herbage, D & Freyria, A.M. (2001). Native and DPPA cross-linked collagen sponges seeded with fetal bovine spiphyseal chondrocytes used for cartilage tissue engineering. *Biomaterials,* Vol. 22, No. 1, pp. (9-18)

Robinson, J.J (1997). Comparative Biochemical Analysis of Sea Urchin Peristome and Rat Tail Tendon Collagen. *Comparative Biochemistry and Physiology Part B: Biochemistry and Molecular Biology,* Vol. 117, No. 2, pp. (307-313)

Saitoa, H., Taguchic,T., Kobayashic,H., Kataokac, K., Tanakac, J., Murabayashia, S. & Mitamuraa, Y. (2004). Physicochemical properties of gelatin gels prepared using citric acid derivative. *Material Science and Engineering C ,* Vol. C24, No. 6-8, pp. (781-785)

Samuel, C.S., Coghlan, J.P. & Bateman, J.F. (1998).Effects of relaxin, pregnancy and parturition on collagen metabolism in the rat public symphysis. *Journal of Endocrinology,* Vol. 159, No.1, pp. (117–125)

Schacht, E.H. (2004). Polymer chemistry and hydrogel systems. *Journal of physics: Conference Series,* Vol. 3, pp. (22-28)

Seifter, S., & Harper, E. (1971). Collagenases, In*: The Enzymes* Vol. 3,*P.* Boyer, Academic Press, NewYork

Silver, F.H. & Garg,A.K. (1997). Collagen. Characterization, Processing, and Medical Applications. *Drug Targeting and Delivery,* Vol. 7, pp. (319 – 346)

Sinha,V.R. & Trehan, A. (2003). Biodegradable Microspheres for Protein Delivery. *Journal of Controlled Release,* Vol. 90, No. 3, pp. (261 – 280)

Sisson, K., Zhang, C., Farach-Carson, M.C., Chase, D.B. & Rabolt,J.F. (2009). Evaluation of Cross-Linking Methods for Electrospun Gelatin on Cell Growth and Viability. *Biomacromolecules, Vol. 10, No. 7, pp. (1675-1680)*

Song, E., KimS.Y., Chun,T., Byun, H.J & Lee,Y.M. (2006). Collagen Scaffolds derived from a marine source and their biocompatibility. *Biomaterials,* Vol 27, No. 15, (2951-2961)

Sung, H.W., Chang, W.H., Ma, C.Y. & Lee, M.H. (2003).Crosslinking of biological tissues using genipin and/or carbodiimide. *Journal of Biomedical Materials Research Part A,* Vol. 64A, No. 3, pp. (427-438)

Sutter, M., Siepmann,J., Hennink, W.E. & Jiskoot, W.(2007). Recombinant gelatin hydrogels for the sustained release of proteins. *Journal of Controlled Release,* Vol. 119, No.3, pp. (301-312)

Suzuki, S., Kawai, K., Ashoori, F., Morimoto, N., Nishimura, Y. & Ikada, Y. (2000). Long-term follow-up study of artificial dermis composed of outer silicone layer and inner collagen sponge. *British Journal of Plastic Surgery*, Vol. 53, No.8, pp. (659 –666)

Shingleton, W.D., Hodges, D.J., Brick, P. & Cawston,T.E. (1996). Collagenase: a Key Enzyme in Collagen Turnover. *International Journal of Biochemistry & Cell Biology*, Vol. 74, pp. (759 – 775)

Shoulders, M.D. & Raines, R.T. (2009). Collagen structure and stability. *Annual Review of Biochemistry*, Vol. 78, pp. (929-958)

Spira, M., Liu, B., Xu, Z., Harrell, R. & Chanhadeh, H. (2004). Human amnion collagen for soft tissue augmentation-biochemical characterizations and animal observations. *Journal of Biomedical Materials Research*, Vol. 28, No. 1, pp. (91-96)

Starin, W.A. (1918). The Antigenic Properties of Gelain. *The Journal of Infectious Diseases*, Vol. 23, No. 2, pp. (139-158)

Stone, K.R., Steadman, J.R., Rodkey, W.G. & Li, S.T. (1997). Regeneration of Meniscal Cartilage With Use of a Collagen Scaffold. Journal of Bone and Joint Surgery, Vol. 79-A, No. 12, pp. (1770-1777)

Sztuka, K. & Kolodziejska, I. (2008). Effect of transglutaminase and EDC on biodegradation of fish gelatin and gelatin-chitosan film. *European Food Research & Technology*, Vol. 226, No. 5, pp. (1127-1133)

Tangsadthakun, C., Kanokpanont, S., Sanchavanakit, N., Banaprasert, T. & Damrongsakkul, S. (2006). Properties of Collagen/Chitosan Scaffolds for Skin Tissue Engineering. *Journal of Metals, Materials and Minerals*, Vol. 16, No. 1, pp. (37-44)

Taylor, P.M., Cass, A.E.G. & Yacoub, M.H. (2006). Extracellular matrix scaffolds for tissue engineering heart valves. *Process in Pediatric Cardiology*, Vol. 21, No. 2, pp. (219-225)

Tedder, M.E., Liao,J., Weed,B., C. Stabler, C., H. Zhang, H., A. Simionescu,A. & Simionescu,D. (2009). Stabilized collagen scaffolds for heart valve tissue engineering. *Tissue Engineering Part A*, Vol. 15, No. 6, pp. (1257-1268)

Tefft, S., Bentz, H., & Estridge, T.D. (1997). Collagen and heparin matrices for growth factor delivery. *Journal of Control Release*, Vol.48, No. 1, pp. (29–33)

Touyama, R.,Takeda, Y., Inoue, K., Kawamura, I., Yatsuzuka, M., Ikumoto, T., Shingu, T., Yokoi, T.I.& Inouye, H. (1994). Studies on the blue pigments produced from genipin and methylamine. I. Structures of the brownish-red pigments, intermediates leading to the blue pigments. *Chemical and Pharmaceutical Bulletin*, Vol. 42, pp. (668-673)

Toricai, A. & Shibata, H. (1999). Effect of ultraviolet radiation on photodegradation of collagen. *Journal of Applied Polymer Science*, Vol. 73, No. 7, pp. (1259-1265)

Trengove,N.J., Stacey,M.C., MacAuley,S., Bennett,N., Gibson,J., Burslem,F., Murphy,G. & Schultz,G. (1999). Analysis of the Acute and Chronic Wound Environments: the Role of Proteases and Their Inhibitors. *Wound Repair and Regeneration*, Vol. 7, pp. (442 – 452)

Tsai, C.C., Huang, R.N., Sung, H.W. & Liang, H.C. (2000). In vitro evaluation of the genotoxicity of a naturally occurring agent (genipin) for biologic tissue fixation. *Journal of Biomedical Materials Research*, Vol. 52, No. 1, pp. (58-65)

Tucci, M.G. & Ricotti, G. (2001). Chitosan & Gelatin as Engineered Dressing for Wound Repair. *Journal of Bioactive andCompatiblePolymers*, Vol. 16, pp. (144-157)

Van Den Bulcke, A.I., Bogdanov, B., De Rooze, N., Schacht,E.H., Cornellssen, M.& Berghmans, H. (2000). Structural and Rheological Properties of Methacrylamide Modified Gelatin Hydrogels. *Biomacromolecules*, Vol. 1, pp. (31-38)

Van Luyn, M.J.A., van Wachem, P.B., Dijkstra, P.J., L.H.H., Damink, O & Feijen, J. (1995). Calcification of subcutaneously implanted collagen in relation to cytotoxicity, cellular interactions and crosslinking. *Journal of Materials Scinecne: Materials in Medicine*, Vol. 6, No. 5, pp. (288–296)

Van Wachem,P.B., Zeeman,R., Dijkstra,P.J., Feijen, J., Hendriks, M., Cahalan, P.T. & van Luyn, V.J. (1999). Characterization and biocompatibility of epoxy-crosslinked dermal sheep collagens. *Journal of Biomedical Materials Research*, Vol.47, No. 2, pp. (270–277)

Van Wachem ,P.B., van Luyn, M.J.A., Brouwer, L.A., Engbers, G.H.M., Krijgsveld, J., Zaat, S.A.J., Dankert, J. & Feijen,J. (2000). In vitro and in vivo evaluation of gelatin-chrondroitin sulphate hydrogels for controlled release of antibacterial proteins. *Biomaterials*, Vol. 21, pp. (1763-1772)

Vargas, G.,Acevedo, J.L.,Lopez,J. & Romero,J. (2008). Study of cross-linking of gelatin by ethylene glycol diglycidyl ether. *Materials Letters*, Vol. 62, pp. (3656-3658).

Vlierberhe,V.S., Dubruel, P., Lippens, E., Cornelissen, M. & Schacht, E. (2009). Correlation Between Cryigenic Parameters and Physico-Chemical Properties of Porous Gelatin Cryogels. *Journal of Biomaterial Science*, Vol. 20, pp. (1417-1438)

Wahl , D.A. & Czernuszka, J.T. (2006). Collagen-hydroxyapatite composites for hard tissue repair. *European Cells and Materials*, Vol. 11, pp. (43-56)

Wall, S.J., Bevan,D., Thomas,D.W., Harding,K.G., Edwards,D.R & Murphy,G. (2002). Differential Expression of Matrix Metalloproteinases During Impaired Wound Healing of the Diabetes Mouse. *Journal of Investigative Dermatology*, Vol. 119, pp. (91 – 98)

Wang, X., Yu, X., Yan, Y. & Zhang, R.(2008). Liver tissue responses to gelatin and gelatin/chitosan gels. *Journal of Biomedical Materials Research A*, Vol. 87, No. 1, pp. (62-80)

Wang, X.H., Li, D.P., Wang, W.J., Feng, Q.L., Cui, F.Z., Xu, Y.X., Song, X.H. & Van Der Werf, M.. (2003). Crosslinked collagen/chitosan matrix for artificial livers. *Biomaterials*, Vol. 24, pp. (3213-3220)

Welgus ,H.G., Jeffrey,J.J., Stricklin,G.P., Roswit,W.T. & Eisen,A.Z. (1980). Characteristics of the Action of Human Skin Fibroblast Collagenase on Fibrillar Collagen. *Journal of Biological Chemistry*, Vol. 255, pp. (6806 – 6813)

Welgus, H.G., Kobayashi,D.K. & Jeffrey, J.J. (1983). The Collagen Substrate Specificity of Rat Uterus Collagenase. *Journal of Biological Chemistry*, Vol. 258, pp. (14162 – 14165)

Weiss, J.B. (1976). Enzymic Degradation of Collagen. *International Review of Connective Tissue Research*, Vol. 7, pp. (101 – 157)

Westney, O.L., Bevan-Thomas, R., Palmer, J.L., Cespedes, R.D. & McGuire, E.J. (2005). Transurethral collagen injections for male intrinsic sphincter deficiency: the University of Texas-Houston experience. *The Journal of Urology*, Vol. 174, No. 3, pp. (994–997)

Woessner, J.F. (1991).Matrix Metalloproteinases and Their Inhibitors in Connective Tissue Remodeling. *The Journal of the Federation of Americal Societies for Experimental Biology*, Vol. 5, pp. (2145 – 2154)

Wong, C., Shital, P., Chen, R., Owida, A. & Morsi, Y. (2010). Biomimmetic alactrospun gelatin-chitosan polyurethane for heart valve leaflets. *Journal of Mechanics in Medicine and Biology*, Vol. 10, No. 4, pp. (563-576)

Yamauchi, M. & Shiiba, M. (2008). Lysine Hydroxylation and Crosslinking of Collagen, In: *Post-translational Modifications of Proteins*, Kannicht, C., Springer, Humana Press, ISBN: 9781588297198, New York

Yan, L.P., Wang, Y.J., Ren, L., Wu, G., Caridade, S.G., Fan, J.B., Wang, L.Y, Ji, P.H., Oliveira, J.M., Oliveira, J.T., Mano, J.F. & Reis, R.L. (2010). Genipin-cross-linked collagen /chitosan biomimetic scaffolds for articular cartilage tissue engineering applications. *Journal of Biomedical Materials Research Part A*, Vol. 95A, No. 2, pp. (465-475)

Yannas, I.V.(1992). Tissue regeneration by use of collagen–glycosaminoglycan co-polymers. *Clinical Materials*, Vol. 9, No. 3-4, pp. (179–187)

Yao, C.H., Lui B.S., Hsu S.H., Chen Y.S.(2005). Cavarial Bone Response to Tricalcium Phosphate-Genipin Crosslinked Gelatin Composite. *Biomaterials*, Vol. 26, pp. (3065-3074)

Yoshida, H., Sasajima, T., Goh, K., Inaba, M. Otani, N. & Kubo, Y. (1996). Early results of a reinforced biosynthetic ovine collagen vascular prosthesis for small arterial reconstruction. *Surgery Today*, Vol. 26, No. 4, pp. (262-266)

Yoshizaki, T., Sato,H. & Furukawa,M. (2002). Recent Advances in the Regulation of Matrix Metalloproteinase 2 Activation: From Basic Research to Clinical Implication (Review). *Oncology Reports*, Vol. 9, pp. (607 – 611)

Ye, Q., Xing, Q., Ren, Y., Harmsen, M.C. & Bank, R.A. (2010). ENDO180 andMT1-MMP are involved in the phagocytosis of collagen scaffolds by macrophages and is regulated by interferon-gamma. *European Cells and Materials*, Vol. 20, pp. (197-209)

Yuan, Y., Zhang, P., Yanq, Y., Wang, X, Gu, X. (2004). The interaction of Schwann cells with chitosan membranes and fibers in vitro. *Biomaterials*, Vol. 25, No. 18, (4273–4278)

Yuan, S.X., Wei, T.T. (2004). New Contact Lens Based on Chitosan/Gelatin Composites. *Journal of Bioactive and Compatible Polymers*, Vol. 19, No. 6, pp. (467-479)

Zeeman, R., Dijkstra,P.J., Van Wachem,P.B., Van Luyn,M.J.A., Hendriks,M., Cahalan,P.T. & Feijen,J. (1999). Successive Epoxy and Carbodiimide Crosslinking of Dermal Sheep Collagen. *Biomaterials*, Vol. 20, pp. (921 – 931)

Zhang, F., Xu, S. & Wang, Z. (2010). Pre-treatment optimization and properties of gelatin from freshwater fish scales. *Food and Bioproducts Processing*, doi: 10.1016/j.fbp.2010.05.003 (Article in press)

Zhang,X, Do, M.D., Casey,P., Sulistio, A., Qiao, G.G., Lundin, L. , Lillford, P. & Kosarju, S. (2010). Chemical crosslinking of gelatin with natural phenolic compounds as studied by high-resolution NMR spectroscopy. *Biomacromolecules*, Vol. 11, No. 4, pp. (1125–1132)

2

Bioactive Ceramics as Bone Morphogenetic Proteins Carriers

Sayed Mahmood Rabiee
Babol University of Technology
Iran

1. Introduction

Bone tissue is the component of the skeletal system that provides the supporting structure for the body. Bone has a complex morphology; it is a specialized connective tissue composed of a calcified matrix and an organic matrix. The tissue can be organized in either the dense (compact) or spongy form (cancellous), with pore sizes within the wide range of 1-100 μm (Lane et al., 1999). Although the shape of bone varies in different parts of the body, the physicochemical structure of bone for these different shapes is basically similar. The biochemical composition of bone is precisely composed of two major phases at the nanoscale level namely, organic and inorganic as a good example for a composite. These phases have multiple components which consist of, in decreasing proportions, minerals, collagen, water, non-collagenous proteins, lipids, vascular elements, and cells (Murugan & Ramakrishna, 2005). An overall composition of the bone is given in Table 1.

Inorganic Phases	Wt%	Bioorganic phases	Wt%
Calcium Phosphates (biological apatite)	~ 60	Collagen type I	~ 20
Water	~ 9	None-collagenous proteins	~ 3
Carbonates	~ 4	Primary bone cells	Balance
Citrates	~ 0.9	Other traces	Balance
Sodium	~ 0.7		
Magnesium	~ 0.5		
Other traces	Balance		

Table 1. The biochemical composition of bone (Murugan & Ramakrishna, 2005).

The mineral fraction of bone consists of significant quantities of non-crystalline calcium phosphate compounds and predominantly of a single phase that closely resembles that of crystalline hydroxyapatite ($Ca_{10}(PO_4)_6(OH)_2$) (Hench & Wilson, 1993; Dorozhkin, 2010a). Biological hydroxyapatite also contains other impurity ions as Cl, Mg, Na, K, and F and trace elements like Sr and Zn (LeGeros, 2002). The apatite in bone mineral is composed of small platelet-like crystals of just 2 to 4 nm in thickness, 25 nm in width, and 50 nm in length (Dorozhkin & Epple, 2002). Bone mineral non-stoichiometry is primarily due to the presence of divalent ions, such as CO_3^{2-} and HPO_4^{2-}, which are substituted for the trivalent PO_4^{3-} ions. Substitutions by CO_3^{2-} and HPO_4^{2-} ions produce a change of the Ca/P ratio, resulting in Ca/P ratio which may vary between 1.50 to 1.70, depending on the age and bone site (Raynaud et al., 2002). When a loss of bony tissue occurs as a result of trauma or by the excision of diseased, healing requires the implantation of bone substitutes. There is a high clinical request for synthetic bone substitution materials, due to the drawbacks such as a prolonged operation time and donor site morbidity in about 10–30% of the cases associated with biological bone grafts (Giannoudis et al., 2005; Beaman et al., 2006; Chu et al., 2007). Biological grafts are generally associated with potential infections. In order to avoid the problems associated with biological bone grafting, there has been a continuous interest in the use of synthetic bone substitute materials. Bioactive ceramics such as calcium phosphates offer alternatives to synthetic bone substitute (Vallet-Regı & lez-Calbet, 2004; Best et al., 2008; Rabiee et al., 2008a). These biomateials with a porous structure not only possess good biocompatibility but also allow the ingrowth of tissues and penetration of biological fluids and form a chemical bond with bone (Lu & Leng, 2005; Rabiee et al. 2008b). Moreover, the Calcium phosphates are freely formed and easily fabricated to satisfy the demands for huge bone and large quantities of bone for bone substitute. For these reasons, the Calcium phosphates have been considered as useful materials for bone repair and replacement. To fabricate a bioactive ceramic bone substitute with various porous configuration, the evidence of tissues ingrowth and biological responses provide obvious advantages in tissue-implant fixation and controlled biodegradation rate for both short-term and long-term implantation purposes (Karageorgiou & Kaplan, 2005, Rabiee et al. 2008b). Many processing technologies have been employed to obtain porous calcium phosphates as bone filler (Rabiee et al., 2007; Best etal. 2008). For example, porous calcium phosphates can be obtained by merging the slurry with a polymer sponge-like mold or polymer beads before sintering. During the sintering, the polymer is completely burnt out, which results in a porous structure. The use of highly porous calcium phosphate induces bone formation inside the implant and increases degradation. Cortical bone has pores ranging from 1 to 100 µm (volumetric porosity 5 to 10%), whereas trabecular bone has pores of 200 to 400 µm (volumetric porosity 70 to 90%). Porosity in bone provides space for nutrients supply in cortical bone and marrow cavity in trabecular bone. Microporosity covers pores sizes smaller than 5 µm for penetration of fluids and Pores larger than 10 µm can be considered as macropores. Macroporous dimensions are reported to play a role in osteoinductive behavior of bone substitutes (Karageorgiou & Kaplan, 2005; Rabiee et al., 2009). Because of the influence of bioactive ceramics on cell behaviour, the bone forming cells are often introduced into these porous ceramics to speed-up tissue ingrowth. The surface of bioactive ceramics is a good substrate for seeding cells (Cao et al., 2010; Rungsiyakull et al., 2010). Bone Tissue engineering typically involves coupling osteogenic cells and/or osteoinductive growth factors with bioactive scaffolds (Buma et al., 2004; Mistry & Mikos, 2005). Some studies have investigated the bone forming capacities of growth factors loaded synthetic bone substitutes. In terms of growth factors, most research has focused on the use of the bone morphogenic proteins (BMPs) (Mont et al. 2004; Termaat et al., 2005). They are signalling molecules which can induce de novo bone formation at orthotopic and heterotropic sites (Boix et al., 2005). Current examination of alternatives to grafting techniques suggests three possible new approaches to inducing new bone formation: implantation of certain cytokines such as BMPs in combination with appropriate delivery systems at the target site (Liu et al., 2007; Niu et al., 2009); transduction of genes encoding cytokines with osteogenic capacity into cells at repair sites; and transplantation of cultured osteogenic cells derived from host bone marrow (Chu et al., 2007). BMPs have crucial roles in growth and regeneration of skeletal tissues (Nie & Wang, 2007). One primary role of BMPs is to regulate the key elements in the bone induction cascade required for regeneration of skeletal tissues (Schneider et al., 2003). BMPs are bone matrix protein that stimulate mesenchymal cell chemotaxis and proliferation, and promotes the differentiation of these cells into chondrocytes and osteoblasts (Calori et al., 2009; Nie & Wang, 2007). This osteoinductive action of BMPs is well established to be beneficial during the repair bone defects (Termaat et al., 2005). BMPs act locally and therefore must be delivered directly to the site of regeneration via a carrier (Hartman et al., 2005; Chu et al., 2007). Bioactive ceramics can act as vehicle for factor delivery to the surrounding tissues. Future research should be investigated the potentials of these constructs to find a successful alternative for biological bone substitute.

2. Bioactive ceramics

Bioactive ceramics are used in a number of different applications in implants and in the repair and reconstruction of diseased or damaged body parts. Most medical applications of bioactive ceramics relate to the repair of the skeletal system and hard tissue. They include several major groups such as calcium phosphate ceramics, bioactive glasses and glass-ceramics.

2.1 Calcium phosphate ceramics

Calcium phosphate ceramics are very popular implants for medical applications because of their similarity to hard tissue. These bioceramics have been synthesized and used for manufacturing various forms of implants, as well as for solid or porous coatings on other implants. Calcium phosphate compounds exist in several phases. Most of these compounds are used as raw material for synthesis of bioactive ceramics. Different types of calcium phosphate are employed to fabricate implants to accommodate bone tissue regeneration. Table 2 lists the main Ca-P compounds for biomedical applications (Vallet-Reg1 & lez-Calbet, 2004). The atomic ratio of Ca/P in calcium phosphates can be varied between 2 and 1 to produce compounds ranged from calcium tetraphosphate(TTCP) $Ca_4P_2O_9$, hydroxyapatite (HA) $Ca_{10}(PO_4)_6(OH)_2$, octacalcium phosphate (OCP) $Ca_8H_2(PO_4)_6.5H_2O$, tricalcium phosphate (TCP) $Ca_3(PO_4)_2$ to dicalcm phosphate dihydrate (DCPD) $CaHPO_4.2H_2O$ or dicalcum phosphate anhydrus (DCPA) $CaHPO_4$. (Raynaud et al., 2002; Vallet-Reg1 & lez-Calbet, 2004; Dorozhkin, 2010b). Due to their high solubility, the calcium phosphates compounds with a Ca/P ratio less than 1 are not suitable for biological implantation. Hydroxyapatite with Ca/P ratio of 1.667 is much more stable than other calcium phosphates. Under physiological conditions, calcium phosphates degrade via dissolution–reprecipitation mechanisms (Raynaud et al., 2002).

When the dissolution of calcium phosphate is higher than the rate of mineral reprecipitation and tissue regeneration, it is not suitable as a good bone substitute. The dissolution process is dependent on the nature and their thermodynamic stability of calcium phosphate substrate, for example (in order of increasing solubility), HA > TCP > OCP > DCPD or DCPA (Bohner, 2000; Dorozhkin, 2010a). In an ideal situation, a biodegeradable bone substitute is slowly resorbed and replaced by natural bone. TCP with Ca/P ratio of 1.5 is a biodegradable and more resorbed than HA. The use of a mixture of HA and β-TCP, as biphasic calcium phosphate (BCP), has been attempted as bone substitute. The dissolution and resorption rate of BCP can be controlled with ratio of β-TCP/HA (Detsch et al., 2008; De Gabory et al., 2010).

Name	Ca/P	Formula	Acronym
Calcium Dihydrogen Phosphate	0.5	$Ca(H_2PO_4)_2H_2O$	MCP
Dicalcum phosphate dihydrate	1	$CaHPO_4.2H_2O$	DCPD
Dicalcum phosphate anhydrous	1	$CaHPO_4$	DCPA
Octacalcium phosphate	1.33	$Ca_8H_2(PO_4)_6.5H_2O$	OCP
Tricalcium phosphate	1.5	$Ca_3(PO_4)_2$	TCP
Hydroxyapatite	1.67	$Ca_{10}(PO_4)_6(OH)_2$	HA
Tetracalcium phosphate	2	$Ca_4O(PO_4)_2$	TTCP

Table 2. Varius calcium phosphate with their respective Ca/P atomic ratios (Vallet-Regı & lez-Calbet, 2004).

The major limitation to use calcium phosphates is their mechanical properties. Calcium phosphates are used primarily as fillers and coatings (Ooms et al., 2003) because they are brittle with poor fatigue resistance (Teoh, 2000).

2.2 Calcium phosphate cements

Calcium phosphate cements (CPCs) are of interest for bone tissue engineering purposes. Different studies with CPCs have shown that they are highly biocompatible and osteoconductive materials, which can stimulate tissue regeneration (Bohner, 2000; Carey et al., 2005; Ginebra et al., 2006). The main difference between cements when compared to other bioactive ceramics, in the form of ceramic granules or bulk materials, is the injectability and in-situ hardening. Calcium phosphate cements consist of a powder phase and an aqueous liquid, which are mixed together to form a paste that sets after being implanted within the body. Brown and Chow prepared the first CPBC in 1985 contained TTCP and DCPA or DCPD as the solid phase (Brown & Chow, 1985). After mixing with water, the cement components results precipitation of apatite (AP: Ca_{10-x} $(HPO_4)_x(PO4)_{6-x}(OH)_{2-x}$, where $0 \le x \le 2$) (Ginebra et al., 2006; Rabiee et al., 2010). There are a variety of different combinations of calcium compounds which are used in the formulation of these bone cements. In general there are two types of CPC: apatite cements and brushite cements. Brushite cement has a lower mechanical strength but a faster biodegradability than the apatite cement. Both types of cement can be applied for bone tissue engineering purposes. (Carey et al., 2005; Rabiee et al., 2010). CPCs as drug delivery systems, where the drugs can be incorporated throughout the whole cement volume. CPCs are suitable materials for local delivery systems in osseous tissue since they can simultaneously promote bone regeneration and prevent infectious diseases by releasing therapeutic agents. Recent advances in CPC technology have resulted in the enhancement of the handling, application and osteoconductive properties of these cements. These improvements have permitted CPCs to be assayed as carriers for local delivery of drugs and biologically active substances (Ginebra et al., 2006). Drugs, such as antibiotics, antitumors, and growth factors, have been administered to defect regions to induce therapeutic effects (Ginebra et al., 2006; Chu et al. 2007). The success of this idea was favored by the easy incorporation of pharmaceutical and biological substances into the cement solid or liquid phases, the intimate adaptation of the cement paste to bone defects and permits the release of the entrapped substance to the local environment.

2.3 Bioactive glasses & glass-ceramics

Bioactive glasses and glass-ceramics have the ability to bind to hard tissues as was discovered by Hench in 1969 (Hench, 2006). They are used as implants to repair or replace parts of the body; long bones, vertebrae, joints, and teeth. Their clinical success is due to formation of a stable, mechanically strong interface with bone (Hench & Wilson, 1993; Cao et al., 2010). Bioactive materials are typically made of compositions from the Na_2O-CaO, MgO-P_2O_5-SiO_2 system. The composition of the first bioglass Hench made was in weight percent 25% Na_2O, 25% CaO, 5% P_2O_5 and 45% SiO_2 and noted as Bioglass 45S5. Melting and sol- gel processing are two methods for producting glasses. Sol-gel processing has been successfully used in the production of a variety of materials for both biomedical and nonbiomedical applications (Hench, 2006; Ravarian et al., 2010). Sol-gel processing, an alternative to traditional melt processing of glasses, involves the synthesis of a solution (sol), typically composed of metal-organic and metal salt precursors followed by the formation of a gel by chemical reaction or aggregation, and lastly thermal treatment for drying, organic removal, and sometimes crystallization (Saravanapavan & Hench, 2003). Sol-gel-derived bioactive glasses were used because they exhibit high specific area, high osteoconductive properties, and a significant degradability. The sol-gel approach to making bioactive glass materials has produced glasses with enhanced compositional range of bioactivity. When in contact with body fluids or tissues, bioactive glasses develop reactive layers at their surfaces resulting in a chemical bond between implant and host tissue (Hench, 2006). Hench has described a sequence of five reactions that result in the formation of a hydroxy-carbonate apatite (HCA) layer on the surface of these bioactive glasses (Hench, 2006). The dissolution of the glass network, leading to the formation of a silica-rich gel layer and subsequent deposition of an apatite-like layer on the glass surface, was found to be essential steps for bonding of glass to living tissues both through in vivo and in vitro studies (Cao et al., 2010). The use of bioactive glass for load-bearing applications is restricted because of its brittleness. One possibility to overcome this drawback is to crystallize the glass to obtain a glass-ceramic. Glass- ceramics are polycrystalline ceramics made by transformation of the glass into ceramic. The formation of glass ceramics is influenced by the nucleation and growth of small crystals. The nucleation of glass is carried out at temperatures much lower than the melting temperature. Professor Kokubo and his coworkers developed a glass-ceramic containing apatite and wollastonite in a glass matrix (Kokubo et al., 1986). Apatite-wollastonite (A-W) glass-ceramic is one of the most important glass ceramics for use as a bone substitute. The apatite crystals form sites for bone growth; the long wollastonite crystals reinforce the glass (Liu et al. 2004). Drug and growth factor loading of bioactive glasses and glass ceramics is possible using the sol–gel method. Ziegler et al. introduced Growth factors into a bioactive glass and observed an initial burst of 10%, followed by a delayed boost between day 3 and 8, depending on the type of growth factor (Ziegler et al., 2002).

3. Bone morphogenetic proteins

Bone morphogenetic proteins (BMPs) induce new bone formation by directing mesenchymal stem cells. They are biologically active osteoinductive cytokines that with significant clinical potential. The key steps are proliferation of cells, and finally differentiation into cartilage and then bone. Proliferation was maximal on day 3, chondroblast differentiation was on day 5, and chondrocytes were on day 7. The cartilage hypotrophied on day 9 with vascularization and osteogenesis. On days 10 to 12 maximal alkaline phosphatase activity, a marker of bone formation was observed. Hematopoietic differentiation was observed in the ossicle on day 21. BMP were first characterized in 1965 by Urist as a biologically activator and he has led to various studies for identification of a variety of growth factors that play roles in osteogenesis. The most studied of these are the insulin-like growth factor (IGF), epidermal growth factor (EGF), fibroblast growth factor (FGF), platelet-derived growth factor (PDGF), and the transforming growth factor (TGF) group, of which, the BMPs form a subgroup. There are 15 members of BMPs family in table 3 and Among members of the BMPs, BMP2, 4, and 7 possess a strong ability to induce bone formation (Termaat et al., 2005; Nie & Wang, 2007; Calori et al., 2009).

BMP designation	Generic Name
BMP1	bone morphogenetic protein 1
BMP2	bone morphogenetic protein 2
BMP3	bone morphogenetic protein 3 (osteogenic)
BMP4	bone morphogenetic protein 4
BMP5	bone morphogenetic protein 5
BMP6	bone morphogenetic protein 6
BMP7	bone morphogenetic protein 7 (osteogenic protein 1)
BMP8A	bone morphogenetic protein 8a
BMP8B	bone morphogenetic protein 8b (osteogenic protein 2)
BMP9	growth differentiation factor 2 (GDF2)
BMP10	bone morphogenetic protein 10
BMP11	growth differentiation factor 11 (GDF11)
BMP12	growth differentiation factor 7 (GDF7)
BMP13	growth differentiation factor 6 (GDF6)
BMP14	growth differentiation factor 5 (GDF5)
BMP15	bone morphogenetic protein 15

Table 3. The BMPs Family. (Termaat et al., 2005).

4. Bioactive ceramic as carrier for bone marrow cells: case study

This experiment focuses on a tissue engineering strategy for bone regeneration using bone marrow carried by a bioactive ceramic scaffold. To fabricate a bioactive ceramic with porous configuration, the evidence of tissues ingrowth and biological responses provide obvious advantages in tissue-implant fixation and controlled biodegradation rate for both short-term and long-term implantation purposes (Klein et al., 1984; Rabiee et al., 2008c). Many processing technologies have been employed to obtain porous bioceramics as bone substuitute. The method of casting foams has shown suitability to manufacture strong and reliable macro-porous bioceramics that have great potential to replace bone tissue (Rabiee et al., 2007, 2008c). Results obtained with bone substitutes are currently less reliable than with autologous cancellous bone grafting which remains the preferred method for healing bone defects. Bone marrow stromal cells haved proved their ability to induce bone formation (Liu et al., 2007b). So the association of autologous bone marrow and porous bioceramic might be a successful hybrid biomaterial for bone substitute (Liu et al., 2007). The porous sample was fabricated by polyurethane foam reticulate method. The macrostructure of the scaffold was controlled by the porous structure of the polymer substrate. After sintering the ceramic resembled the polymer matrix texture, giving rise to a structure characterized by several macropores, whose size (100 μm <macropores size<200 μm) can assure osteoconduction after implantation (Fig. 1). The total porosity of the porous body was evaluated from the density value calculated as weight/volume and amounted to 64±5%. Details of the preparation method can be found in Ref. (Rabiee et al., 2009).

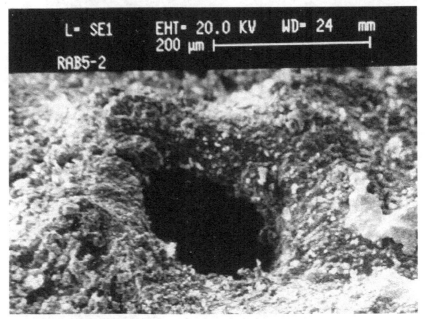

Fig. 1. SEM micrograph of a macropore in sintered bioactive ceramic.

Synthetic porous ceramic were supplied in the form of cylindrical specimens with a mean diameter of 3.4 ±0.5 mm and a mean length of 6.3±0.7 mm. Under general anesthesia, bone marrow was harvested from one medullar midshaft of the rabbit femur and diluted with 1 cc of saline. The porous ceramic were immersed in the solution for 5 min before implantation. A cavity of 3.5 mm in diameter and 7 mm in depth was drilled manually in the femoral condyles under general anaesthetic conditions and antibiotic protection. After carefully washing with a physiological saline solution, the cavities were filled with porous bioactive ceramic (BC) on one side and with porous bioactive ceramic contain Bone marrow

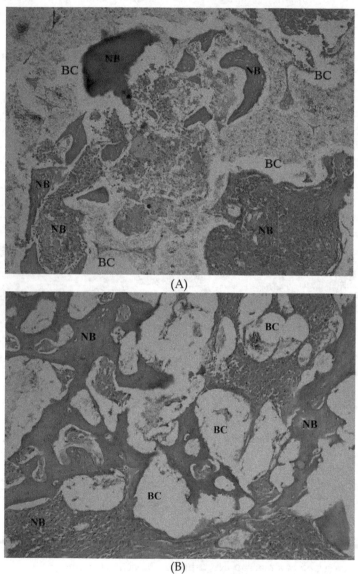

(A)

(B)

Fig. 2. Histological section of implants were harvested 3 months after implantation and stained with hematoxylin and eosin at 100x magnification. (A) bioactive ceramic, (B) bioactive ceramic with bone marrow cells. BC=bioactive ceramic, NB= newly formed bone.

(BCBM) on the other side. After 1, 2, 3 and 6 months, animals were killed by an overdose of thiopental sodium and the femoral condyles were removed. Experiments were performed according to the European Guidelines for Care and Use of Laboratory Animals (European Directive 86/609/CEE). During the experiment, all rabbits remained in good health and did not show any wound complications. No inflammatory signs or adverse tissue reaction could be observed. After 3 months, revealed the bridging of the BC and BCBM by host bone. Fig. 2 shows in vivo test results after 3 months. Histological investigations show a higher presence of newly formed bone and a higher osteogenesis in BCBM compared to BC after 3 & 6 months. In general, osteoblasts occurred evidently one month postoperatively, bone marrows began to develop in new bone tissues two months postoperatively, and bone tissues tended to be mature with the development of osteocytes and bone marrows over three months postoperatively.

Ideally, an implant, when placed in an osseous defect, should induce a response similar to that of fracture healing, where by the defect is initially filled with a blood clot which is invaded by mesenchymal cells, osteoblasts and fibroblasts within 2 weeks, followed by extensive bone and osteoid formation at 6 weeks, with complete healing/repair of the cancellous structure by 12 weeks (Orr et al., 2001). [

An equivalent amount of host bone was found in the BC and BCBM treated sites (Fig. 3). No significant difference was seen between BCBM and BC, at month 1 and month 2, but in Group 3 and 6 months, osteoid surface was higher in BCBM than in BC alone (p<0.05). BCBM have a stable biomechanical environment conducive to the formation of callus. Data from several sources show the exact effect of bone ingrowth on compressive strength and elastic modulus (Orr et al., 2001; Rabiee et al., 2008b). The porous implant with tissue ingrowth acts a composite structure. The implanted block consists of the mineral matrix of the block, fibrovascular tissue and bony tissue. All of these parameters effect on the compressive strength and modulus.

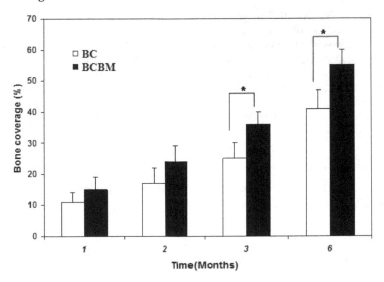

Fig. 3. Histomorphometry of the amount of bone coverage in BC and BCBM at 1, 2, 3 and 6 months after implantation. *p<0.05.

Results from mechanical compressive strength and elastic modulus of implanted specimens are presented in Table 4. BC specimens possessed an elastic modulus of 299±21 MPa prior to implantation. Elastic moduli of BC and BCBM became weaker after implantation (Table 4). BC moduli were significantly higher than those of the control at all time points, but no significant difference was apparent between BCBM and control 3 and 6 months after implantation. One example of the influence of a high modulus of elasticity of an implant material on surrounding bone is the dramatic bone loss around certain joint replacement prostheses. This bone loss has been attributed to the stress shielding resulting from the large disparity between the stiffness of the implant and the host bone (Orr et al., 2001).

Time of implantation	Compressive strength (MPa)		Elastic modulus (MPa)	
	BC	BCBM	BC	BCBM
Before implantatiom	6(0.5)	-	299(21)	-
1 months	5.2(0.94)	5.73(1)	268(33)	232(21)
2 months	4.8(0.9)	5.56(1.02)	232(20)	205(19)
3 months	5(0.3)	5.96(0.62)	206(22)	188(16)
6 months	5.1(0.5)	5.76(1.05)	195(17)	171(14)
AC	4.7(0.6)		169(23)	

Table 4. Mechanical properties of BC and BCBM. BC= Bioactive ceramic without bone marrow; BCBM= Bioactive ceramic with bone marrow; AC= anatomic control.

After implantation, BC and BCBM were partly degraded and their compressive mechanical properties decreased or remained at the same level. This could have resulted from two opposing reactions, with the matrix degrading slowly at the same time the amount of bone related to the reduced implant size was increasing. The first results of in vivo tests on rabbits showed good biocompatibility and osteointegration of the synthetic bioactive ceramic with bone marrow, with higher osteoconductive properties and earlier bioresorption, compared to similar synthetic bioactive ceramic without bone marrow samples. Bone marrow improved mechanical properties and bone growth. Bone ingrowth and degradation of the bioactive ceramic allow bone remodeling, which is a prerequisite for a good bone substitute.

5. Acknowledgments

The author would like to thank Prof. Moztarzadeh and Dr Mortazavi for their technical assistance, and Dr Sharifi for organizing the surgery.

6. References

Beaman, F.D., Bancroft, L.W., Peterson, J.J. & Kransdorf, M.J. (2006). Bone Graft Materials and Synthetic Substitutes. *Radiologic Clinics of North America*, Vol. 44, No. 3, pp. 451-461.

Best, S.M., Porter, A.E., Thian, E.S. & Huang, J. (2008). Bioceramics: Past, present and for the future. *Journal of the European Ceramic Society*, Vol. 28, No. 7, pp. 1319-1327.

Bohner, M. (2000). Calcium orthophosphates in medicine: from ceramics to calcium phosphate cements. *Injury*. Vol. 31, pp. 37-47.

Buma, P., Schreurs, W. & Verdonschot, N. (2004). Skeletal tissue engineering from in vitro studies to large animal models. *Biomaterials*, Vol. 25, No. 9, pp.1487–95.

Boix, T., Gómez-Morales, J., Torrent-Burgués, J., Monfort, A., Puigdomènech, P. & Rodríguez-Clemente, R. (2005). Adsorption of recombinant human bone morphogenetic protein rhBMP-2m onto hydroxyapatite. *Journal of Inorganic Biochemistry*, Vol. 99, No. 5, pp. 1043-1050

Brown,W.E., Chow,L.C. (1985). Dental restorative cement pastes. U. S. Patent No. 4518430.

Calori, G.M., Donati, D., Bella C.D. & Tagliabue, L. (2009). Bone morphogenetic proteins and tissue engineering: future directions. *Injury*, Vol. 40, pp. 67-S76

Cao, B., Zhou, D., Xue, M., Li, G., Yang, W., Long, Q. & Ji, L. (2010). Study on surface modification of porous apatite-wollastonite bioactive glass ceramic scaffold. *Applied Surface Science*, Vol. 255, No. 2, pp. 505-508.

Carey, L.E., Xu, H.H.K., Simon Jr, C.G., Takagi, S. & Chow, L.C. (2005). Premixed rapid-setting calcium phosphate composites for bone repair. *Biomaterials*, Vol. 26, pp. 5002–5014.

Chu, T.M.G., Warden, S.J., Turnera, C. H. & Stewart, R.L. (2007). Segmental bone regeneration using a load-bearing biodegradable carrier of bone morphogenetic protein-2. *Biomaterials*, Vol. 28, pp. 459–467.

De Gabory, L., Bareille, R., Stoll, D., Bordenave, L. & Fricain, J. (2010). Biphasic calcium phosphate to repair nasal septum: The first in vitro and in vivo study. *Acta Biomaterialia*, Vol., No. 3, pp. 909-919.

Detsch, R., Mayr, H. & Ziegler, G. (2008). Formation of osteoclast-like cells on HA and TCP ceramics, *Acta Biomaterialia*, Vol. 4, No. 1, pp. 139-148.

Dorozhkin, S.V. & Epple, M. (2002). Biological and medical significance of calcium phosphates. *Angewandle Chemie International Edition*, Vol. 41, pp. 3130-3146.

Dorozhkin, S.V. (2010a). Amorphous calcium (ortho)phosphates. *Acta Biomaterialia*, Vol. 6, No. 12, pp. 4457-4475.

Dorozhkin, S.V. (2010b), Bioceramics of calcium orthophosphates. *Biomaterials*, Vol. 31,Vol. 7, pp. 1465-1485.

Giannoudis, P.V., Dinopoulos, H. & Tsiridis, E. (2005). Bone substitutes: An update. *Injury*, Vol. 36, No. 3, pp. S20-S27.

Ginebra, M.P., Traykova, T.& Planell, J.A. (2006). Calcium phosphate cements as bone drug delivery systems: A review. *Journal of Controlled Release*, Vol. 113, No. 2, pp. 102-110.

Hartman, E.M., Vehof, J.W.M., Spauwen, P.H.M. & Jansen, J.A. (2005). Ectopic bone formation in rats: the importance of the carrier. *Biomaterials*, Vol. 26, No. 14, pp. Pages 1829-1835.

Hench, L.L. (2006). The story of Bioglass, *Journal of Materials Science: Materials in Medicine*, Vol. 17, pp. 967-978.

Hench, L.L. & Wilson J. (1993). An introduction to bioceramics, World Scientific Publishing Co.; Singapore. pp. 245-251.

Karageorgiou, V. & Kaplan, D. (2005). Porosity of 3D biomaterial scaffolds and osteogenesis. *Biomaterials*, Vol. 26, No. 27, pp. 5474-5491.

Klein, C., Driessen, A.A. & De Groot, K. (1984). Relationship between the degradation behavior of calcium phosphate ceramics and their physical chemical characteristics and ultra structural geometry. *Biomaterials*, Vol. 5, pp. 157–160.

Kokubo, T., Ito, S., Sakka S. & Yamamuro, T. (1986). Formation of a high-strength bioactive glass-ceramic in the system $MgO-CaO-SiO_2-P_2O_5$, *Journal of Materials Science*, Vol. 21, No. 2, pp. 536–540.

Lane, J. M.; Tomin, E., & Bostrom, M.P.G. (1999). Biosynthetic bone grafting. *Clinical Orthopaedics and Related Research*, Vol.65, pp. 107–117.

LeGeros, R.Z. (2002). Properties of osteoconductive biomaterials: calcium phosphates. *Clinical Orthopaedics and Related Research*, Vol. 395, pp. 81–98.

Liu, X., Ding, C. & Chu, P.K. (2004). Mechanism of apatite formation on wollastonite coatings in simulated body fluids. *Biomaterials*, Vol. 25, No. 10, pp. 1755-1761.

Liu, Y., Enggist, L., Kuffer, A.F., Buser, D. & Hunziker, E.B. (2007a). The influence of BMP-2 and its mode of delivery on the osteoconductivity of implant surfaces during the early phase of osseointegration, *Biomaterials*, Vol. 28, pp. 2677–2686

Liu, Y., Cooper, P.R., Barralet J.E. & Shelton, R.M. (2007b). Influence of calcium phosphate crystal assemblies on the proliferation and osteogenic gene expression of rat bone marrow stromal cells. *Biomaterials*, Vol. 28, No. 7, pp. 1393-1403.

Lu, X. & Leng, Y. (2005). Theoretical analysis of calcium phosphate precipitation in simulated body fluid. *Biomaterials*, Vol. 26, pp.1097-1108.

Mistry, A.S. & Mikos, A.G. (2005). Tissue engineering strategies for bone regeneration. *Advances in Biochemical Engineering/Biotechnology*, Vol. 94, pp.1–22.

Mont, M.A., Ragland, P.S., Biggins, B., Friedlaender, G., Patel, T., Cook S, Etienne, G., Shimmin, A., Kildey, R., Rueger, D.C. & Einhorn, T.A. (2004). Use of bone morphogenetic proteins for musculoskeletal applications. An overview. (2004). *Journal of Bone and Joint Surgery*, Vol. 86, pp. 41–55.

Murugan, R. & Ramakrishna, S. (2005). Development of nanocomposites for bone grafting. *Composites Science and Technology* Vol.367, pp. 2385–2406.

Nie, H., & Wang, C. (2007). Fabrication and characterization of PLGA/HAp composite scaffolds for delivery of BMP-2 plasmid DNA. *Journal of Controlled Release*, Vol. 120, No. 1-2, pp. 111-121.

Niu, X., Feng, Q., Wang, M. Guo, X. & Zheng, Q. (2009). Porous nano-HA/collagen/PLLA scaffold containing chitosan microspheres for controlled delivery of synthetic peptide derived from BMP-2. *Journal of Controlled Release*, Vol. 134, No. 2, pp. 111-117.

Ooms, E.M., Wolke, J.G.C., Van de Heuvel, M.T., Jeschke, B. & Jansen, J.A. (2003). Histological evaluation of the bone response to calcium phosphate cement implanted in cortical bone. *Biomaterials*, Vol. 24, No. 6, pp. 989–1000.

Orr, T.E., Villars, P.A., Mitchell, S.L., Hsu, H.P. & Spector, M. (2001). Compressive properties of cancellous bone defects in a rabbit model treated with particles of natural bone mineral and synthetic hydroxyapatite. *Biomaterials*, Vol. 22, pp. 1953-1959.

Rabiee, S.M., Moztarzadeh, F., Salimi-Kenari, H. & Solati-Hashjin, M. (2007). Preparation and properties of a porous calcium phosphate bone graft substitute, *Materials Science- Poland*. Vol. 25, No. 4, pp. 1019-1027.

Rabiee, S. M., Moztarzadeh, F., Solati-Hashjin, M. & Salimi-Kenari, H. (2008a). Porous tricalcium phosphate as a bone substitute. *American Ceramic Society Bulletin*, Vol. 87, No.2, pp.43-45.

Rabiee, S.M., Mortazavi, S.M.J., Moztarzadeh, F., Sharifi, D., Sharifi, Sh., Salimi-Kenari, H., Solati-Hashjin, M. & Bizari, D. (2008b). Mechanical behavior of a new biphasic calcium phosphate bone graft. *Biotechnology and Bioprocess Engineering*. Vol. 13, pp. 204-209.

Rabiee, S.M., Moztarzadeh, F., Salimi-Kenari, H., Solati-Hashjin, M. & Mortazavi, S.M.J. (2008c). Study of Biodegradable Ceramic Bone Graft Substitute, *Advances in Applied Ceramics*, Vol.107, No.4, pp.199-202.

Rabiee, S.M., Mortazavi, S.M.J., Moztarzadeh, F., Sharifi, D., Fakhrejahani, F., Khafaf, A., Houshiar Ahmadi, S.A., Ravarian, R. & Nosoudi, N. (2009). Association of a Synthetic Bone Graft and Bone Marrow Cells as a Composite Biomaterial. *Biotechnology and Bioprocess Engineering*. Vol. 14, pp. 1-5.

Rabiee, S.M., Moztarzadeh, F. & Solati-Hashjin, M. (2010). Synthesis and characterization of hydroxyapatite cement. *Journal of Molecular Structure*, Vol. 969, pp. 172–175.

Ravarian, R., Moztarzadeh, F., Solati-Hashjin, M., Rabiee, S.M., Khoshakhlagh, P. & Tahriri, M. (2010). Synthesis, characterization and bioactivity investigation of bioglass/hydroxyapatite composite, *Ceramics International*, Vol. 36, No. 1, pp. 292-297.

Raynaud, S., Champion, E., Bernache-Assollant, D. & Thomas, P. (2002). Calcium phosphate apatites with variable Ca/P atomic ratio I. Synthesis, characterisation and thermal stability of powders. *Biomaterials*, Vol. 23, pp. 1065-72.

Rungsiyakull, C., Li, Q., Sun, G., Li,W. & Swain, M.V. (2010). Surface morphology optimization for osseointegration of coated implants. *Biomaterials*, Vol. 31, No. 27, pp. 7196-7204.

Schneider, A., Taboas, J.M., McCauley L.K. & Krebsbach, P.H. (2003). Skeletal homeostasis in tissue engineered bone. *Journal of Orthopaedic Research*, Vol. 21, No. 5, pp. 859-864.

Saravanapavan, P. & Hench, L.L. (2003). Mesoporous calcium silicate glasses. II. Textural characterisation. Journal of Non-Crystalline Solids, Vol. 318, No. 1-2, pp. 14-26.

Teoh, S.H. (2000). Fatigue of biomaterials: a review. *International Journal of Fatigue*, Vol. 22, No. 10, pp. 825-837.

Termaat, M.F., Den Boer, F.C., Bakker, F.C., Patka, P. & Haarman, H.J. (2005). Bone morphogenetic proteins. Development and clinical efficacy in the treatment of fractures and bone defects. *Journal of Bone and Joint Surgery*, Vol. 87, No. 6, pp.1367–78.

Vallet-Regı, M., lez-Calbet, J.M.G. (2004). Calcium phosphates as substitution of bone tissues, *Progress in Solid State Chemistry*, Vol. 32, pp. 1–31.

Ziegler, J., Mayr-Wohlfahrt, U., Kessler, S., Breitig, D. & Günther K.P. (2002). Adsorption and release properties of growth factors from biodegradable implants. *Journal of Biomedical Materials Research*, Vol. 59, pp. 422–428.

3

Hydrogel Scaffolds Contribute to the Osteogenesis and Chondrogenesis in the Small Osteochongral Defects

Miroslav Petrtyl et al.*
Laboratory of Biomechanics and Biomaterial Engineering, Department of Mechanics, Faculty of Civil Engineering, Czech Technical University in Prague
Czech Republic

1. Introduction

Hyaline cartilage shows only a limited response to self-repair (Hunter, 1743). Many people are stricken with degenerative osteochondral defects. Modern therapies of osteochondral defects are focused (for example) on the transplantation of osteochondral autografts, rushed spongiosa with collagen, chondrocytes and many others. The insertion of a crushed autologous bone graft has been reported as a possible therapy. However, the regenerative biomechanical (material) quality was less than 70% of healthy cartilage for fragments and controls (Kleemann et al., 2006). The transplantation of autologous osteochondral 3D-cylinders is one of several surgical therapies (Horas, 2003). During operations osteochondral defects are filled with material of a natural histological structure. However, the subchondral bone plates are interrupted and the biomechanical stability between the original tissue and the transplanted tissue is different. Provision of a long-term functional stability of inanimate implants in live surroundings is a complex and quite uneasy task. The development of replacements for a human subchondral bone and articular cartilage follows the path of a proposal and investigation of such materials whose mechanical properties are very similar to the biomechanical properties of a bone/cartilage tissue and whose biophysical and biochemical interactions with the surrounding living tissue neither cause necroses, nor lead to any initiation of other pathological processes. The biophysical and biochemical fixation of replacements and/or scaffolds to the tissue depends dominantly: (a) on the biomechanical properties and biochemical environments of the implants and the tissue; (b) on the stress–strain distributions in the tissue and the replacement, (c) on the organization and stability of

Jaroslav Lisal[1], Ladislav Senolt[2], Zdenek Bastl[3], Zdenek Krulis[4], Marketa Polanska[2], Hana Hulejova[2], Pavel Cerny[5] and Jana Danesova[1]
[1]Laboratory of Biomechanics and Biomaterial Engineering, Department of Mechanics, Faculty of Civil Engineering, Czech Technical University in Prague
[2] Institute of Rheumatology, The First Faculty of Medicine, Charles University in Prague
[3] J. Heyrovsky Institute of Physical Chemistry, Academy of Sciences of the Czech Republic
[4] Institute of Macromolecular Chemistry, Academy of Sciences of the Czech Republic
[5] ORTOTIKA, s.r.o., Prague, Czech Republic

collagen molecules adsorbed to modified surfaces of COC-blend replacements and (d) on the chondrogenesis on the hydrogel scaffold.

Our activities were aimed at forming new articular cartilage and subchondral bone using biocompatible and bioconductive polymer replacements.

2. Methods

Finding the optimal biomechanical, biophysical and biochemical conditions for chondrogenesis is a very complicated and difficult task. The aim of our research is to assess the principal conditions improving the treatment of osteochondral defects. We have been focused preferentially on the application of biomaterials with material properties close to the natural properties of the relevant tissue. Special attention has been focused on the surface modification of the COC-blend by the action of nitrogen and/or oxygen microwave plasma, the application of type I collagen, the application of chitosan and the influence of the vertical position of replacements in the localities of osteochondral defects.

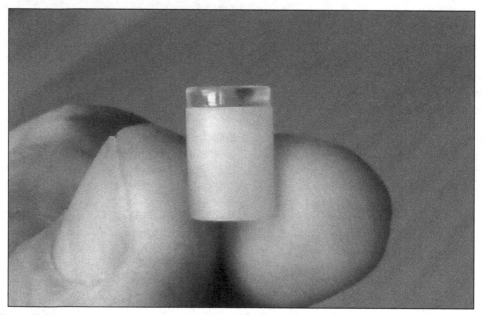

Fig. 1. Bi-component replacement of the subchondral bone (in the distal part, nontransparent material) and the articular cartilage scaffold (partly, in the proximal part, transparent hydrogel)

The presumed concept applies a substitute consisting of two supporting polymer components (see Fig. 1.). One of them (the lower element) is composed of a polycycloolefinic (blend) material (with the modulus of elasticity $E = 0.5$–3 GPa, the diameter of 8 mm, and the length of 10–12 mm, Krulis et al., 2006), while the upper hydrogel scaffold element of poly (2-hydroxyethylmethacrylate) has the relative modulus of deformation $E_{r/def} = 1.5$ MPa, the diameter of 8 mm and the thickness of the upper plate of 1.1– 1.3 mm, Fig. 2. The COC-blend substance was made with spherical/ellipsoidal pores (with a diameter of 0.6–1.5 µm), Fig. 3.

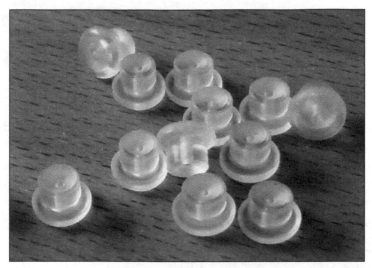

Fig. 2. Poly (2-hydroxyethylmethacrylate) scaffolds – upper parts of hybrid replacements

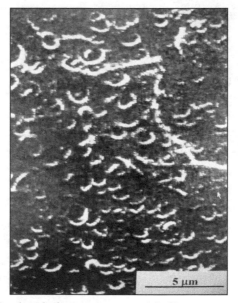

Fig. 3. Surface of COC-blend with designed pores with diameters ranging from 0.6 to 1.5 μm

In order to improve the bonding between the polymer blend and collagen, the surface of the polymer matrix was modified by the action of a nitrogen and/or oxygen microwave plasma. The plasmatic modification resulted in a significant increase of surface hydrophilicity demonstrated by a decrease of water contact angle.

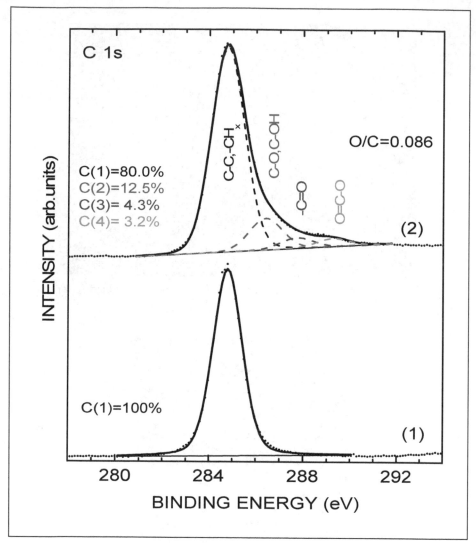

Fig. 4. Spectra of C 1s electrons of (1) unmodified and (2) plasma-modified surface of polymer blend

The plasma modification was carried out in a MW reactor equipped with the SLAN I OV 425 (Plasma Consult) magnetron operand at 300 W, 80 Pa, a gas flow of 15 scm/min and with exposure times of 15 min. For water contact angle measurements, the SEE System was used (Milli-Q water droplet volume 2 μL).

After optimizing conditions for the surface modification with regard to achieving the highest hydrophilicity of the surface, the samples were examined by the XPS method with the aim of identifying their chemistry and the population of individual chemical groups present on the surface. After plasmatic treatment (Spirovova et al., 2007), the components with higher values of binding energy occurred in the C 1s spectra of electrons (see Fig. 4.).

The aging of modified surfaces was also studied by XPS and by water contact angle measurements. The adsorption of collagen I on untreated and treated polymers was studied by XPS and AFM methods. XPS measurements were carried out using the ESCA 310 spectrometer. Electrons were excited by Al Kα monochromatized radiation. For the visualization of surface topography, the AFM Nanoscope IIIa (Digital Instruments) in the tapping mode was used.

The upper components of the replacement were made of poly-hydroxyethylmethacrylate with chitosan without any additional plasma surface treatment. Osteochondral defects (depth: 12 mm, diameter: 8 mm) were created in each lateral and medial tibial condyle of the right and left knees in 6 adult pigs. Histological analyses of the cartilage matrix were accomplished after 6 and 4 months.

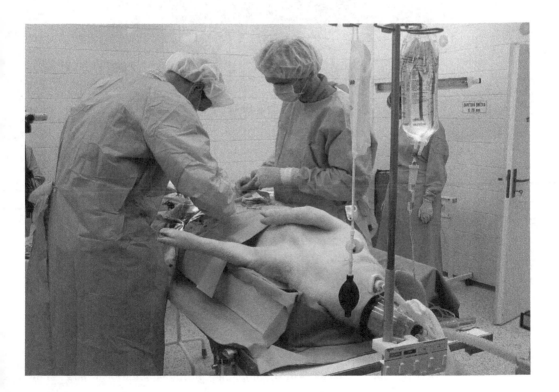

Fig. 5. Total operative time was less than eight minutes per two osteochondral defects in knee joint

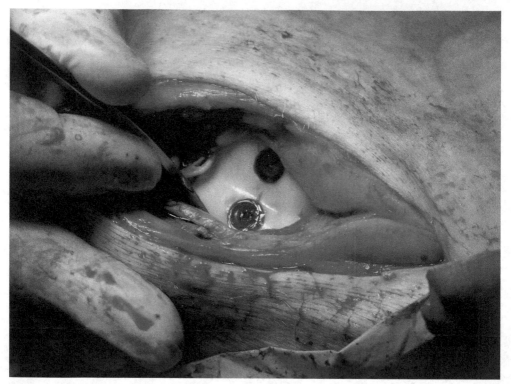

Fig. 6. Implantation of replacements. The lower hydrogel scaffold has been allocated approximately 1 mm under the articular surface and the upper one has been allocated ca 2.5 mm under the articular surface

3. Results

The replacements developed and plasmatically modified/unmodified under in vivo conditions have been proven as bioactive, bioconductive and biotolerant materials. It is well known that collagen adsorption promotes cell adhesion and proliferation.

The measured spectra of C 1s electrons showed the presence of components belonging to C–O, C=O and O–C=O functionalities (see Fig. 4.). For examining the collagen adsorption, table samples whose surface composition did not change with time were used. The presence of adsorbed collagen was indicated by the presence of the spectrum of N 1s electrons in the spectrum and its morphology was visualized by the AFM method. It was observed that on untreated, hydrophobic smooth polymer surfaces comparable or larger amounts of collagen are adsorbed than on hydrophilic surfaces, but immobilized collagen tends to form aggregates on hydrophobic surfaces. On hydrophilic, plasma-modified surfaces, more homogeneous coverage by collagen is observed.

The developed subchondral bone around the COC blend had the same quality as a natural healthy one (Petrtyl et al., 2008). The new subchondral bone mineralized perfectly. The mediator C+TGF films (made from type I collagen and from growth hormones TGF-β) applied on the COC-blend surface contribute to the creation of stable encapsulation (Fig. 7.,

Fig. 8.). Verifying the C+TGF films on the COC surface (in vitro) showed very good cell proliferation and cell differentiation. The modified surface exhibits enhanced adsorption of collagen and improvement of its adhesion. Stronger bonding explains a higher quantity, better organization and better stability of collagen molecules adsorbed on oxidized surfaces. The polymer replacements installed into artificially executed osteochondral defects of porcine tibial condyles, including both modified and non-modified implants, demonstrated a perfect tolerability and appeared to heal into the existing subchondral bone without any displacement or evidence for necrosis. Histological findings and morphological changes of osteochondral samples did not demonstrate any pathological features. The top surfaces of the bi-component replacements were overgrown with viable new articular cartilage (Fig. 7.) or with articular cartilage and partly with fibrocartilage (Fig. 9.).

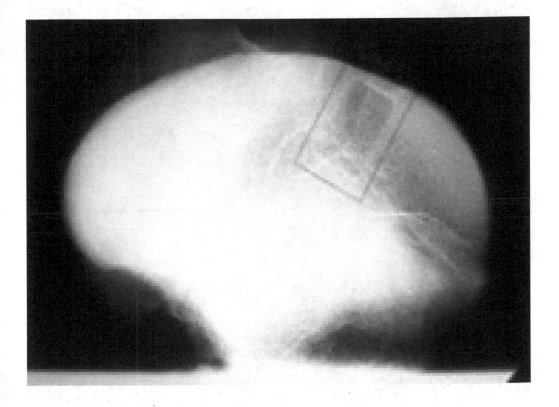

Fig. 7. X-ray stability analyses of replacement + scaffold with the new articular cartilage. Excellent stability of replacement in the subchondral bone without necrosis

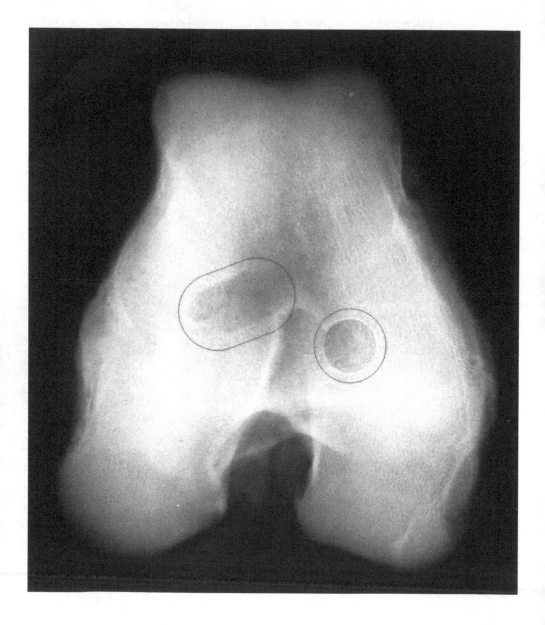

Fig. 8. X-ray analyses of the encapsulated COC-blend replacements in the subchondral bone by collagen (I. type)

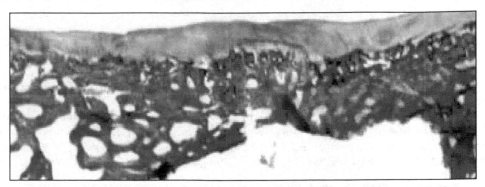

Fig. 9. Tissue bridge from articular cartilage and subchondral/spongy bone across the HEMA scaffold

The biomechanical in vivo environments have particularly potent regulatory effects on chondrogenesis, both in terms of proliferation and the new matrix synthesis. The matrix synthesis is regulated by mechanical stimuli and depends on the initial high stability of subchondral bone COC-blend replacements.

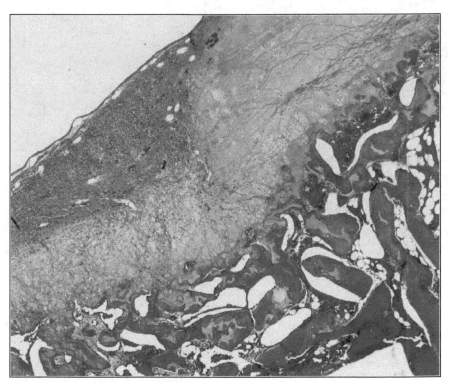

Fig. 10. Top surfaces of the hydrogel scaffold were overgrown with subchondral bone (the lower layer), with viable new articular cartilage (the medial layer) and partly by fibrocartilage (the upper small part)

4. Discussion

The leading strategies in the treatment of osteochondral defects are to minimize the operative trauma by minimally invasive procedures, to stimulate chondro/osteogenesis and/or to regenerate the tissues. Operative approaches are becoming ever smaller. Current and future concepts are based on a better understanding of biomechanical conditions and local mechanisms of healing, tissue regeneration and prophylaxis.

The local application of growth factors is investigated in clinical practice and has a great potential in treatment. The reason for a limited acceptance in clinical use may be that the applied proteins are expensive and with limited availability, and considerable quantities have to be implanted locally (Raschke, Fuchs & Stange, 2006).

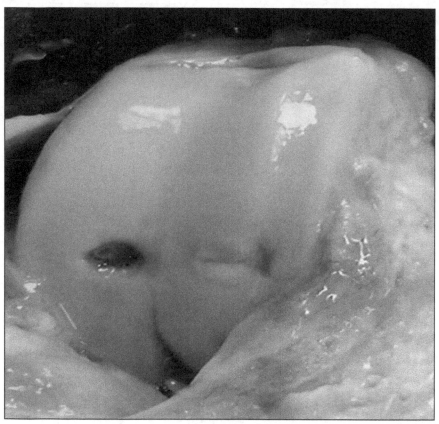

Fig. 11. New articular cartilage after 12-week chondrogenesis (the right tibial condyle) and the control defect (the left tibial condyle)

Other relatively new innovative techniques include *the stem cell therapy*. The application of autologous stem cells taken out and re-transplanted can also be used for healing (Raschke, Fuchs & Stange, 2006). However, this manner of treatment depends on the appropriate biomechanical and biochemical conditions of the tissue. The healing of osteochondral defects is controlled both mechanically and biologically. The processes of osteo/chondrogenic differentiation are slightly promoted by mechanical effects (Bader et al., 2006). The cells are very sensitive to small strains. The physiological balance between the microstrain magnitude and biochemical stimulation can be easily disrupted when the subchondral/spongy bone is pathologically a soft one. In the case of an unstable subchondral bone and spongy bone, the articular surface of cartilage is affected by small sags (Petrtyl et al., 2008).

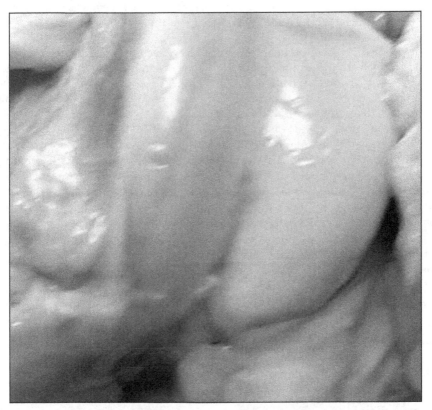

Fig. 12. Chondrogenesis after 20 weeks (in both the left and right tibial condyles). The application of chitosan (0.3% liquid, pH 5.5), TGF-β (1.2 mg/1 ml PBS) type I collagen (0.3%), surface plasmatic modification of COC-blend

The regeneration of osteochondral defects treated with crushed bone grafts is in verified cases accompanied by the presence of soft regenerated tissue (Kleemann et al., 2006). The regeneration of osteochondral defects treated with crushed bone grafts remains incomplete still after three months. However, the inserted bone graft can be completely absorbed. After six months, the connective tissue within the defect is transformed into a bone and fibrocartilage tissue through enchondral ossification. The surface of the regenerated joint area is rough and irregular. The regenerate mechanical quality was 61%–70% of healthy cartilage for treatment and control, respectively. Although this method was reported as successful in the clinical treatment, it failed to enhance the quality of regenerated defects in the case of a sheep study (Kleemann et al., 2006). It must be noted that the stability of biomaterials substituting pathological subchondral/spongy bone tissues is the fundamental condition for the regeneration of osteochondral defects.

Osteoarthrosis is the result of pathological biological processes and high biomechanical effects that destabilize the natural tissue degradation and synthesis of articular cartilage (Dieppe, 1998). The decrement of hyaluronic acid (HA, hyaluronate) concentrations and the descent of its molecular mass are the principal causes of chondral defects. The application of intraarticular injections of hyaluronan upgrades the quality of articular cartilage through the synovial liquid (Balasz & Delinger, 1993). This is a therapeutic experiment for effective temporary elimination of pains (Petrella, Di Silvestro & Hidebrandt, 2002; Dahlberg, Lohmander & Ryd, 1994). Good clinical results have been obtained after the treatment of deep chondral defects in the knee with autologous chondrocytes implantation using 3D hyaluronan-based scaffolds (Hyalograft C), (Podskubka et al., 2010). Some scaffolds can effectively increase the initial bearing capacity of newly created tissue. It is also the fundamental condition for successful chondrogenesis.

From the previous small/non-invasive methods of treatments it is apparent that the quality of microstructures and continuous biomechanical properties of the subchondral bone play an important role in the morphology and the quality of chondrogenesis. Chondrogenesis depends very sensitively on the initial stability of biomaterials implanted into the subchondral bone. Vertical displacements and rotations of COC-blend replacements shortly after implantations must be eliminated. The initial integrity of biomaterials substituting the subchondral bone, the initial bearing capacity and the vertical position of these replacements have a major influence on chondrogenesis. The initial biomechanical stiffness of materials (substituting the subchondral bone) has a fundamental influence on the quality of new articular cartilage.

5. Conclusion

With regard to these initial requirements, acceleration of the stability of COC-blend replacements in the subchondral bone is a requisite of advisable conditions for the tissue genesis.

The stability of COC-blend replacements in the subchondral bone can be ensured by:

1. plasmatic modification of the COC-blend surface by the action of a nitrogen and/or oxygen microwave plasma;
2. surface spherical/ellipsoidal pores with the diameter of < 0.5, 1.5 > μm in the COC-blend;
3. application of both type I collagen (0.3%) and growth hormones TGF-β (1.2 mg/1 ml PBS) on the COC-blend surface;
4. application of chitosan (0.3% liquid, pH 5.5) on the hydrogel surface.

The bearing capacities of subchondral bone COC-blend replacements considerably contribute to the genesis of a new extracellular cartilage matrix (Fig. 11. and Fig. 12.). Histological analyses demonstrated the healing process with partial (12 weeks) or complete (20 weeks) spongy bone + cartilage bridging (in vivo) (Fig. 9. and Fig. 10.).

The COC-blend copolymers and hydrogel [poly (2-hydroxyethylmethacrylate)] scaffolds can be suggested as a reliable reconstructive alternative for local osteochondral defects and effective support for the creation of new hyaline cartilage having an articular surface without fibrillation.

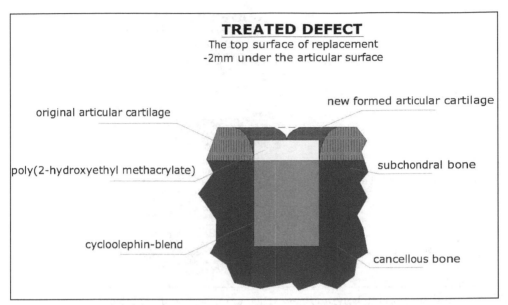

Fig. 13. New articular cartilage is formed over the hydrogel scaffold. Its surface is approximately 1–1.5 mm above the tide

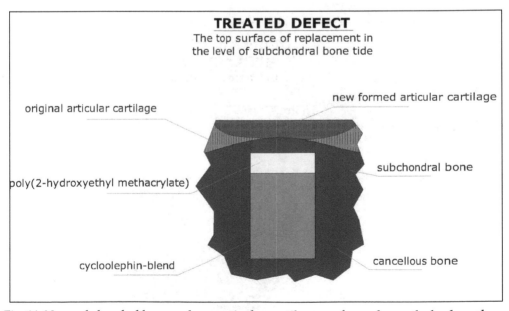

Fig. 14. New subchondral bone and new articular cartilage are formed over the hydrogel scaffold. The top plane of hydrogel surfaces is allocated approximately 0.5 mm under the indigenous level of the tidemark

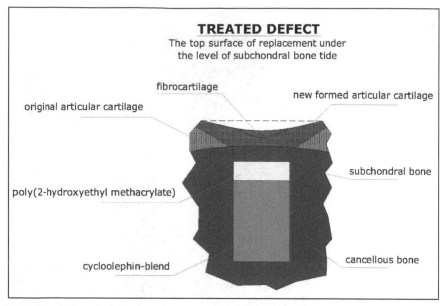

Fig. 15. New subchondral bone and new articular cartilage with peripheral fibrocartilage are formed over the hydrogel scaffold. The surface of hydrogel scaffold is allocated approximately 2 mm under the indigenous level of the tidemark. The articular surface has a sag profile

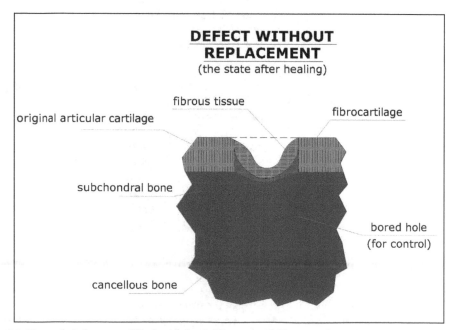

Fig. 16. Control defects are filled with both fibrous and fibrocartilage tissues

With regard to the conditions mentioned previously, the new articular cartilage is formed over the hydrogel scaffold when its surface is approximately 1–1.5 mm above the tidemark (see Fig. 13.). If the hydrogel surfaces are allocated approximately 0.5 mm under the indigenous level of the tidemark, then a new subchondral bone and new articular cartilage are formed over the hydrogel scaffold (Fig. 14.). A new subchondral bone and new articular cartilage with peripheral fibrocartilage are also formed over the hydrogel scaffold when the top surface of the hydrogel scaffold is allocated approximately 2 mm under the indigenous level of the tidemark. The articular surface has a sag profile (Fig. 15.). Control defects are filled with both fibrous and fibrocartilage tissues (Fig. 16.).

6. Acknowledgment

This research has been supported by the GAČR grant No. 106/06/0761 and by the MŠMT grant No.: VZ-6840770012. An extraordinary acknowledgement belongs to Professor C. Povýšil, Dr. Sc., M.D., from the Institute of Pathology of the First Faculty of Medicine, Charles University in Prague, and to MVDr. S. Špelda, PhD, from the Military Hospital and Faculty of Medicine in Hradec Králové.

7. References

Bader, D.L.; Pingguan-Murphy, B., van de Logt, V. & Knight, M. (2006). Intracellular signalling pathways of chondrocytes in 3D constructs subjected to physiological loading, *Proceedings of The Interaction of Mechanics and Biology in Knee Joint Restoration and Regeneration*, Center for Musculoskeletal Surgery, Charité, Berlin, June 2006

Balasz, E.A. & Denlinger, S.L. (1993). Viscosupplementation: a new concept in the treatment of osteoarthritis, Journal of Rheumatology, Vol. 20, Suppl. 39, pp. 3-9, ISSN 1499-2752

Dahlberg, L.; Lohmander, L.S. & Ryd, L. (1994). Intraarticular injections of hyaluronan in patients with cartilage abnormalities and knee pain, *Arthritis and rheumatism*, Vol. 37, No. 4, (April 1994), pp. 521-528, ISSN 0004-3591

Dieppe, p. (1998). Osteoarthritis, *Acta Orthopaedica Scandinavica*, Vol. 69, No. S281, pp. 2-5, ISSN 0001-6470

Horas, U.; Pelinkovic, D.; Herr, G.; Aigner, T. & Schnettler, R. (2003). Autologous chondrocyte implantation and osteochondral cylinder transplantation. *Journal of Bone and Joint Surgery (American)*, Vol. 85, No. 2, (February 2003), pp. 185-192, ISSN 1535-1386

Hunter, W. (1743). On the structure and diseases of articulating cartilage, In: *Phil Trans Roy Soc*, 42B, 514–521

Kleemann, R. (2006). Mechanical influences on cartilage regeneration, *Proceedings of The Interaction of Mechanics and Biology in Knee Joint Restoration and Regeneration*, Center for Musculoskeletal Surgery, Charité, Berlin, June 2006

Krulis, Z.; Stary, Z.; Horak, Z. & Petrtyl, M. (2006). Thermoplastic polymer composition for skeletal replacements and method of production, Patent Application No. 2006-70, Industrial Property Office, Prague, Czech Republic

Petrella, R.J.; DiSilvestro, M.D. & Hidebrand, C. (2002). Effects of hyaluronate sodium on pain and physical functioning in osteoarthritis of the knee: a randomized, double-blind, placebo-controlled clinical trial, *Arch. Intern. Med.*, Vol. 162, No. 2, (February 2002), pp. 292-298, ISSN 0003-9926

Petrtyl, M.; Senolt, L.; Hulejova, H.; Cerny, P.; Krulis, Z.; Bastl, Z. & Horak, Z. (2008). Treatment of osteoarthritis by hybrid polymer replacement, *Proceedings of 6th International Workshop for Musculoskeletal and Neuronal Interactions - ISMNI*, Cologne, Germany, May 2008

Podskubka, A.; Vaculik, J.; Povysil, C.; Masek, M. & Sprindrich J. (2010). Autologous chondrocytes implantation in the treatment of the knee chondral defects, Findings in one, three and five years, *Ortopedie*, Vol. 4, No. 3, pp. 25

Raschke, M.J.; Fuchs, T. & Stange, R. (2006). Future concepts in healing stimulation, *Proceedings of The Interaction of Mechanics and Biology in Knee Joint Restoration and Regeneration*, Center for Musculoskeletal Surgery, Charité, Berlin, June 2006

Spirovova, I.; Janda, P.; Krulis, Z.; Petrtyl, M. & Bastl, Z. (2007). Surface modification of COC-LLDPE copolymer by ion beams, plasma, ozone and excimer laser radiation, *Proceedings of Abstr. 12th European Conference on Applications of Surface and Interface Analysis*, Brussels, Belgium, September 2007

4

Development and Applications of Varieties of Bioactive Glass Compositions in Dental Surgery, Third Generation Tissue Engineering, Orthopaedic Surgery and as Drug Delivery System

Samit Kumar Nandi[1], Biswanath Kundu[2] and Someswar Datta[2]
[1]*Department of Veterinary Surgery and Radiology, West Bengal University of Animal and Fishery Sciences, Kolkata,*
[2]*Bioceramics and Coating Division, Central Glass and Ceramic Research Institute, Kolkata,*
India

1. Introduction

Bioactive glass is composed mainly of silica, sodium oxide, calcium oxide and phosphates. The bone-bonding reaction results from a series of reactions in the glass and its surface (Hench & Wilson, 1984). When granules of bioactive glass are inserted into bone defects, ions are released in body fluids and precipitate into a bone-like apatite on the surface, promoting the adhesion and proliferation of osteogenic cells (Ohtsuki et al., 1991; Neo et al., 1993) which is partially replaced by bone after long time implantation (Neo et al., 1994). The ion leaching phenomenon involves the exchange of monovalent cations from the glass, such as Na+ or K+, with H3O+ from the solution, and thus causes an increase in the pH of the solution. It is known that osteoblasts prefer a slightly alkaline medium (Ramp *et al.*, 1994; Kaysinger & Ramp, 1998), but it is also known that severe changes in pH can inhibit osteoblast activity and cause cell necrosis or apoptosis (Brandao-burch et al., 2005; Frick et al., 1997; El-ghannam et al., 1997). Bioactive glass with a macroporous structure has the properties of large surface areas, which are favourable for bone integration. The behaviour of bioactive glass is dependent on the composition of the glass (Brink, 1997; Brink et al., 1997), the surrounding pH, the temperature, and the surface layers on the glass (Andersson et al., 1988; Gatti & Zaffe, 1991). The porosity provides a scaffold on which newly-formed bone can be deposited after vascular in growth and osteoblast differentiation. The porosity of bioglass is also beneficial for resorption and bioactivity (De Aza et al., 2003). In push-out tests the strength of the chemical bond between bioactive glass and the host tissue has been measured to be at least ten times higher than the contact osteogenesis (Anderson et al., 1992). Its high modulus and brittle nature makes its applications limited, but it has been used in combination with poly-methylmethacrylate to form bioactive bone cement and with metal implants as a coating to form a calcium-deficient carbonated calcium phosphate layer. Certain bioactive glass are strong enough to function in stress-bearing sites in the head and neck (e.g., mandible replacement); however, such implants cannot be easily contoured in the operating room, and screws cannot be easily placed into bioactive glass blocks because they defy drilling and have a tendency to fragment during creation of screw holes.

2. Bioactive glass materials

Legendary Prof. L. L. Hench of University of Florida, USA discovered in 1969 that some compositions of glasses can bond chemically with bone when implanted to living tissues. Many researchers later on discovered some other ceramics, glass-ceramics and composites also have the same property (De Groot, 1983, 1988; De Groot et al., 1990; De Groot & LeGeros, 1988; Ducheyne et al., 1980; Gross et al., 1988; Gross and Strunz, 1985; Hench, 1987, 1988; Hench & Ethridge, 1982; Hench et al., 1971; Hench & Wilson, 1984; Holand et al., 1985; Hulbert et al., 1987; Jarcho, 1981; Kitsugi et al., 1989; Kokubo et al., 1986; Kokubo et al., 1982; Nakamura et al., 1985; Wilson et al., 1981; Yamamuro et al., 1990b; Yamamuro et al., 1988; Yoshii et al., 1988). He defined these glasses as 'bioactive glass' and since then it has been used mostly as a reconstructive material for damaged hard tissues such as bone (Hench, 2006; Hench et al., 1971). Some more specialized compositions of bioactive glass will bond to soft tissues and bone (Wilson & Nolletti, 1990; Wilson et al., 1981; Yamamuro et al., 1990a). General characteristics of these bioactive glasses are a time-dependent, kinetic modification of the surface that occurs when implanted *in vivo* (Gross et al., 1988; Hench, 1988), the surface forms biologically active hydroxycarbonate apatite (HCA) layer providing bonding interface with tissues. The advantage is that it is possible to design this glass to get a controlled rate of degradation and bonding to the tissue. The HCA phase that forms on these implants is very similar chemically and structurally to the mineral phase in bone and thus responsible for interfacial bonding. These bioactive materials develop an adherent interface with tissues that resists significant mechanical forces. In some cases this interfacial strength of adhesion is equivalent to or greater than the cohesive strength of the implant material or the tissue bonded to bioactive implant. The rapid reaction at the surface leads to a fast bonding with the living tissues, but, due to the mainly two-dimensional structure of the glass network, the mechanical properties are relatively low. It may be noted that small changes in the composition can lead to very different properties and thus has added advantage of its versatility in contact with different living tissues, on range of properties depending on the implantation site of the prosthesis.

Certain compositional range of bioactive glass containing SiO_2, Na_2O, CaO, and P_2O_5 like ordinary soda-lime-silica glasses in specific proportions shows bonding to bone (Table 1).Three key compositional features of these glasses distinguish them from traditional Na_2O-CaO-SiO_2 glasses: (1) less than 60 mol. % SiO_2, (2) high-Na_2O and high-CaO content, and (3) high-CaO/P_2O_5 ratio. As known, SiO_2/Al_2O_3 act as glass network former, $CaO/MgO/P_2O_5$ is the network modifier and Na_2O/K_2O is the fluxing agent. These compositional features made the surface highly reactive when exposed to aqueous medium. Very popular 45S5 bioactive silica glasses are based upon 45 wt. % SiO_2, S as the network former, and a 5 to 1 molar ratio of Ca to P. Glasses with very lower molar ratios of Ca to P (in the form of CaO and P_2O_5) do not bond to bone (Hench and Paschall, 1973). Different substitutions in the 45S5 compositions of 5-15 wt. % B_2O_3 for SiO_2, or 12.5 wt. % CaF_2 for CaO or crystallizing the various bioactive glass compositions to form glass-ceramics were found to have no measurable effect on the ability of the material to form a bone bond (Hench & Paschall, 1973). But, addition of small 3 wt. % Al_2O_3 to the 45S5 formula prevents bonding

Development and Applications of Varieties of Bioactive Glass Compositions in Dental Surgery, Third Generation Tissue Engineering, Orthopaedic Surgery and as Drug Delivery System

71

Sl. No.	Name of the composition	All are in weight %											
		SiO_2	P_2O_5	CaO	Ca $(PO_3)_2$	CaF_2	MgO	MgF_2	Na_2O	K_2O	Al_2O_3	B_2O_3	Ta_2O_5 /TiO_2
1.	45S5 Bioglass ® (Hench et al., 1971)	45	6	24.5	-	-	-	-	24.5	-	-	-	-
2.	45S5.4F Bioglass ® (Hench et al., 1986; Hench et al., 1971)	45	6	14.7	-	9.8	-	-	24.5	-	-	-	-
3.	45B15S5 Bioglass ® (Hench and Paschall, 1974; Hench et al., 1975)	30	6	24.5	-	-	-	-	24.5	-	-	15	-
4.	52S4.6 Bioglass ® (Hench and Clark, 1982)	52	6	21	-	-	-	-	21	-	-	-	-
5.	55S4.3 Bioglass ® (Hench and Clark, 1982)	55	6	19.5	-	-	-	-	19.5	-	-	-	-
6.	KGC Ceravital ® (Gross et al., 1988)	46.2	-	20.2	25.5	-	2.9	-	4.8	0.4	-	-	-
7.	KGS Ceravital ® (Gross et al., 1988)	46	-	33	16	-	-	-	5	-	-	-	-
8.	KGy213 Ceravital ® (Gross et al., 1988)	38	-	31	13.5	-	-	-	4	-	7	-	6.5
9.	A/W glass-ceramic (Kokubo et al., 1986)	34.2	16.3	44.9	-	0.5	4.6	-	-	-	-	-	-
10.	MB glass-ceramic (Holand et al., 1985)	19-52	4-24	9-3	-	-	5-15	-	3-5	3-5	12-33	-	-
11.	S45P7 (Andersson et al., 1988)	45	7	22	-	-	-	-	24	-	-	2	-
12.	S53P4 (Zehnder et al., 2004)	53	4	20	-	-	-	-	23	-	-	-	-
13.	13-93 (Fu et al., 2008)	53	4	20	-	-	5	-	6	12	-	-	-
14.	4-Mar (Zhang et al., 2008)	50.5	1	22.5	-	-	6	-	5	15	-	-	-
15.	18-04 (Zhang et al., 2008)	54.5	4	20	-	-	4.5	-	15	-	-	2	-
16.	23-04 (Zhang et al., 2008)	56.25	1	20	-	-	4.5	-	5	11.25	-	2	-
17.	H2-02 (Munukka et al., 2008)	53	2	22	-	-	4.5	-	6	11	0.5	1	-

Sl. No.	Name of the composition	All are in mole %												
		SiO_2	P_2O_5	CaO	$Ca(PO_3)_2$	CaF_2	MgO	MgF_2	Na_2O	K_2O	Al_2O_3	B_2O_3	Ta_2O_5/TiO_2	ZnO
18.	CEL-2 (Vitale-Brovarone et al., 2009)	45	3	26	-	-	7	-	15	4	-	-	-	-
19.	55S (Loty et al., 2001)	55	4	41	-	-	-	-	-	-	-	-	-	-
20.	H (Linati et al., 2005)	46.2	2.6	26.9	-	-	-	-	24.3	-	-	-	-	-
21.	HZ5 (Linati et al., 2005)	44.4	2.5	25.9	-	-	-	-	23.4	-	-	-	-	3.8
22.	HZ10 (Linati et al., 2005)	42.5	2.4	4.8	-	-	-	-	22.5	-	-	-	-	7.8
23.	HZ20 (Linati et al., 2005)	38.8	2.2	22.6	-	-	-	-	20.5	-	-	-	-	15.9

Table 1. Different compositions of bioactive glass materials

(Andersson et al., 1990; Greenspan & Hench, 1976; Gross et al., 1988; Gross and Strunz, 1985; Hench & Clark, 1982; Hench & Paschall, 1973). Gross and co-workers found that a range of low-alkali (0-5 wt. %), bioactive silica glass-ceramics (Ceravital ®) also bond to bone (Gross et al., 1981; Gross et al., 1988; Gross et al., 1986a; Gross et al., 1986b; Gross & Strunz, 1985; 1980). Also small additions of Al_2O_3, Ta_2O_5, TiO_2, Sb_2O_3 or ZrO_2 inhibit bone bonding (Table 1). A two-phase silica-phosphate glass-ceramic composed of apatite ($Ca_{10}(PO_4)_6(OH1F_2)$) and wollastonite ($CaO.SiO_2$) crystals (termed A/W glass-ceramic by the Kyoto University team, Japan) and a residual SiO_2 glassy matrix, also bonds with bone with very high interfacial bond strength (Kitsugi et al., 1989; Kokubo et al., 1986; Kokubo et al., 1982; Nakamura et al., 1985; Yamamuro et al., 1988; Yoshii et al., 1988). But, addition of Al_2O_3 or TiO_2 to the A/W glass-ceramic inhibits bone bonding, while a second phosphate phase, β-whitlockite ($3CaO.P_2O_5$) does not. Multiphase machinable bioactive silica phosphate glass-ceramic containing phlogopite ($(Na,K)Mg_3(AlSi_3O_{10})F_2$), mica and apatite crystals, developed by the Freidrich Schiller University, Jena, Germany, bonds to bone despite presence of alumina in the composition (Holand et al., 1985). Al^{3+} ions incorporated within the crystal phase did not alter the surface reaction kinetics of the material (Vogel et al., 1990). Some other compositions of bioactive glass have been developed at Abo Akademi, Turku, Finland, for coating onto dental alloys (Andersson et al., 1988; Andersson et al., 1990; Kangasniemi & Yti-Urpo, 1990).

Prof. Hench has recently published the history leading to the development of bioactive glass from the discovery of classical 45S5 Bioglass® composition to successful clinical applications and tissue engineering (Hench, 2006). High amounts of Na_2O and CaO as well as relatively high CaO/P_2O_5 ratio make the glass surface highly reactive in physiological environments (Hench, 1991). Other bioactive glass compositions developed over few years contain no sodium or have additional elements incorporated in the silicate network such as fluorine (Vitale-Brovarone et al., 2008), magnesium (Vitale-Brovarone et al., 2005; Vitale-Brovarone et al., 2007), strontium (Gentleman et al., 2010; O'Donnell & Hill, 2010; Pan et al., 2010), iron (Hsi et al., 2007), silver (Balamurugan et al., 2008; Bellantone et al., 2002; Blaker et al., 2004;

Development and Applications of Varieties of Bioactive Glass Compositions in Dental Surgery, Third Generation
Tissue Engineering, Orthopaedic Surgery and as Drug Delivery System

73

Delben et al., 2009), boron (Gorriti et al., 2009; Liu et al., 2009a; Liu et al., 2009b; Munukka et al., 2008), potassium (Cannillo & Sola, 2009) or zinc (Aina et al., 2009; Haimi et al., 2009). Introduction of Ag_2O into bioactive glass compositions minimize the risk of microbial contamination by antimicrobial activity of the leaching Ag^+ ions has been reported (Blaker et al., 2004; Saravanapavan et al., 2003). In the reports synthesis by sol-gel process also allowed tailoring of the textural characteristics of the matrix in order to obtain a controlled Ag^+ delivery system. Introduction of B_2O_3 into the CaO–SiO_2 system on the other hand enhanced the bioactivity, for more soluble boric compounds increased the supersaturating of Ca ions in the SBF (simulated body fluid) solution and water-corrosive borosilicate glass forms Si–OH groups that act as nucleation sites for the apatite layer (Ryu et al., 2003). Zn-substituted bioactive glass creates a template for osteoblast proliferation and differentiation by the interaction between the Zn and inorganic phosphate at the surface of the bioactive glass. Addition of Zn has synergistic effect on cell attachment which also maintains the pH of SBF within the physiological limit by forming zinc hydroxide in the solution. Limited amounts of Zn in the bioactive glass system stimulate early cell proliferation and promote differentiation as assessed by the *in vitro* biocompatibility experimentation. Now, compositional dependence of bone bonding and soft-tissue bonding for the Na_2O-CaO-P_2O_5-SiO_2 glasses (constant 6 wt. % of P_2O_5) is presented in Fig. 1. Compositions at the middle of the diagram form a bond with bone (region A). Region A is termed as the bioactive-bone bonding boundary. Silica glasses within region B (such as bottle, window or slide glasses of microscope) behave as nearly inert materials and elicit a fibrous capsule at the implant-tissue interface. Glasses within region C are resorbable and disappear within maximum 1 day of implantation. Glasses within region D are not technically realistic and have not been tested as implants. The collagenous constituent of soft tissues can strongly adhere to the bioactive silica glasses which lie within the compositional range marked as E (Fig. 1).

Very briefly, bioactive glass can be made either by conventional melt-quenching (Chen et al., 2008b; Guarino et al., 2007; Hench & Polak, 2002; Hutmacher et al., 2007; Jones, 2007; Jones, 2009; Misra et al., 2006) or by modern sol-gel method (Balamurugan et al., 2007; Radha & Ashok, 2008). Sol-gel process involves synthesis of solution (sol), typically composed of metal-organic and metal salt precursors followed by formation of gel by chemical reaction or aggregation and finally thermal treatment for drying, organic removal and sometimes crystallization (Olding et al., 2001). This particular method is a low temperature preparative method and glasses produced by this method may have some porous structure too with high specific surface area (Sepulveda et al., 2001). There are diversified application potential of different bioactive glass which have been discussed many authors and will be presented in the subsequent sections. But, bone tissue engineering is a very exotic future clinical application of these materials. Both micron-sized and nano-scale particles deployed recently (Brunner et al., 2006; Delben et al., 2009; Vollenweider et al., 2007) are considered to be the part of this application field which also include fabrication of composite materials, e.g., combination of biodegradable polymers and bioactive glass (Liu et al., 2008; Lu et al., 2003; Misra et al., 2010a; Misra et al., 2010b; Misra et al., 2008; Yang et al., 2001). Bioactive glass-ceramics on the other hand belong to the group of Class A bioactive materials which are characterized by both osteoconduction (growth of bone at the implant surface) and osteoinduction (activation and recruitment of osteoprogenitor cells by the material itself stimulating bone growth on the surface of the material) (Hench, 2006; Hench, 1998; Jones, 2007; Thompson & Hench, 1998). In contrast, Class B bioactive materials exhibit only osteoconductivity. A recent review summarizing research on Ca-Si-based ceramics is also available (Wu, 2009). As far as bioactive glass-ceramics are concerned, these are partially crystallized glasses produced by heating the parent bioactive glass above its crystallization temperature, usually at about 610-630° C (Boccaccini, 2005; Boccaccini et al., 2007; Brunner et al., 2006; Jones, 2007). Glass-ceramics obtained by a sintering process, it is found that during the incidence of crystallization and densification, the microstructure of the parent glass shrinks, porosity is reduced and the solid structure gains mechanical strength (Thompson & Hench, 1998). But, brittleness and low fracture toughness remain a major problem of these materials. The limited strength and low fracture toughness (i.e., resistance to fracture crack propagation) of bioactive glass has so far prevented their use for load-bearing implants (Boccaccini, 2005; Hench, 2006; Thompson & Hench, 1998; Thompson, 2005). Subsequently, the repair and regeneration of large bone defects at load-bearing anatomical sites remains a clinical/orthopedic challenge (Fu et al., 2010; Kanczler & Oreffo, 2008).

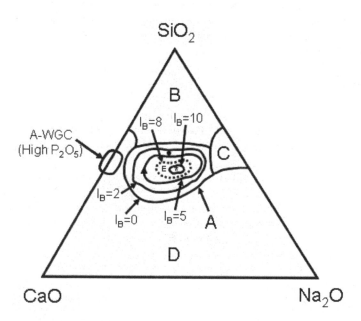

Fig. 1. Compositional dependence of bone bonding and soft tissue bonding of bioactive glass and glass ceramics. All compositions in region A have a constant 6 wt. % of P_2O_5. A-WGC (apatite-wollastonite glass-ceramic) has higher P_2O_5 content (Table 1). Region E (soft tissue boding) is inside the dashed line where $I_B > 8$ [* 45S5 Bioglass ®, ▲ Ceravital®, • 55S4.3 Bioglass ®, and (---) soft-tissue bonding; $I_B = 100/t_{0.5bb}$, where $t_{0.5bb}$ is the time to have more than 50% of the implant surface bonded to the bone and I_B is bioactivity index, i.e. the level of bioactivity of a specific material can be related to the time for more than 50% of the interface to be bonded (Hench, 1988; Hench, 1991)]

Development and Applications of Varieties of Bioactive Glass Compositions in Dental Surgery, Third Generation
Tissue Engineering, Orthopaedic Surgery and as Drug Delivery System

75

2.1 Reaction kinetics

When a bioactive glass is immersed in an aqueous solution, like SBF (simulated body fluid) or TBS (tris buffer solution), there are three distinguishing reactions could be identified (Andersson et al., 1992; Hench, 1991, 1996, 1998; Hench & Andersson, 1993) (Fig. 2):

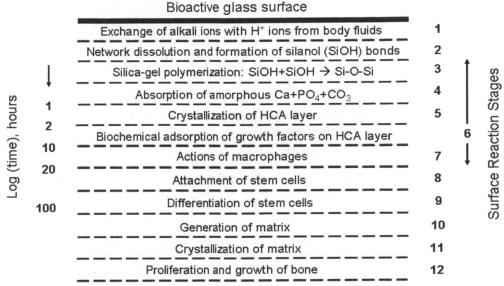

Fig. 2. Sequence of interfacial reactions kinetics involved in forming a bond between bone and a bioactive glass [modified after (Hench, 1998) and (Gerhardt & Boccaccini, 2010)].

1. Leaching and formation of silanols: Glass network releases alkali or alkaline earth elements exchanging cations with H^+ or H_3O^+ cations proceeding from the solution. These modifying ions lead to high values of the interfacial pH, usually more than 7.4.
2. Dissolution of the glass network: -Si-O-Si-O-Si- bonds break through the action of hydroxyl ions. Breakdown of the silica network releases locally silicic acid [$Si(OH)_4$]. If there is more than 60% of silica, the dissolution rate decreases as this increases the number of bridging oxygens in the structure of the glass. The hydrated silica (Si-OH) formed on the glass surface by these reactions undergoes rearrangement by polycondensation of neighboring silanols, resulting in a silica rich gel layer.
3. Precipitation: Calcium and phosphate ions released from the glass together with those from solution form a calcium-phosphate rich layer (CaP) on the surface. This phosphate is initially amorphous, then crystallizes to a hydroxycarbonate apatite (HCA) structure by incorporating carbonate anions from solution within the amorphous CaP phase. The mechanism of nucleation and growth of HCA appears to be the same *in vivo* and *in vitro* and is accelerated by the presence of hydrated silica. These stages do not depend on the presence of the tissue and they are observed in distilled water as well as SBF or tris-buffer solution. The following additional series of reactions is needed to get a bond with the tissue:
4. Absorption of biological moieties in the SiO_2-HCA layer
5. Action of macrophages

6. Attachment of stem cells
7. Differentiation of stem cells
8. Generation of matrix
9. Mineralisation of matrix

This model as proposed by Prof. Hench is widely accepted but has some limitations too. As for example the first stage of the reaction relies on the rapid exchange of the Na^+ ions released from the glass with the protons of the solution, although bioactive glass have been produced without sodium. The index as given in Fig. 1 is also not predictive of the influence of the silica mole fraction on the reactivity of the glass. Some parameters like network connectivity based on the inorganic polymer model for glasses could be considered to describe the behavior of a bioactive glass (Bovo, 2007). The closer the glass composition to the boundary of Fig. 1, the slower is the bonding rate. Usually, the thickness of the bonding zone is proportional to I_B. As the thickness of this zone increases, the failure strength decreases. Further, it was found that if they break after implantation and the broken surfaces stay in contact with SBF, they may self-repair fusing themselves through their apatite surface layers (Bovo, 2007). Again, bioactive glass produced by Ebisawa et al. with a molecular formula of $CaO.SiO_2$ (Ebisawa et al., 1990) could not account for the bioactivity, the model of which proposed by Prof. Hench (Hill, 1996).

Concepts such as cross-link density or network connectivity can be applied to describe their structure if silicate glasses are considered to be inorganic polymers of silicon cross-linked by oxygen (Ray, 1978). The network connectivity of a glass is defined as the average number of additional cross-linking bonds (more than two) for elements other than oxygen that form the network backbone. The calculation of network connectivity of a glass network is based on the relative numbers of network-forming oxide species (those which contribute "bridging" or cross-linking oxygen species) and network-modifying species (those which result in the formation of "non-bridging" species) present (Wallace et al., 1999). The network connectivity of a glass can be used to predict various physical properties of the glass, including its solubility (Hill, 1996). The silicate structural units in a glass of low network connectivity are probably of low molecular mass and are capable of going into solution. Thus, glass solubility increases as network connectivity is reduced. So, glasses of low network connectivity are potentially bioactive (Wallace et al., 1999). Lockyer et al. determined the effect of substituting sodium oxide for calcium oxide on some glass properties (Lockyer et al., 1995). Most studies on bioactive glass systems have been carried out on a weight per cent basis. But, mole per cent substitutions are known to have more significance on a structural level. Weight percent basis has the effect of hiding the composition-property relationships of bioactive glass as there is no account taken of the degree of disruption of the glass network (Lockyer et al., 1995; Strnad, 1992). Fig. 3 represents a highly disrupted glass network. It can be seen that for every mole of calcium oxide removed from the glass network, one mole of sodium oxide must be added in order to maintain the same number of non-bridging oxygen species and, thus the same network connectivity value. So, a substitution on weight per cent basis produces a change in the relative number of non-bridging oxygen species and bridging oxygen species, with consequent change in network connectivity. Work carried out by Wallace et al. uses the concepts of network connectivity for the purposes of designing bioactive glass compositions for control of the physical, chemical and biological properties of bioactive glass (Wallace et al., 1999).

Development and Applications of Varieties of Bioactive Glass Compositions in Dental Surgery, Third Generation
Tissue Engineering, Orthopaedic Surgery and as Drug Delivery System

77

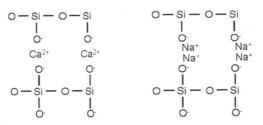

Fig. 3. Representation of glass structure (Wallace et al., 1999)

2.2 Fabrication

Properties of bioactive glass and glass-ceramics are dependent on fabrication methods and the heat-treatment used. Many scaffold fabrication techniques have been reported in the literature, e.g., foam replication methods, salt or sugar leaching, thermally induced phase separation, microsphere emulsification sintering, electrospinning for nano-fibrous structures, computer aided rapid prototyping techniques (Yang et al., 2002; Yun et al., 2007), textile and foam coating methods (De Diego et al., 2000; Francis et al., 2010; Mohamad Yunos et al., 2008) and biomimetic approach (Oliveira et al., 2003; Taboas et al., 2003). All of these methods were done to optimize the structure, properties and mechanical integrity of scaffolds. The design and incorporation of nano-topographic features on the scaffold surface architecture, in order to mimic the nanostructure of natural bone, is also becoming a significant area of research in bone tissue engineering (Berry et al., 2006; Jones, 2009; Stevens & George, 2005; Webster & Ahn, 2007). Also, comprehensive reviews of the general state-of-the art in scaffold manufacturing and optimization are available (Boccaccini & Blaker, 2005; Guarino et al., 2007; Hutmacher et al., 2007; Mohamad Yunos, 2008; Rezwan et al., 2006; Yang et al., 2001).

Pores of bioactive glass and glass-ceramics could be formed by the addition of suitable porogens, such as polymeric materials and foaming agents (Karlsson et al., 2000). Rainer et al. prepared bioactive glass foams for mimicking bone tissue engineering scaffolds using *in situ* foaming of bioactive glass-loaded polyurethane foam (Rainer et al., 2008). Inspired by this fabrication technique, the bioactive materials were prepared with three-dimensional processing and showed promising applications in reconstructive surgery tailored to each single patient. Polyethylene glycol 4000 ($HO(C_2H_4O)$-nH) with particles sizes of 5-500 μm was used as foaming agent for preparing porous bioactive glass ceramic (Lin et al., 1991). This group has also reported the compatibility of porous bioactive glass ceramic with animal tissues. The microstructures of the implant were distributed uniformly in the material, which provided channels for bone in-growth and improved the microscopic bioresorption. Organic polymers were found to be an alternate attractive choice for generating desired pores and porosity due to the complete degradation at temperatures above 600° C. These organic polymers are abundant in natural environment, also available as biomass such as dry and wet woods and crops. This can be obtained from wastes in many related industries too such as food processing and wood finishing manufactures (Sooksaen et al., 2008). It was reported that textural properties (pore size, pore volume, pore structure) of biomaterials may have complex influences on the development of the apatite layer in bioactive glass. Increasing the specific surface area and pore volume of bioactive glass may greatly accelerate the apatite formation and therefore enhance the bioactive behavior (Vallet-Regí et al., 2003).

Sl. No.	Glass composition or system	Reference	Fabrication method adopted	Particle size of starting glass powder
1	45S5	(Ochoa et al., 2009)	Polymer foam replication	< 5 μm
2	SiO_2-CaO-CaF_2-Na_2O-K_2O-P_2O_5-MgO	(Vitale-Brovarone et al., 2008)	Polymer foam replication	< 32 μm
3	SiO_2-P_2O_5-CaO-MgO-Na_2O-K_2O	(Vitale-Brovarone et al., 2009b; Vitale-Brovarone et al., 2007)	Polymer foam replication	< 30 μm
4	SiO_2-P_2O_5-CaO-MgO-Na_2O-K_2O	(Renghini et al., 2009)	Polymer foam replication	-do-
5	45S5	(Chen et al., 2008a)	Polymer foam replication	10-20 μm
6	SiO_2-Na_2O-CaO-MgO	(Vitale-Brovarone et al., 2005)	Starch consolidation	< 100 μm
7	SiO_2-P_2O_5-B_2O_3-CaO-MgO-K_2O-Na_2O	(Moimas et al., 2006)	Compaction and sintering of melt-spun fibers	75 μm (fibre diameter)
8	SiO_2-CaO-Na_2O-K_2O-P_2O_5-MgO-CaF_2	(Baino et al., 2009)	Polymer porogen bakeout	< 106 μm
9	45S5	(Boccaccini et al., 2007)	Polymer foam replication	20-50 μm
10	SiO_2-Na_2O-K_2O-MgO-CaO-P_2O_5	(Fu et al., 2007)	Slip casting	255-325 μm
11	SiO_2-Na_2O-K_2O-MgO-CaO-P_2O_5	(Fu et al., 2008)	Polymer foam replication	< 5-10 μm
12	SiO_2-Na_2O-K_2O-MgO-CaO-P_2O_5	(Fu et al., 2010)	Freeze casting	< 5 μm
13	SiO_2-CaO-K_2O	(Vitale Brovarone et al., 2006)	Polymer porogen burn-off	< 106 μm
14	SiO_2-TiO_2-B_2O_3-P_2O_5-CaO-MgO-K_2O-Na_2O	(Haimi et al., 2009)	Compaction and sintering of melt-spun fibers	75 μm (fibre diameter)
15	45S5	(Deb et al., 2010)	Polymer porogen bakeout	45-90 μm
16	45S5	(Bretcanu et al., 2008)	Polymer foam replication	< 5 μm
17	SiO_2-Na_2O-K_2O-MgO-CaO-P_2O_5; 45S5	(Brown et al., 2008)	Densification and sintering of melt-spun fibers	25-40 μm (fibre diameter)

18	45S5	(Chen et al., 2006b)	Polymer foam replication	$\approx 5\ \mu m$
19	45S5	(Chen et al., 2006a)	Polymer foam replication	5-10 μm
20	45S5	(Chen et al., 2007)	Polymer foam replication	$\approx 10\ \mu m$
21	SiO_2-P_2O_5-CaO-MgO-Na_2O-K_2O	(Vitale-Brovarone et al., 2010)	Polymer burn-off, foam replication	Not applicable
22	45S5	(Vargas et al., 2009)	Polymer foam replication	< 5 μm
23	SiO_2-Na_2O-CaO-P_2O_5-B_2O_3-TiO_2	(Ghosh et al., 2008)	Polymer porogen bakeout	Not applicable
24	SiO_2-Na_2O-CaO-P_2O_5-B_2O_3-TiO_2	(Nandi et al., 2009)	Polymer porogen bakeout	Not applicable
25	SiO_2-CaO-P_2O_5-Al_2O_3	(Mahmood et al., 2001)	Manual free-forming of melt- spun fibers	8-30 μm (fibre diameter)
26	SiO_2-CaO-Na_2O-P_2O_5-K_2O-MgO-B_2O_3	(Mantsos et al., 2009)	Polymer foam replication	Not applicable
27	SiO_2-CaO-Na_2O-K_2O-MgO-P_2O_5-B_2O_3	(Miguel et al., 2010)	Densification and sintering of melt-spun fibers	75 μm (fibre diameter)

Table 2. Summary of recent studies performed on silicate bioactive glass-ceramic scaffolds

2.3 Clinical relevance

For bioactive glass-ceramics, recent developments related to bone tissue engineering scaffolds have been used to remove the gap of load-bearing large bone defects by inter-playing between architectures and components carefully designed from comprehensive levels, i.e., from the macro-, meso-, micrometer down to the nanometer scale (Deville et al., 2006), including both multifunctional bioactive glass composite structures and advanced bioactive glass-ceramic scaffolds exhibiting oriented microstructures, controlled porosity and directional mechanical properties (Baino et al., 2009; Bretcanu et al., 2008; Fu et al., 2010; Fu et al., 2008; Vitale-Brovarone et al., 2010). As summarized in Table 2 [reproduced from (Gerhardt & Boccaccini, 2010)], most of the studies have mainly investigated the mechanical properties, in vitro and cell biological behavior of glass-ceramic scaffolds (Baino et al., 2009; Boccaccini et al., 2007; Bretcanu et al., 2008; Brown et al., 2008; Chen et al., 2007; Chen et al., 2006a; Chen et al., 2008a; Chen et al., 2006b; Deb et al., 2010; Fu et al., 2010; Fu et al., 2007; Fu et al., 2008; Ghosh et al., 2008; Haimi et al., 2009; Klein et al., 2009; Kohlhauser et al., 2009; Mahmood et al., 2001; Mantsos et al., 2009; Miguel et al., 2010; Moimas et al., 2006; Nandi et al., 2009; Ochoa et al., 2009; Renghini et al., 2009; Vargas et al., 2009; Vitale-Brovarone et al., 2009a; Vitale-Brovarone et al., 2010; Vitale-Brovarone et al., 2009b; Vitale-Brovarone et al., 2008; Vitale-Brovarone et al., 2004; Vitale-Brovarone et al., 2005; Vitale-Brovarone et al., 2007; Vitale Brovarone et al., 2006). Scaffolds with compressive strength (Baino et al., 2009; Fu et al., 2010) and elastic modulus values (Fu et al., 2010; Fu et al., 2008) in magnitudes far above that of cancellous bone and close to the lower limit of cortical bone have been realized.

3. Bioactive glass in dental surgery and cranio-maxillofacial augmentation

The increasing need for biomedical devices, required to face dysfunctions of natural tissues and organs caused by traumatic events, diseases and simple ageing, has drawn attention onto new materials that could be able to positively interact with the human body. Biomaterials play a significant role in dental, craniofacial and maxillofacial reconstruction. Their ever-increasing ease of use, long 'shelf-life' and safety enables them to be used efficiently and play an important role in reducing operating times (Gosain & Persing, 1999; Chim & Gosain, 2009). The ideal biomaterial in such reconstruction should be biocompatible with surrounding tissue without elucidating a foreign body reaction, radiolucent, easily shaped or molded, strong enough to endure trauma, stable over time, able to maintain volume, and osteoactive (Gosain & Persing, 1999; Damien & Parsons, 1991; Costantino et al., 1992; Jackson & Yavuzer, 2000; Gosain, 2003).

Abnormality of the craniofacial skeleton may bring in from various causes, including tumor resection, severe infection, trauma, or congenital deformity. Restoring appropriate contour and support in the cranio-orbital region following loss or removal of bone may be quite challenging to the Craniofacial and Neurosurgeons. Since the late 1800's when Muller described using calvarial bone grafts for reconstruction, they have remained the gold standard [Muller, 1890]. Autologous bone grafting provides a rich amount of native tissue that has a high possibility of osseous integration with little risk of rejection or infection long-term, in addition to safety and security (Manson et al., 1986). Although autogenous bone is the ideal material to primarily reconstruct large skull bone defects (Barone & Jimenez, 1997; Goodrich et al., 1992; Weber et al., 1987), it has some drawbacks in reconstruction including donor site morbidity, prolonged operating times, limited availability, and difficulty to contour (Nickell et al., 1972; Whitaker et al., 1979; Jackson et al., 1983). In the pediatric surgery, bone grafts may be relatively easily contoured and curved while, in adults, it is often difficult to achieve the precise three dimensional contours normally found in the cranio-orbital region (Ducic, 2001). Research was then initiated by reconstructive surgeons to find alternative means of reconstruction with alloplasts. In reality, alloplast reconstruction of the calvarium dates back to the year 2000 B. C. in ancient Peru when a gold plate was used to disguise a trephination defect (Grana et al., 1954). Since then, various alloplasts have been used in craniofacial reconstruction. The most commonly utilized material has been methylmethacrylate. Although, it suffers from several potential drawbacks including lack of osseointegration, secondary infection, plate fracture, erosion of the underlying recipient bone, necrosis of surrounding tissues during setting as it forms during an exothermic reaction with temperatures reaching 110° C, and difficulty shaping once polymerization occurs (Ducic , 2002; Costantino et al., 2000; Smith et al., 1999).

In the past century, other metallic materials, such as silver, tantalum, stainless steel or titanium and calcium phosphate based materials like hydroxyapatite cement, calcium orthophosphate cements, porous granular hydroxyapatite, marine coral-based calcium carbonate were used for reconstruction purposes. The present endeavor deals with the application of bioactive glass based material in dental, craniofacial and maxillofacial reconstruction. Bioactive glass (BG) is biocompatible, osteoconductive, form a strong bond with living tissue via the formation of a hydroxyapatite layer on their surface (Meffert et al., 1985; Schepers et al., 1991; Hench et al., 1971) and have been used to repair hard tissues in a variety of craniofacial, maxillofacial, and periodontal applications (Hench, 1991). It has also been established that BG has good mechanical properties and a higher bioactivity in comparison to hydroxyapatite (Mardare et al., 2003; Ghosh et al., 2008)

Development and Applications of Varieties of Bioactive Glass Compositions in Dental Surgery, Third Generation
Tissue Engineering, Orthopaedic Surgery and as Drug Delivery System

81

BG particulate, for example, is used in a variety of dental procedures (Shapoff et. al., 1997), and many BG compositions can be formed into scaffolds for tissue engineering (Jones et al., 2007). Surface reactivity, however, is not their only mechanism of action as BG also releases ions that promote the osteoblast phenotype (Effah Kaufmann et al., 2000; Jell et al., 2008). In vitro studies have established that BG stimulates osteoprogenitors to differentiate to mature osteoblasts that produce bone-like nodules (Tsigkou et al., 2007; 2009). Bioactive glass was used in dentistry as a bioactive material in endosseous ridge maintenance implants (ERMI) as early as in 1986. Dicor® was the first glass-ceramic that allowed the manufacture of inlays and crowns where the major crystalline phase in the glass ceramic was mica (Grossman, 1991). A new glass-ceramic was developed by sol-gel technique having resemblance with commercial leucite based fluorapatite dental glass-ceramic. The produced material has prospective application in dental restorations and it is anticipated to exhibit better control of composition, microstructure and properties due to the intrinsic advantages of the sol-gel preparation method (Chatzistavrou et al., 2009). Recent studies indicated that rhenanite glass-ceramics can be utilized in dentistry (Holand et al., 2006). In a study, bioactive glass coated titanium alloy dental implants were compared with hydroxyapatite implants in human jaw bone and observed that bioactive glass coated implants were as equally successful as hydroxyapatite in achieving osseointegration and supporting final restorations (Mistry et al., 2011). Bioglass was mixed with phosphoric acid and irradiated with CO_2 laser could occlude the dentinal tubule orifices with calcium-phosphate crystals where the application of CO_2 laser potentially improved the mechanical organization of these crystals (Bakry et al., 2011). In another study, radio-opaque nanosized bioactive glass was used for root canal application particularly for dressing or filling material (Mohn et al., 2010). A modified bioglass formula was used as a pulp capping agent where the incidence of properly positioned dentin bridge formation was higher and the incidence of extruded dentin bridge formation was reduced (Stanley et al., 2001). A new treatment for localized aggressive periodontitis using enamel matrix proteins and bioactive glass resulted in the successful treatment of intrabony defects (Miliauskaite et al., 2007; Zietek et al., 1998). Bioactive glass was used in the treatment of intrabony defects in patients with generalized aggressive periodontitis (Mengel et al., 2006), in patients with moderate to advanced periodontitis with excellent outcome in mandibular molar Class II furcations (Yukna et al., 2001), molar furcation invasions (Anderegg et al., 1999), periodontal intrabony defects (Zamet et al., 1997) and in experimental periodontal wound healing in animal model (Karatzas et al., 1999). The effects of a recombinant mouse amelogenin (rM179) on the growth of apatite crystals nucleated on a bioactive glass (45S5 type Bioglass) surface were investigated with a view to gaining a better understanding of the role of amelogenin protein in tooth enamel formation and of its potential application in the design of novel enamel-like biomaterials (Wen et al., 1999). A fibre-reinforced bioglass composite is a promising material for dental applications where fibre significantly increases strength and toughness (Gheysen et al., 1983). PerioGlas, a silicate-based synthetic biomaterial was used for regeneration of peri-implant infrabony defects where new bone eventually reaches the implant, and osseointegration occurs with incorporation of the PerioGlas particles (Johnson et al., 1997). Bioactive glass has been used in cranio-maxillofacial reconstruction especially on the repair of periodontal and alveolar ridge defects (Quinones & Lovelace, 1997; Han et al., 2002; Sy, 2002; Throndson & Sexton, 2002; Norton & Wilson, 2002; Knapp et al., 2003) although its use is also extended for successful reconstruction of other areas of the head and neck (Scotchford et al., 2011). Bioactive glass has been utilized for the repair of orbital floor fractures with maintenance of globe position (Kinnunen et al., 2000; Aitasalo et al., 2001) and elevation of the floor of the maxillary sinus floor (Tadjoedin et al., 2002) in combination with autogenous iliac bone. Bioactive glass particles (Nova Bone, Porex Surgical) mixed with autogenous bone particles has also been used to cranial vault reconstruction (Gosain, 2003), in clinical studies in the treatment of cystic defects, ridge augmentations, apical resections, extraction sites, periodontal osseous defects and sinus lifts and augmentation (Furusawa T, Mizunuma, 1997; Low et al., 1997; Lovelace et al., 1998; Galindo-Moreno et al., 2008; Klongnoi et al., 2006). Bioactive glass posed some complications when used as a ceramic implant for contour restoration of the facial skeleton.

4. Bioglass as bone graft substitute

The management of fractures remains an incessant challenge for trauma and orthopedic surgeons. Although, majority of fractures heal uncomplicated, 5–10% of patients meet problems due to bone defects or impaired fracture healing, or a combination of both (Einhorn, 1995). Bone grafts fill voids and offer support, and therefore may augment the biological repair of the defect. Bone grafting is a widespread surgical procedure, carried out in approximately 10% of all skeletal reconstructive surgery cases (Schnettler & Markgraf, 1997).

Bone healing differs from any other soft tissue since it heals through the generation of new bone rather than by forming fibrotic tissue. Osteogenesis, osteoinduction, osteoconduction and adequate blood and nutrient supply are the four critical elements of bone regeneration along with the final bonding between host bone and grafting material which is called osteointegration (Hing, 2004). Osteoprogenitor cells living within the donor graft, may survive during transplantation, could potentially proliferate and differentiate to osteblasts and eventually to osteocytes which represent the "osteogenic" potential of the graft (Cypher & Grossman, 1996; Giannoudis et al., 2005). "Osteoinduction" conversely is the stimulation and activation of host mesenchymal stem cells from the surrounding tissue, which differentiate into bone-forming osteoblasts. This process is mediated by a cascade of signals and the activations of several extra and intracellular receptors the most important of which belong to the TGF-beta superfamily (Urist, 1965; Cypher & Grossman, 1996). Osteoconduction describes the facilitation and orientation of blood-vessel and the creation of the new Haversian systems into the bone scaffold [Burchardt, 1983; Constantino & Freidman, 1994]. At last, "osteointegration" describes the surface bonding between the host bone and the grafting material (Constantino & Freidman, 1994).

The most desirable form of bone substitute is the autologous bone graft for their superior osteoconduction, ease of incorporation, lack of immunological reactions, contains living bone cells that offer osteogenesis and growth factors that stimulate osteoinduction (Cypher & Grossman, 1996; Naber et al., 1972; Marciani et al., 1977). However, massive replacements of bone are not easily achieved by bone autografts as autogenous bone is limited in availability, and may result in the donar site morbidity (Mankin et al., 1976). Moreover, harvesting the autograft requires an additional surgery at the donar site that can result in its own 8–39% risk of complications, such as inflammation, risk of extensive blood loss infection, nerve and urethral injury, pelvic instability, cosmetic disadvantages and chronic pain (Banwart et al., 1995; Constantino & Freidman, 1994; Patka et al., 1998; Younger & Chapman, 1989; Summers & Eisenstein, 1989; Ross et al., 2000; Seiler & Johnson, 2000;

Development and Applications of Varieties of Bioactive Glass Compositions in Dental Surgery, Third Generation
Tissue Engineering, Orthopaedic Surgery and as Drug Delivery System

83

Skaggs et al., 2000). Furthermore, autografting is normally not recommended for elderly or pediatric patients or for patients with malignant or infectious disease (Bridwell et al., 1994; Gau et al., 1991; McCarthy et al., 1986). An allograft is preferred in some cases but the possible immune response and disease transmission may be detrimental for the recipient (Asselmeier et al., 1993; Stevenson & Horowitz, 1992; Chapman et al., 1997; Gazdag et al., 1995), so their use is suboptimal.

Despite the benefits of autografts and allografts, the limitations of each have necessitated the pursuit of alternatives biomaterials. The ideal bone composite material with composition and mechanical properties equivalent to that of bone should have adequate biocompatibility, tailorable biodegradability, ability to initiate osteogenesis; in short, the graft should closely mimic the natural bone. Biodegradability together with biocompatibility and suitable mechanical properties are found only in a small group of materials. The aim of the present chapter was to provide a comprehensive overview of literature data of bioactive glass as bone substitutes for use in trauma and orthopedic surgery.

Bioactive glasses exhibit osteoinductive and osteoconductive properties (Giannoudis et al., 2005) and can be manufactured into microspheres, fibers and porous implants. They are bioactive, as they interact with the body. Bioactivity depends upon the SiO_2 content; the bonding between bone and glass is most excellent if the bioactive glass contains 45–52% SiO_2 (Valimaki & Aro, 2006). The combination of hydroxyapatite with bioglass result in better composite bioactivity and biocompatibility compared to hydroxyapatite alone (Cholewa-Kowalska et al., 2009). They have significantly greater mechanical strength when compared to calcium phosphate preparations. After contact with body fluids, a silicate- rich layer is formed leading to mechanical strong graft–bone bonding. Above this, a hydroxyapatite layer will form, which directs new bone formation together with protein absorption. The extracellular proteins magnetize macrophages, mesenchymal stem cells and osteoprogenitor cells. Consequently, the osteoprogenitor cells proliferate into matrix-producing osteoblasts (Valimaki & Aro, 2006; Hench & Paschall, 1973). Mechanical properties of bioactive glass are not optimal, and therefore other ceramic components are sometimes added to the bioactive glass for reinforcement. Mechanical capability and biological absorbability of $SiO(2)$-CaO bioactive glass may also be improved by incorporating $Na(2)O$ into bioactive glass, which can result in the formation of a hard yet biodegradable crystalline phase from bioactive glass when sintered by sol-gel process (Chen et al., 2010). In another study, mechanical properties of potassium fluorrichterite $(KNaCaMg(5)Si(8)O(22)F(2))$ glass-ceramics may be improved by either increasing the concentration of calcium (GC5) or by the addition of $P(2)O(5)$ (GP2) that has potential as a load bearing bioceramic for fabrication of medical devices intended for skeletal tissue repair (Bhakta et al., 2010; Bandyopadhyay-Ghosh et al., 2010). A new porous bioactive glass has been developed by foaming with rice husks and sintering at 1050 degrees C for 1 hour that provides sufficient mechanical support temporarily while maintaining bioactivity, and that can biodegrade at later stages is achievable with the developed 45S5 bioglass-derived scaffolds (Wu et al., 2009).

In experimental cancellous bone defects in rat models, bioactive glass was found biocompatible, and the filler effect was greater with bioactive glass than with autogenous bone (Heikkila et al., 1995). Bioglass was found to trigger new bone formation by allogenic demineralized bone matrix, and the biocompatibility of the glass was verified by the absence of adverse cellular reactions (Erdemli et al., 2010; Pajamaki et al., 1993a, 1993b).

Biocompatibility and osteogenesis of biomimetic bioglass-collagen composite scaffolds alone and in combination with phosphatidylserine were also studied and confirmed that the composite scaffolds fulfill the basic requirements of bone tissue engineering scaffold and have the potential to be applied in orthopedic and reconstructive surgery (Marelli et al., 2010; Xu et al., 2011). Addition of hyaluronic acid and mesenchymal stem cell in the aforesaid scaffold further enhanced the healing of the bone defect (Xu et al., 2010). Bone-bonding response significantly enhanced with the micro-roughening of the bioactive glass surface, but the glass composition affected the intensity of the response (Itala et al., 2003). Bioactive glass have shown no or only mild inflammatory responses in the surrounding tissue in histological in vivo studies and in 6 months, the glass fiber scaffolds are completely resorbed (Moimas et al., 2006). In an experimental critical size bone defect model in goat, porous bioactive glass promoted bone formation over the extension of the defect and offers interesting potential for orthopedic reconstructive procedures (Nandi et al., 2009). Bioglass has been investigated extensively in bone tissue engineering but there has been relatively little previous research on its application to soft-tissue engineering. In a study, bioactive glass incorporated into scaffold was able to increase neovascularization that is extremely beneficial during the engineering of larger soft-tissue constructs (Day et al., 2004). Irrespective of soft and hard tissue healing necessitates enhanced neovascularization which can be induced by localized low concentration bioglass delivery and may offer an alternative approach to costly growth factors and their potential side-effects in bone regeneration (Leu et al., 2009).

The first reports on clinical applications of bioactive glass materialize in the 1980s (Reck, 1981). Screw augmentation with bioactive glass was evaluated in 37 Weber type B ankle fractures with no information of screw loosening within a period of 2 years (Andreassen et al., 2004). Bioactive glass have been clinically used in vertebroplasty (Middleton et al., 2008; Palussiere et al., 2005), treatment of an unstable distal radius fracture (Smit et al., 2005), tympanoplastic reconstruction (Reck, 1983), as filling material in benign tumour surgery (Heikkila et al., 1995), for reconstruction of defects in facial bones [Suominen & Kinnunen, 1996], for treatment of periodontal bone defects (Villaca et al., 2005; Leonetti et al., 2000), in obliteration of frontal sinuses (Suonpaa et al., 1997; Peltola et al., 2000a, 2000b), in repairing orbital floor fractures (Kinnunen et al., 2000; Aitasalo et al., 2001), in lumbar fusion (Ido et al., 2000), reconstruction of the maxillary sinus (Scala et al., 2007), in cementless metal-backed acetabular cups (Hedia et al., 2006) and for reconstruction of the iliac crest defect after bone graft harvesting (Asano et al., 1994). The combination of a thermoplastic, viscous carrier with a granular bioglass scaffold allowed for the delivery of allergenic mesenchymal stem cells in a clinically manageable form that enhanced bone formation at early stages of canine alveolar repair (Mylonas et al., 2007).

5. Bioactive glass in drug delivery system

In recent years wide spread research has been initiated with new advanced drug delivery systems with better drug control and prolonged action. The drug delivery process is of paramount importance in assuring that a certain molecule will reach without decomposition or secondary reactions at the right place to perform its task with efficiency. The drug is introduced as part of an inert matrix, from which it should be released in a controlled way and where it should be distributed uniformly. Smart delivery systems that can be utilized

Development and Applications of Varieties of Bioactive Glass Compositions in Dental Surgery, Third Generation
Tissue Engineering, Orthopaedic Surgery and as Drug Delivery System

85

for the delivery of antibiotics, insulin, anti-inflammatory drugs, anticancer drugs, hormones and vaccines are yet to be developed, which are responsive to normal physiological process. Significant consideration is paid on the use of microspheres as carriers for proteins and drugs. The main benefit of microspheres over the more traditional macroporous block orthopaedic scaffolds is that microspheres possess not only better drug-delivery properties, but also the potential to fill the bone defects with irregular and complex shapes and sizes (Wu et al., 2004). The interstitial space between the particles of the microspheres is imperative for effective and functional bone regeneration (Malafaya et al., 2008; Luciani et al., 2008; Hsu et al., 1999), as they permit for both bone and vascular ingrowths. Several difficulties are encountered when macromolecules are incorporated in polymer devices e.g. protein drugs when impregnated may denature within the polymer matrix causing a loss of biological activity and probable changes in immunogenicity (Langer, 1990a, 1980b). This may happen due to degradation of the drug by the solvents or the temperature involved in the fabrication of the polymeric devices. Presently, ceramics have gained major recognition as bone substitute materials in dentistry and medicine as ceramics are biocompatible, resorbable and porous, attempts have been made to exploit them as delivery systems for drugs, chemicals and biologicals (Bajpai & Benghuzzi, 1988; Bajpai, 1994; Lasserre & Bajpai, 1998).

5.1 Drug delivery of antibiotics for treatment of osteomyelitis

Treatment of orthopaedic infections with antibacterial agents by oral or intravenous route often leads the clinicians to be distrustful about patient outcome (Walenkamp, 1997); as the condition is frequently associated with poor vascular perfusion accompanied by infection of the surrounding tissue (Mader et al., 1993). Subsequent to surgical debridement, it is essential to maintain a highly effective concentration of the antibiotic in the infected area for a sufficient period of time (usually 4–6 weeks) to allow the healing process to complete (Kanellakopoulou & Giamarellos-Bourboulis, 2000).

Treatment of osteomyelitis with local biodegradable antibiotic delivery systems has become a common practice in orthopaedic surgery. Biodegradable implants could provide high local bactericidal concentrations in tissue for the prolonged time needed to completely eradicate the infection and the likelihood to match the rate of implant biodegradability according to the type of infection treated (Kanellakopoulou & Giamarellos-Bourboulis, 2000). Biodegradation also makes surgical removal of the implant unnecessary. The implant can also be used initially to obliterate the dead space and, eventually to guide its repair. Porous block of bioactive glass has been studied for drug delivery applications of antibiotics for treatment of osteomyelitis in animal model (Nandi et al., 2009; Kundu et al., 2011). The glass ceramic block exists in two forms: one with porosity of 20-30 % and the other of 70 %. Excellent results were observed in infected arthroplasty after 2 years of treatment and the implanted material triggered osteogenesis so as to produce a complete radiological replacement of the osseous defect (Kawanabe et al., 1998). It has been observed that locally produced pure or bioglass reinforced plaster of Paris, hydroxyapatite and sodium alginate with cephazoline antibiotic are promising biomaterials for treatment of osteomyelitis and mainly because of economical reasons and availability, may be an alternative in clinical practice, especially for developing countries (Heybeli et al., 2003). Glass reinforced hydroxyapatite with sodium ampicillin, a broad spectrum antibiotic has been successfully applied for treatment of periodontitis (Queiroz et al., 2001). Gentamicin sulfate impregnated bioactive SiO_2-CaO-P_2O_5 glass implants are good carriers for local gentamicin release into the local osseous tissue, where they show excellent biocompatibility and bone integration. Moreover, these implants are able to promote bone growth during the resorption process (Mes eguer-Olmo et al., 2006; Arcos et al., 2001). Antimicrobial activity of bioactive glass (BG) as a controlled release device for tetracycline hydrochloride and an inclusion complex formed by tetracycline and b-cyclodextrin has been investigated in mice model where there is prolonged period of release of antibiotic due to presence of cyclodextrin. It has been observed that there was an initial burst of 12%, followed by a sustained release over 80 days and a total release of 22–25%. (Dominguesa et al., 2004). The effectiveness of a degradable and bioactive borate glass has been compared with the clinically used calcium sulfate in the treatment of osteomyelitis of rabbits, as a carrier for vancomycin and proved to have excellent biocompatibility and to be very effective in eradicating osteomyelitis and simultaneously stimulating bone regeneration, avoiding the disadvantages of vancomycin loaded calcium sulphate (Zongping et al., 2009). Chitosan-bonded mixture of borate bioactive glass particles with teicoplanin (antibiotic) combining sustained drug release with the ability to support new bone ingrowth, could provide a method for treating chronic osteomyelitis *in vitro* and *in vivo* (Wei-Tao et al., 2010; Xin et al., 2010). In another study, well-ordered mesoporous bioactive glass impregnated with gentamycin has been carried out *in vitro* as a bioactive drug release system for preparation of bone implant materials vis-à-vis treatment of osteomyelitis (Xia & Chang, 2006; Zhu & Kaskel, 2009). Mesoporous bioactive glass (MBGs) with different compositions impregnated tetracycline has been prepared and their drug release behaviors have been studied (Zhao et al., 2008). Recently, an unique multifunctional bioactive composite scaffold mainly 45S5 Bioglass-based glass–ceramic scaffolds has been investigated with the potential to enhance cell attachment and to provide controlled delivery of gentamicin for bone tissue engineering (Francis et al., 2010). Composite materials composed of borate bioactive glass and chitosan (designated BGC) were investigated *in vitro* and *in vivo* as a new delivery system for teicoplanin in the treatment of chronic osteomyelitis induced by methicillin-resistant *Staphylococcus aureus* (MRSA) and demonstrated that this system is effective in treating chronic osteomyelitis by providing a sustained release of teicoplanin, in addition to participating in bone regeneration (Jia et al., 2010).

5.2 Bioactive glass delivery of growth factors

Bone regeneration is a coordinated cascade of events regulated by several hormones, cytokines and growth factors (Carano & Filvaroff, 2003; El-Ghannam, 2005; Hsiong & Mooney, 2000). Bioactive glass is regarded as high-potential scaffolds due to their osteoconductive properties (Thomas et al., 2005). The bone bonding ability is based on the chemical reactivity of the bioactive glass in which silicon bonds are broken and finally a CaP-rich layer is deposited on top of the glass which crystallizes to hydroxycarbonate apatite (HCA). To improve the biodegradability of this implant, porosity is introduced (Karageorgiou & Kaplan, 2005) which also helps to bone ingrowth, though pore sizes should be large enough. This porosity is occasionally called macroporosity while the bioglass implants can encompass a micro or nanoporosity of their own. Interconnectivity of the pores is of paramount necessity for tissue engineered bone constructs which implies generation of overlapping pore connection into the scaffolds. In bone tissue engineering growth factors are also introduced to accelerate tissue ingrowth. However, due to variation in potency and efficacy of individual growth factors, each study claimed different levels of bone healing. Growth factors like bone morphogenic protein-2&7 (BMP-2&7), transforming growth factor

(TGF-β), basic fibroblast growth factor (bFGF), insulin like growth factor-1&2 (IGF-1&2) and vascular endothelial growth factor (VEGF) are commonly introduced into these scaffolds due to their osteoinductive properties and vascularization (Seeherman & Wozney, 2005; Ginebra et al., 2006; Jansen et al., 2005). This increases the clinical significant amount high above normal values inside the human body and increases the cost of a single implant considerably, therefore diminishing a possible use of the material. The most appropriate technique for growth factor delivery is still under debate. Bioactive glass   stimulates fibroblasts to secrete significantly increased amounts of angiogenic growth factors and can induce infiltration of a significantly increased number of blood vessels into tissue engineering scaffolds (Day, 2005; Day et al., 2004). Therefore it has a number of potential applications in therapeutic angiogenesis (Keshaw et al., 2005).

PLGA polymeric system coated bioactive glass with VEGF has been investigated in the rat critical-sized defect with resultant enhanced angiogenesis and additive bone healing effects (Leach et al., 2006). An additional study in which BMP-4 and VEGF were concertedly delivered confirmed that combination of two growth factors promoted greater bone formation as compared to single factor treatment group (Huang et al., 2005). These results delineate a promising approach to enhance bone healing in hypovascularized defects that commonly occur after removal of bone tumors by radiation therapy. Sol-gel silica-based porous glass (xerogel) was used as a novel carrier material for recombinant human transforming growth factor-β1 (TGF-β1) and is capable of eliciting bone tissue reactivity that may serve as an effective bone graft material for the repair of osseous defects (Nicoll et al., 1997). A delivery system consisting of collagen Type I gel, Recombinant human BMP-2 (rhBMP-2) and 45S5 Bioglass microspheres seem to be a promising system for bone regeneration (Bergeron et al., 2007). Bovine bone morphogenetic protein has been delivered in bioactive glass on demineralized bone matrix grafts in the rat muscular pouch with effective outcome (Pajamaki et al., 1993).

6. Bioglass as coating of implants

In the present days, metallic materials gained considerable dimension as medical and dental devices due to their mechanical properties (Roessler et al., 2002). Implants are usually prepared of metals such as titanium alloys, cobalt alloys and SS 316L (García et al., 2004). The need to diminish costs in public health services has constrained the use of SS as the most economical option for orthopedic implants (Meinert et al., 1998; Fathi et al., 2003), because of its comparative low cost, ease of fabrication, ready availability and reasonable corrosion resistance. However, this material is prone to localized attack in long term use due to the hostile biological effects (Yılmaz et al., 2005). Besides, the corrosion of the metallic implants is imperative because it could adversely affect the biocompatibility and the mechanical integrity. Large concentrations of metallic cations coming from the implant can result in biologically unwanted reactions and might lead to the mechanical failure of the implant. Titanium and Ti-alloys are commonly used materials for *in vivo* applications, due to their good physical and mechanical properties such as low density, high corrosion resistance and mechanical resistance. Nevertheless, titanium and other alloying metal ions as aluminium and vanadium, release from the implants being accumulated in the nearby tissues, due to the aggressive action of the biological fluids (Hodgson et al., 2002; Zaffe et al., 2003; Yue et al., 2002; Finet et al., 2000; Milosev et al., 2000). The lack of interaction with the biological environment prevents the implant from integrating with the surrounding hard tissue.

The perfection of the interface between bone and orthopaedic or dental implants is still considered as a challenge because the formation and maintenance of viable bone closely apposed to the surface of biomaterials are indispensable for the stability and clinical success of non-cemented orthopaedic/dental implants. It has been addressed to create a suitable environment where the natural biological potential for bone functional regeneration can be encouraged and maximized (Carlsson et al., 1994; Wennerberg et al., 1996; Larsson et al., 1996; Buser et al., 1998). Implant osseointegration depends on various factors viz. surface structure, biomechanical factors and biological response (Carlsson et al., 1994; Chappard et al., 1999). At the present time, osseointergation is defined not only as the absence of a fibrous layer around the implant with an active response in terms of integration to host bone, but also as a chemical (bonding osteogenesis) or physico-chemical (connective tissue osteogenesis) bond between implant and bone (Branemårk et al., 1983; Albrektsson, 1993) which in turn, depends on the biomineralization into the surrounding tissue. Biomineralization is normally happens when the bony injury or normal bone tissue in cellular level takes place. The process starts with the osteolysis through the osteoclastic cells from the vicinity as well as from the systemic source. This is instantaneously followed by formation of a protein-rich matrix in the localized area (injury site) which ultimately being mineralized with the inorganic ions viz. calcium and phosphorous from the serum and the localized tissues. Once the nucleation of bone formation takes place at a very faster rate (approx. 10 days), then routinely further bone formation with the incorporation of above-mentioned inorganic ions are found from the serum (Weiner, 1986). Further, implant loosening/migration is an unanswered complication associated with internal fixation. This problem may be overcome by modifying the implant/bone interface for improved osseous integration. Improved osseous integration may be obtained by the use of hydroxyapatite (HAp), b-tri calcium phosphate (b-TCP) and their composite coatings as nominally HAp to enhance the osteoconductivity of metallic implant (Thomas et al., 1987; Filiaggi, et al., 1991; Rivero et al., 1988). These coatings have been shown to promote osseointegration by stimulating bone growth onto the surface (Dey et al., 2011).

Apart from calcium phosphate coating of metallic implants, extensive research has been initiated with bioglass as coatings for metallic implants because of their controlled surface reactivity and good bone bonding ability (Hench and Andersson, 1993; Hench, 1993; Ferraris et al., 1996). These coatings accomplish two purposes: improving the osseointegration of the implants, and shielding the metal against corrosion from the body fluids and the tissue from the corrosion products of the alloys. Unfortunately, most of the attempts to coat metallic implants with bioactive glass have had poor success. The explanation behind is due to poor adhesion of the coating and/or degradation of the glass properties during the coating procedure (typically enameling, or flame or plasma spray coating) (Hench & Andersson, 1993). Bioactive glass can be used to coat titanium alloys by different methods such as conventional enamelling, sputtering techniques, vacuum plasma spray and subsonic thermal spraying technique (STS) (Ferraris et al., 1996; Verné et al., 2000; Jana et al., 1995; Gomez-Vega et al., 2000; Li et al., 2007). These implants can offer several advantages, in terms of the high mechanical properties of the metallic substrate combined with the bioactivity of the coating aside from good protection of the substrate from corrosion. Bioactive glass and nanohydroxyapatite (BG-nHA) on titanium-alloy orthopaedic implants and surrounding bone tissue in vivo was evaluated and observed that these coatings could enhance the osteointegration of orthopaedic implant (Xie et al., 2010). Bioglass coating of the three-dimensional Ti scaffolds by the radio frequency magnetron sputtering technique

Development and Applications of Varieties of Bioactive Glass Compositions in Dental Surgery, Third Generation
Tissue Engineering, Orthopaedic Surgery and as Drug Delivery System

89

determines an in vitro increase of the bone matrix elaboration and may potentially have a clinical benefit (Saino et al., 2010). Biocompatible yttrium-stabilized zirconia (YSZ) in the form of nanoparticles and bioactive Bioglass (45S5) in the form of microparticles were used to coat Ti6Al4V substrates by electrophoretic deposition with potential applications in the orthopedics (Radice et al., 2007). Fluorapatite glass LG112 can be used as a sputtered glass coating on roughened surfaces of Ti6Al4V for possible future use for medical implants (Bibby et al., 2005). However, the Ti-alloys used in the fabrication of prosthetic implants are very reactive, and the glass/metal reactions that occur during firing are unfavorable to adhesion and bioactivity. Thus, coating titanium with bioactive glass is challenging. Besides, tremendous care should be taken in storing and/or shipping HA- or BG-coated Ti6A14V implants due to loss of bonding strength in low and high humidity (Chern et al., 1993). Bioactive glass comprising of SiO_2-Na_2O-K_2O-CaO-MgO-P_2O_5 system has been formulated to coat orthopedic metallic implants by enameling and now have been utilized for coatings on commercial dental implants approximately 100 μm thick (Lopez-Esteban et al., 2003). Due to the peculiar softening properties of these materials, bioactive glass and glass-ceramics do imply a good alternative to hydroxyapatite, commonly used as bioactive coating on metallic prostheses in order to improve their adhesion to the bone. Further, bioglass coated implants exhibited greater bone ingrowth compared to hydroxyapatite coated and control implants in animal model and they maintained their mechanical integrity over time (Wheeler et al., 2001). In a study, multilayered bioactive glass-ceramic coatings on a Ti6Al4V alloy screws was conducted for dental applications with layers of controlled thickness (Verné et al., 2004). A biocompatible composite implant system was developed by coating bioglass onto cobalt-chromium alloy substrates where thin, adherent bioglass coating provides the ability of bonding directly to bone, while the underlying metal substrate gives the composite implants adequate strength to be used in load bearing applications (Lacefield & Hench, 1986). Improvement of the alumina/bone interface in Alumina on alumina total hip arthroplasty can be done by coating with sol-gel derived bioactive glass (Hamadouche et al., 2000). Polyurethane (PUR) and polyurethane/poly(d, l-lactide) acid (PUR/PDLLA) based scaffolds coated with Bioglass particles have potential to be used as bioactive, biodegradable scaffolds in bone tissue engineering (Bil et al., 2007).

7. Bioactive glasses' in biomolecular engineering with special referencing to third generation biomaterials

Third generation biomaterials should be biocompatible, resorbable, and also bioactive eliciting specific cellular responses at the molecular level (Hench & Polak, 2002). Three-dimensional porous structures that stimulate cells' invasion, attachment and proliferation, as well as functionalized surfaces with peptide sequences that mimic the ECM components so as to trigger specific cell responses are being developed (Agrawal & Ray, 2001; Hutmacher et al., 1996; Temenoff & Mikos, 2000).

Tissue engineering applications and development of third generation biomaterials emerged at the same time. Tissue engineering is the promising therapeutic approach that combines cells onto resorbable scaffolds for in situ tissues regeneration and has emerged as an alternative potential solution to tissue transplantation and grafting. Tissue engineering is a multidisciplinary field that applies principles of life sciences and engineering towards the development of biological substitutes employing three fundamental "tools", namely cells, scaffolds and growth factors (GFs) for the restoration, maintenance or improvement of tissue form and function (Langer & Vacanti, 1993). The common limitations associated with the application of allografts, autografts and xenografts include donor site insufficiency, rejection, diseases transfer, harvesting costs and post-operative morbidity (Fernyhough et al., 1992; Banwart et al., 1995; Goulet et al., 1997). Tissue engineering and regenerative medicine has made a new horizon in repairing and restoring organs and tissues using the natural signaling pathways and components such as stem cells, growth factors and peptide sequences among others, in amalgamation with synthetic scaffolds (Hardouin et al., 2000). Apart from the basic tissue engineering triad (cells, signaling and scaffold), angiogenesis and nutrients delivery should be taken into account as they both play vital role to stimulate tissue regeneration. Although tissue engineering emerged as a very dazzling option to overcome many existing problems related to the current use of autografts, allografts and xenografts, its implementation as part of a routine treatment for tissue replacement is controversial. Despite such limitations, tissue engineering is a very promising approach that opens newer vista of study and research in the field of regenerative medicine.

Scaffolds of three-dimensional porous structures need to achieve the following criteria in order to be used in tissue engineering [Spaans et al., 2000; Boccaccini et al., 2008].

- must be biocompatible and bio-resorbable at a controllable degradation and resorption rate as well as provide the control over the appropriation
- must possess well defined microstructure with an interconnected porous network, formed by a combination of macro and micro pores to allow proper tissue ingrowth, vascularization and nutrient delivery.
- must have proper mechanical properties to regenerate bone tissue in load-bearing sites.
- must keep its structural integrity during the first stages of the new bone formation.

The amalgamation of bioactivity and biodegradability is most likely the pertinent characteristics that include third-generation biomaterials. The bioactivation of surfaces with specific biomolecules is an influential means that allows cell guidance and stimulation towards a particular response. The endeavor is to mimic the ECM environment and function in the developed scaffold by coupling specific cues in its surface. Thus, cell behavior including adhesion, migration, proliferation and differentiation into a particular lineage will be influenced by the biomolecules attached to the material surface. In addition, pore distribution, interconnectivity and size are of paramount significance in order to assurance of proper cell proliferation and migration, as well as tissue vascularization and diffusion of nutrients.

The concept of using bioactive glass substrates as templates for in vitro synthesis of bone tissue for transplantation by assessing the osteogenic potential has been investigated (Xynos et al., 2000; Phan et al., 2003; Chen et al., 2008; Brown et al., 2008) and confirmed that Bioglass scaffolds have potential as osteoconductive tissue engineering substrates for maintenance and normal functioning of bone tissue (Bretcanu et al., 2009). Human primary osteoblast-like cells cultured in contact with different bioactive glass suggested that bioglass not only induces osteogenic differentiation of human primary osteoblast-like cells, but can also increase collagen synthesis and release. The newly formulated bioactive gel-glass seems to have potential applications for tissue engineering, inducing increased collagen synthesis (Bosetti et al., 2003; Jones et al., 2007). Bone marrow is a combination of hematopoietic, vascular, stromal and mesenchymal cells capable of skeletal repair/regeneration with the ability of bone marrow cells to differentiate into osteoblasts and osteoclasts which is imperative in tissue regeneration during fracture healing, or for successful osteointegration of implanted prostheses, and in bone remodelling. Bone marrow cell culture systems with bioactive glass seem to be useful and induce osteogenic differentiation and cell mineralization (Bosetti & Cannas, 2005). In another study, bioglass granules in combination with expanded periosteal cells in culture were investigated in rabbit large calvarial defects with increased ossification (Moreira-Gonzalez et al., 2005).

Bioresorbable and bioactive tissue engineering composite scaffolds based on bioactive glass (45S5 Bioglass(R)) particles and macroporous poly(DL-lactide) (PDLLA) and polylactide-co-glycolide (PLAGA) with osteoblasts (HOBs) cells have tremendous potential as scaffolds for guided bone regeneration (Roether et al., 2002; Lu et al., 2005; Yang et al., 2006;), for intervertebral disc tissue repair (Wilda & Gough, 2006; Helen & Gough, 2008). In another study, the cellular response of fetal osteoblasts to bioactive resorbable composite films consisting of a poly-D,L-lactide (PDLLA) matrix and bioactive glass 45S5 particles in the absence of osteogenic factors stimulates osteoblast differentiation and mineralization of the extracellular matrix, demonstrating the osteoinductive capacity of the composite (Tsigkou et al., 2007).

Revision cases of total hip implants are complicated by the considerable amount of bone loss. New materials and/or approaches are desirable to provide stability to the site, stimulate bone formation, and eventually lead to fully functional bone tissue. Porous bioactive glass have been developed as scaffolds for bone tissue engineering. The incorporation of tissue-engineered constructs utilizing these scaffolds seeded with osteoprogenitor cells or culture expanded to form bonelike tissue on the scaffold prior to implantation has been conducted in large, cortical bone defects in the rat (Livingston et al., 2002).

Bioglass-incorporated alginate hydrogels encapsulated with murine embryonic stem cells have potential implications and applications for tissue engineering where bioglass substrates could be used for the production of bioengineered bone both in vitro and in vivo and bioglass-incorporated alginate hydrogels can be injected directly into the defect area (Zhang et al., 2009). One of the major factors in the therapeutic accomplishment of bone tissue engineered scaffolds is the capacity of the construct to vascularise after implantation. For improving vascularization, porous bioactive glass-ceramic construct combination of co-culture human umbilical vein endothelial cells (HUVECS) with human osteoblasts (HOBS) may promote vascularization and facilitate tissue regeneration (Deb et al., 2010).

8. Conclusion

During the past decades, there has been a major breakthrough in development of biomedical materials including various ceramic materials for bone and dental repair as well as implantable drug delivery systems. Both increases in life expectancy and the social obligations to provide a better quality of life appeared to be the vital factors to this development. Significant attention has been paid towards the use of synthetic graft materials in bone tissue and dental repair and development of new implant technologies has led to the design concept of novel bioactive materials. Bioactive glass inducing active biomineralization in vivo have been a high demand in the development of clinical regenerative medicine. Originally, it was thought for bone repair and bone regeneration via tissue engineering (TE), but eventually has become a very attractive biomaterials of choice having implications in: dental, maxillofacial and ear implants, drug delivery system, injectable for treatment of enuresis, to activate genes for maintaining the health of tissues as they age, third generation TE scaffolds for soft connective tissue regeneration and repair, hybrid inorganic/organic bioactive scaffolds, anti-microbial effect for wound dressing, molecular modeling of the interaction of surface sites with amino acids, coating of metallic implants, effective carriers of growth factors, bioactive peptides etc.. In the coming future, bioactive glass may be explored by the scientists/researchers/clinicians in a better way and dimension for wellbeing of human kind.

9. References

Agrawal, CM. & Ray, RB. (2001). Biodegradable polymeric scaffolds for musculoskeletal tissue engineering. *Journal of Biomedical Materials Research*, 55(2): 141-150

Aina, V., Malavasi, G., Fiorio Pla, A., Munaron, L. & Morterra, C. (2009) 'Zinc-containing bioactive glasses: Surface reactivity and behaviour towards endothelial cells', *Acta Biomaterialia*, 5(4): 1211-1222.

Aitasalo, K., Kinnunen, I., Palmgren, J. & Varpula, M. (2001). Repair of orbital floor fractures with bioactive glass implants. *J. Oral. Maxillofac. Surg.*, 59(12):1390-1395.

Albrektsson, T. (1993). On long-term maintenance of the osseointegrated response. *Australian Pros. J.*, 7: 15-24.

Anderegg, C.R., Alexander, D.C. & Freidman, M. (1999). A bioactive glass particulate in the treatment of molar furcation invasions. *J. Periodontol.*, 70(4):384-7.

Anderson, O.H., Liu, G., Kangasniemi, K. & Juhanoja, J. (1992). Evaluation of the acceptance of glass in bone. Journal of Materials Science: *Materials in Medicine*, 3(2):145-150.

Andersson, O.H., Karlsson, K.H., Kangasniemi, K. & Xli-Urpo, A. (1988). Models for physical properties and bioactivity of phosphate opal glasses. *Glastechnische Berichte*, 61(10):300-305.

Andersson, Ö.H., Liu, G., Kangasniemi, K. & Juhanoja, J. (1992) 'Evaluation of the acceptance of glass in bone', *Journal of Materials Science: Materials in Medicine*, 3(2): 145-150.

Andersson, Ö.H., Liu, G., Karlsson, K.H., Niemi, L., Miettinen, J. & Juhanoja, J. (1990) 'In vivo behaviour of glasses in the $SiO_2-Na_2O-CaO-P_2O_5-Al_2O_3-B_2O_3$ system', *Journal of Materials Science: Materials in Medicine*, 1(4): 219-227.

Andreassen, G.S., Hoiness, P.R., Skraamm, I., Granlund, O. & Engebretsen, L. (2004). Use of a synthetic bone void filler to augment screws in osteopenic ankle fracture fixation. *Arch. Orthop. Trauma. Surg.*, 124:161–5.

Arcos, D., Ragel, CV. & Vallet-Regí, M. (2001). Bioactivity in glass/PMMA composites used as drug delivery system. *Biomaterials*, 22(7): 701-708

Asano, S., Kaneda, K., Satoh, S., Abumi, K., Hashimoto, T. & Fujiya, M. (1994). Reconstruction of an iliac crest defect with a bioactive ceramic prosthesis. *Eur. Spine J.*, 3(1):39-44.

Asselmeier, M.A., Caspari, R.B. & Bottenfield, S. (1993). A review of allograft processing and sterilization techniques and their role in transmission of the human immunodeficiency virus. *Am. J. Sports Med.*, 21.170–5.

Baino, F., Verné, E. & Vitale-Brovarone, C. (2009) '3-D high-strength glass-ceramic scaffolds containing fluoroapatite for load-bearing bone portions replacement', *Materials Science and Engineering: C*, 29(6): 2055-2062.

Development and Applications of Varieties of Bioactive Glass Compositions in Dental Surgery, Third Generation
Tissue Engineering, Orthopaedic Surgery and as Drug Delivery System

93

Bajpai, PK. (1994). Using ceramics as drug delivery devices. *Biomedical Engineering - Applications, Basis and Communications*, 6(4): 64-70.

Bajpai, PK. & Benghuzzi HA. (1988). Ceramic systems for long-term delivery of chemicals and biologicals. *Journal of Biomedical Materials Research*, 22(12): 1245-1266.

Bakry, A.S., Takahashi, H., Otsuki, M., Sadr, A., Yamashita, K. & Tagami, J. (2011). CO2 laser improves 45S5 bioglass interaction with dentin. *J. Dent. Res.*, 90(2):246-50.

Balamurugan, A., Balossier, G., Laurent-Maquin, D., Pina, S., Rebelo, A.H.S., Faure, J. & Ferreira, J.M.F. (2008) 'An in vitro biological and anti-bacterial study on a sol-gel derived silver-incorporated bioglass system', *Dental Materials*, 24(10): 1343-1351.

Balamurugan, A., Balossier, G., Michel, J., Kannan, S., Benhayoune, H., Rebelo, A.H.S. & Ferreira, J.M.F. (2007) 'Sol gel derived SiO_2-CaO-MgO-P_2O_5 bioglass system - Preparation and *in vitro* characterization', *Journal of Biomedical Materials Research Part B: Applied Biomaterials*, 83B(2): 546-553.

Bandyopadhyay-Ghosh, S., Faria, P.E., Johnson, A., Felipucci, D.N., Reaney, I.M., Salata, L.A., Brook, I.M. & Hatton, P.V. (2010). Osteoconductivity of modified fluorcanasite glass-ceramics for bone tissue augmentation and repair. *J. Biomed. Mater. Res. A.*, 94(3):760-8.

Banwart, JC., Asher, MA. & Hassanein, RS. (1995). Iliac crest bone graft harvest donor site morbidity. A statistical evaluation. *Spine*, 20(9): 1055-1060.

Barone, C.M. & Jimenez, D.F. (1997). Split-thickness calvarial grafts in young children. *The Journal of craniofacial surgery*, 8(1):43-47.

Bellantone, M., Williams, H.D. & Hench, L.L. (2002). 'Broad-Spectrum Bactericidal Activity of Ag_2O-Doped Bioactive Glass', *Antimicrob. Agents Chemother.*, 46(6): 1940-1945.

Bergeron, E., Marquis, ME., Chrétien, I. & Faucheux, N. (2007). Differentiation of preosteoblasts using a delivery system with BMPs and bioactive glass microspheres. *J. Mater. Sci. Mater. Med.* 18(2): 255-63.

Berry, C.C., Dalby, M.J., Oreffo, R.O.C., McCloy, D. & Affrosman, S. (2006) 'The interaction of human bone marrow cells with nanotopographical features in three dimensional constructs', *Journal of Biomedical Materials Research Part A*, 79A(2): 431-439.

Bhakta, S., Pattanayak, D.K., Takadama, H., Kokubo, T., Miller, C.A., Mirsaneh, M., Reaney, I.M., Brook, I., van Noort, R. & Hatton, P.V. (2010). Prediction of osteoconductive activity of modified potassium fluorrichterite glass-ceramics by immersion in simulated body fluid. *J. Mater. Sci. Mater. Med.*, 21(11):2979-88.

Bibby, JK., Bubb, NL., Wood DJ. & Mummery, PM. (2005). Fluorapatite-mullite glass sputter coated Ti6Al4V for biomedical applications. *J. Mater. Sci. Mater. Med.*, 16(5): 379-85.

Bil, M., Ryszkowska, J., Roether, JA., Bretcanu, O. & Boccaccini, AR. (2007). Bioactivity of polyurethane-based scaffolds coated with Bioglass. *Biomed. Mater.*, 2(2): 93-101.

Blaker, J.J., Nazhat, S.N. & Boccaccini, A.R. (2004) 'Development and characterisation of silver-doped bioactive glass-coated sutures for tissue engineering and wound healing applications', *Biomaterials*, 25(7-8): 1319-29.

Boccaccini, A.R. (2005) 'Ceramics', in Hench, L.L. & Jones, J.R. (Eds.): *Biomaterials, Artificial Organs and Tissue Engineering*, Woodhead Publishing Limited CRC Press, Cambridge, U. K., pp. 26-36.

Boccaccini, A.R. & Blaker, J.J. (2005). 'Bioactive composite materials for tissue engineering scaffolds', *Expert Review of Medical Devices*, Vol. 2, No. 3, pp. 303-317.

Boccaccini, A.R., Chen, Q., Lefebvre, L., Gremillard, L. & Chevalier, J. (2007) 'Sintering, crystallisation and biodegradation behaviour of Bioglass (R)-derived glass-ceramics', *Faraday Discussions*, 136: 27-44.

Boccaccini, AR., Roelher, JA., Hench, LL., Maquet, V. & Jérome, RA. (2008). Composites approach to tissue engineering. 26th Annual Conference on Composites, Advanced Ceramics, Materials, and Structures: B: *Ceramic Engineering and Science Proceedings*, 23(4): 805-816.

Bosetti, M. & Cannas, M. (2005). The effect of bioactive glasses on bone marrow stromal cells differentiation. *Biomaterials*, 26(18): 3873-9.

Bosetti, M., Zanardi, L., Hench, L. & Cannas, M. (2003). Type I collagen production by osteoblast-like cells cultured in contact with different bioactive glasses. *J. Biomed. Mater. Res. A.*, 64(1): 189-95.

Bovo, N. (2007) 'Structure-properties relationships in bioactive glasses for PAA-based polyalkenoate cements': *Departament de Ciència dels Materials i Enginyeria Metallúrgica*, Universitat Politècnica de Catalunya, Barcelona, Spain.

Brandao-Burch, A., Utting, JC., Orriss, IR. & Arnett, TR. (2005). Acidosis inhibits bone formation by osteoblasts in vitro by preventing mineralisation. *Calcified Tissue International*, 77: 167-174.

Branemårk, PI., Adell, R., Albrektsson, T., Lekholm, U., Lundkvist, S. & Rockler, B. (1983). Osseointegrated titanium fixtures in the treatment of endentulosness. *Biomaterials*, 4: 25-28.

Bretcanu, O., Misra, S., Roy, I., Renghini, C., Fiori, F., Boccaccini, AR. & Salih, V. (2009). In vitro biocompatibility of 45S5 Bioglass-derived glass-ceramic scaffolds coated with poly(3-hydroxybutyrate). *J. Tissue Eng. Regen. Med.*, 3(2): 139-48.

Bretcanu, O., Samaille, C. & Boccaccini, A. (2008) 'Simple methods to fabricate Bioglass andlt;sup>®</sup>-derived glass–ceramic scaffolds exhibiting porosity gradient', *Journal of Materials Science*, 43(12): 4127-4134.

Bridwell, KH., O'Brien, MF., Lenke, LG., Baldus, C. & Blanke, K. (1994). Posterior spinal fusion supplemented with only allograft bone in paralytic scoliosis. Does it work? *Spine*, 19: 2658 – 66.

Brink, M. (1997). The influence of alkali & alkaline earths on the working range for bioactive glasses. *Journal of biomedical materials research*, 36(1):109-117.

Brink, M., Turunen, T., Happonen, R.P. & Yli-Urpo, A. (1997). Compositional dependence of bioactivity of glasses in the system Na_2O-K_2O-MgO-CaO-B_2O_3-P_2O_5-SiO_2. *Journal of biomedical materials research*, 37(1):114-121.

Brown, R.F., Day, D.E., Day, T.E., Jung, S., Rahaman, M.N. & Fu, Q. (2008) 'Growth and differentiation of osteoblastic cells on 13-93 bioactive glass fibers and scaffolds', *Acta Biomaterialia*, Vol. 4(?): 387-396.

Brunner, T.J., Grass, R.N. & Stark, W.J. (2006) 'Glass and bioglass nanopowders by flame synthesis', *Chemical Communications*, 13: 1384-1386.

Burchardt, H. (1983). The biology of bone graft repair. *Clin. Orthop. Relat. Res.*, 174: 28–42.

Development and Applications of Varieties of Bioactive Glass Compositions in Dental Surgery, Third Generation
Tissue Engineering, Orthopaedic Surgery and as Drug Delivery System

95

Buser, D., Nydegger, T., Hirt, HP., Cochran, DL. & Nolte, LP. (1998). Removal torque values of titanium implants in the maxilla of miniature pigs. *Int. J. Oral Maxillofac. Implants*, 13: 611-619.

Cannillo, V. & Sola, A. (2009) 'Potassium-based composition for a bioactive glass', *Ceramics International*, 35(8): 3389-3393.

Carano, RA. & Filvaroff, EH. (2003). Angiogenesis and bone repair, *Drug Discov. Today* 8: 980–989.

Carlsson, L., Regner, L., Johansson, C., Gottlander, M. & Herberts, P. (1994). Bone response to hydroxyapatite-coated and commercially pure titanium implants in the human arthritic knee. *J. Orthop. Res.*, 12: 274-285.

Chapman, M.W., Bucholz, R. & Cornell, C. (1997). Treatment of acute fracture with collagen-calcium phosphate graft material. *J. Bone Joint Surg.*, 79-A: 143-147.

Chappard, D., Aguado, E., Huré, G., Grizon, F. & Basle, MF. (1999). The early remodeling phases around titanium implants: a histomorphometric assessment of bone quality in a 3- and 6-month study in sheep. *Int. J. Oral. Maxillofac. Implants*, 14: 189-196.

Chatzistavrou, X., Hatzistavrou, E., Kantiranis, N., Papadopoulou, L., Kontonasaki, E., Chrissafis, K., Petros, K., Konstantinos, M., Paraskevopoulos, A. & Boccaccini, R. (2009). Novel glass-ceramics for dental application by sol-gel technique. *Key Engineering Materials*, 396-398: 153-156.

Chen, Q., Rezwan, K., Armitage, D., Nazhat, S. & Boccaccini, A. (2006a) 'The surface functionalization of 45S5 Bioglass (R)-based glass-ceramic scaffolds and its impact on bioactivity', *Journal of Materials Science: Materials in Medicine*, 17(11): 979-987.

Chen, Q.Z., Efthymiou, A., Salih, V. & Boccaccini, A.R. (2008a) 'Bioglass®-derived glass–ceramic scaffolds: Study of cell proliferation and scaffold degradation in vitro', *Journal of Biomedical Materials Research Part A*, 84A (4): 1049-1060.

Chen, Q.Z., Li, Y., Jin, L.Y., Quinn, J.M. & Komesaroff, PA. (2010). A new sol-gel process for producing Na(2)O-containing bioactive glass ceramics. *Acta Biomater.*, 6(10):4143-53.

Chen, Q.-Z., Rezwan, K., Françon, V., Armitage, D., Nazhat, S.N., Jones, F.H. & Boccaccini, A.R. (2007) 'Surface functionalization of Bioglass®-derived porous scaffolds', *Acta Biomaterialia*, 3(4): 551-562.

Chen, Q.Z., Thompson, I.D. & Boccaccini, A.R. (2006b). '45S5 Bioglass®-derived glass-ceramic scaffolds for bone tissue engineering', *Biomaterials*, 27(11): 2414-2425.

Chen, X., Meng, Y., Li, Y. & Zhao, N. (2008b). 'Investigation on bio-mineralization of melt and sol-gel derived bioactive glasses', *Applied Surface Science*, 255(2): 562-564.

Chern, LJ., Liu, ML. & Ju, CP. (1993). Environmental effect on bond strength of plasma-sprayed hydroxyapatite/bioactive glass composite coatings. Technical note. *Dent. Mater.*, 9(4): 286-7.

Chim, H. & Gosain, A.K. (2009). Biomaterials in craniofacial surgery: experimental studies and clinical application. *The Journal of craniofacial surgery*, 20(1):29-33.

Cholewa-Kowalska, K., Kokoszka, J., Laczka, M., Niedźwiedzki, L., Madej, W. & Osyczka, A.M. (2009). Gel-derived bioglass as a compound of hydroxyapatite composites. *Biomed. Mater.*, 4(5):055007.

Constantino, P.D. & Freidman, C.D. (1994). Synthetic bone graft substitutes. *Otolaryngol. Clin. North Am.*, 27: 1037–73.

Costantino, P.D., Friedman, C.D., Jones, K., Chow, L.C. & Sisson, G.A. (1992). Experimental hydroxyapatite cement cranioplasty. *Plastic and reconstructive surgery*, 90(2):174-185.

Costantino, PD., Chaplin, JM., Wolpoe, ME., Catalano, PJ., Sen, C., Bederson, JB. & Govindaraj, S. (2000). Applications of fast-setting hydroxyapatite cement: cranioplasty. *Otolaryngol Head Neck Surg.*, 123(4): 409-412.

Cypher, T.J. (1996). Grossman JP. Biological principles of bone graft healing. *J. Foot Ankle Surg.*, 35: 413–7.

Damien, C.J. & Parsons, J.R. (1991). Bone graft and bone graft substitutes: a review of current technology and applications. *J. Appl. Biomater.*, 2(3):187-208.

Day, R.M., Boccaccini, A.R., Shurey, S., Roether, J.A., Forbes, A., Hench, L.L. & Gabe, S.M. (2004). Assessment of polyglycolic acid mesh and bioactive glass for soft-tissue engineering scaffolds. *Biomaterials*, 25(27):5857-66.

Day, RM. (2005). Bioglasss stimulates the secretion of angiogenic growth factors and angiogenesis. *Tissue Eng.*, 11(5-6): 768-77.

Day, RM., Boccaccini, AR., Shurey, S., Roether, JA., Forbes, A., Hench, LL. & Gabe, SM. (2004). Assessment of polyglycolic acid mesh and bioactive glass for soft tissue engineering scaffolds. *Biomaterials*, 25 (27): 5857–66.

De Aza, P.N., Luklinska, Z.B., Santos, C., Guitian, F. & De Aza, S. (2003). Mechanism of bone-like formation on a bioactive implant in vivo. *Biomaterials*, 24(8):1437-1445.

De Diego, M.A., Coleman, N.J. & Hench, L.L. (2000). 'Tensile properties of bioactive fibers for tissue engineering applications', *Journal of Biomedical Materials Research*, 53(3): 199-203.

De Groot, K. (1983). *Bioceramics of Calcium Phosphate*. CRC Press, Boca Raton, FL.

De Groot, K. (1988). 'Effect of porosity and physico-chemical properties on the stability, resorption and strength of calcium phosphate ceramics', in Ducheyne, P. & Lemons, J. (Eds.): *Bioceramics: Material Characteristics Versus In Vivo Behaviour*, Annals of New York Academy of Sciences, New York.

De Groot, K. & LeGeros, R.Z. (1988) 'Significance of porosity and physical chemistry of calcium phosphate ceramics', in Ducheyne, P. & Lemons, J. (Eds.): *Bioceramics: Material Charactersitics Versus In Vivo Behaviour*, Annals of New York Academy of Sciences, New York, pp. 268-277.

De Groot, K., Klein, C.P.A.T., Wolke, J.G.C. & De Blieck-Hogervorst, J. (1990) 'Chemistry of calcium phosphate bioceramics', in Yamamuro, T., Hench, L.L. & Wilson, J. (Eds.): *Handbook of Bioactice Ceramics*, CRC Press, Boca Raton, FL, pp. 3-15.

Deb, S., Mandegaran, R. & Di Silvio, L. (2010) 'A porous scaffold for bone tissue engineering/45S5 Bioglass and lt;supandgt;®and lt;/supandgt; derived porous scaffolds for co-culturing osteoblasts and endothelial cells', *Journal of Materials Science: Materials in Medicine*, 21(3): 893-905.

Delben, J., Pimentel, O., Coelho, M., Candelorio, P., Furini, L., Alencar dos Santos, F.b., de Vicente, F.b. & Delben, A. (2009) 'Synthesis and thermal properties of nanoparticles of bioactive glasses containing silver', *Journal of Thermal Analysis and Calorimetry*, 97(2): 433-436.

Deville, S., Saiz, E., Nalla, R.K. & Tomsia, A.P. (2006) 'Freezing as a Path to Build Complex Composites', *Science*, 311(5760): 515-518.

Dey, A., Nandi, SK., Kundu, B., Kumar, C., Mukherjee, P., Roy, S., Mukhopadhyay, AK., Sinha, MK. & Basu, D. (2011). Evaluation of hydroxyapatite and β-tri calcium phosphate microplasma spray coated pin intra-medullary for bone repair in a rabbit model. *Ceramic International*, 37 (4): 1377-1391

Dominguesa, ZR., Cortes, ME., Gomes, TA., Diniz, HF., Freitas, CS. Gomes, JB., Faria, AMC. & Sinisterra, RD. (2004). Bioactive glass as a drug delivery system of tetracycline and tetracycline associated with b-cyclodextrin. *Biomaterials*, 25 (2004): 327–333

Ducheyne, P., Hench, L.L., Kagan, A., 2nd, Martens, M., Bursens, A. & Mulier, J.C. (1980) 'Effect of hydroxyapatite impregnation on skeletal bonding of porous coated implants', *J. Biomed. Mate.r Res.*, 14(3): 225-37.

Ducic, Y. (2001). Three-dimensional alloplastic orbital reconstruction in skull base surgery. *The Laryngoscope*, 111(7):1306-1312.

Ducic, Y. (2002). Titanium mesh and hydroxyapatite cement cranioplasty: a report of 20 cases. *J. Oral Maxillofac. Surg.*, 60(3):272-276.

Ebisawa, Y., Kokubo, T., Ohura, K. & Yamamuro, T. (1990) 'Bioactivity of CaO SiO$_2$-based glasses: *In vitro* evaluation', *Journal of Materials Science: Materials in Medicine*, 1(4): 239-244.

Effah Kaufmann, E.A., Ducheyne, P. & Shapiro, I.M. (2000). Evaluation of osteoblast response to porous bioactive glass (45S5) substrates by RT-PCR analysis. *Tissue Eng.*, 6(1):19–28.

Einhorn, T.A. (1995). Enhancement of fracture-healing. *J. Bone Joint Surg. Am.*, 77:940–56.

El-Ghannam, A. (2005). Bone reconstruction: from bioceramics to tissue engineering, *Expert Rev. Med. Devices*, 2: 87–101.

El-Ghannam, A., Ducheyne, P. & Shapiro, IM. (1997a). Formation of surface reaction products on bioactive glass and their effects on the expresssion of the osteoblastic phenotype and the deposition of mineralized extracellular matrix. *Biomaterials*, 18: 295-303.

Erdemli, O., Captug, O., Bilgili, H., Orhan, D., Tezcaner, A. & Keskin, D. (2010). In vitro and in vivo evaluation of the effects of demineralized bone matrix or calcium sulfate addition to polycaprolactone-bioglass composites. *J. Mater. Sci. Mater. Med.*, 21(1):295-308.

Fathi, MH., Salehi, M., Saatchi, A., Mortazavi, V. & Moosavi, SB. (2003). In vitro corrosion behavior of bioceramic, metallic, and bioceramic-metallic coated stainless steel dental implants. *Dent. Mater.*, 19(3): 188-198.

Fernyhough, JC., Schimandle, JJ., Weigel, MC., Edwards, CC. & Levine, AM. (1992). Chronic donor site pain complicating bone graft harvesting from the posterior iliac crest for spinal fusion. *Spine*, 17(12): 1474-1480.

Ferraris, M., Rabajoli, P., Brossa, F. & Paracchini, L. (1996). Vacuum plasma spray deposition of titanium particle/glass-ceramic matrix biocomposites. *Journal of the American Ceramic Society*, 79(6): 1515-1520.

Filiaggi, M., Pilliar, RM. & Coombs, NA. (1991). Characterization of the interface in the plasma-sprayed HA coating/Ti-6AI-4V implant system. *Journal of Biomedical Materials Research*, 25: 1211-29.

Finet, B., Weber, G. & Cloots, R. (2000). Titanium release from dental implants: An in vivo study on sheep. *Materials Letters*, 43(4):159-165.

Francis, L., Meng, D., Knowles, J.C., Roy, I. & Boccaccini, A.R. (2010) 'Multi-functional P(3HB) microsphere/45S5 Bioglass®-based composite scaffolds for bone tissue engineering', *Acta. Biomaterialia*, 6(7): 2773-2786.

Frick, KK., Jiang, L., & Bushinsky, DA. (1997). Acute metabolic acidosis inhibits the induction of osteoblastic egr-1 and type 1 collagen. *Am. J. Physiol. (Cell Physiol.)*, 272: C1450-C1456

Fu, Q., Rahaman, M.N., Bal, B.S. & Brown, R.F. (2010) 'Preparation and in vitro evaluation of bioactive glass (13–93) scaffolds with oriented microstructures for repair and regeneration of load-bearing bones', *Journal of Biomedical Materials Research Part A*, 93A (4): 1380-1390.

Fu, Q., Rahaman, M.N., Bal, B.S., Huang, W. & Day, D.E. (2007) 'Preparation and bioactive characteristics of a porous 13–93 glass, and fabrication into the articulating surface of a proximal tibia', *Journal of Biomedical Materials Research Part A*, 82A (1): 222-229.

Fu, Q., Rahaman, M.N., Sonny Bal, B., Brown, R.F. & Day, D.E. (2008) 'Mechanical and in vitro performance of 13-93 bioactive glass scaffolds prepared by a polymer foam replication technique', *Acta Biomaterialia*, 4(6): 1854-1864.

Furusawa, T. & Mizunuma, K. (1997). Osteoconductive properties and efficacy of resorbable bioactive glass as a bone-grafting material. *Implant dentistry*, 6(2):93-101.

Galindo-Moreno, P., Avila, G., Fernández-Barbero, J.E., Mesa, F., O'Valle-Ravassa, F. & Wang, H.L. (2008). Clinical and histologic comparison of two different composite grafts for sinus augmentation: a pilot clinical trial. *Clin. Oral. Implants Res.*, 19(8):755-9.

García, C., Ceré, S. & Durán, A. (2004). Bioactive coatings prepared by sol-gel on stainless steel 316L. *Journal of Non-Crystalline Solids*, 348: 218-224

Gatti, A.M. & Zaffe, D. (1991). Short-term behaviour of two similar active glasses used as granules in the repair of bone defects. *Biomaterials*, 12(5):497-504.

Gau, YL., Lonstein, JE., Winter, RB., Koop, S. & Denis, F. (1991). Luque—Galveston procedure for correction and stabilization of neuromuscular scoliosis and pelvic obliquity: a review of 68 patients. *J. Spinal Disord*. 4: 399—410.

Gazdag, A.R., Lane, J.M., Glaser, D. & Forster, R.A. (1995). Alternatives to autogenous bone graft: efficacy and indications. *J. Am. Acad. Orthop. Surg.*, 3: 1-8.

Gentleman, E., Fredholm, Y.C., Jell, G., Lotfibakhshaiesh, N., O'Donnell, M.D., Hill, R.G. & Stevens, M.M. (2010) 'The effects of strontium-substituted bioactive glasses on osteoblasts and osteoclasts in vitro', *Biomaterials*, 31(14): 3949-3956.

Gerhardt, LC. & Boccaccini, A.R. (2010) 'Bioactive glass and glass-ceramic scaffolds for bone tissue engineering', *Materials*, 3(7): 3867-3910.

Gheysen, G., Ducheyne, P., Hench, L.L. & de Meester, P. (1983). Bioglass composites: a potential material for dental application. *Biomaterials*, 4(2):81-4.

Ghosh, SK., Nandi, SK., Kundu, B., Datta, S., De, DK., Roy, SK. & Basu, D. (2008) 'In vivo response of porous hydroxyapatite and β-tricalcium phosphate prepared by aqueous solution combustion method and comparison with bioglass scaffolds', *Journal of Biomedical Materials Research Part B: Applied Biomaterials*, 86B (1): 217-227.

Giannoudis, P.V. (2005). Dinopoulos H, Tsiridis E. Bone substitutes: an update. *Injury*, 36(Suppl. 3): S20–7.

Ginebra, MP., Traykova, T. & Planell, JA. (2006). Calcium phosphate cements as bone drug delivery systems: a review, *J. Control. Release.*, 113: 102–110.

Gomez-Vega, JM., Saiz, E., Tomsia, AP., Marshall, GW. & Marshall, SJ. (2000). Bioactive glass coatings with hydroxyapatite and Bioglass particles on Ti-based implants. 1. Processing. *Biomaterials*, 21(2): 105-111.

Goodrich, J.T., Argamaso, R. & Hall, C.D. (1992). Split-thickness bone grafts in complex craniofacial reconstructions. *Pediatric neurosurgery*, 18(4):195-201.

Gorriti, MF., López, JMP., Boccaccini, AR., Audisio, C. & Gorustovich, A.A. (2009) 'In vitro Study of the Antibacterial Activity of Bioactive Glass-ceramic Scaffolds', *Advanced Engineering Materials*, 11(7): 67-B70.

Gosain, A.K. (2003). Biomaterials in facial reconstruction. *Operative Techniques in Plastic and Reconstructive Surgery*, 9(1):23-30.

Gosain, A.K. & Persing, J.A. (1999). Biomaterials in the face: benefits and risks. *The Journal of craniofacial surgery*, 10(5):404-414.

Goulet, JA., Senunas, LE., DeSilva, GL. & Greenfield, ML. (1997). Autogenous iliac crest bone graft. Complications and functional assessment. *Clinical Orthopaedics and Related Research*, 339: 76-81.

Grana, F., Rocca, ED. & Grana, L. (1954). Las trepanaciones craneanas en el Peru en a epoca prehispanica. Lima, Peru: Imprenta Santa Maria,

Greenspan, DC. & Hench, LL. (1976). 'Chemical and mechanical behavior of bioglass-coated alumina', *J Biomed Mater Res*, 10(4): 503-9.

Gross, U. & Strunz, V. (1985) 'The interface of various glasses and glass ceramics with a bony implantation bed', *J Biomed Mater Res*, Vol. 19, No. 3, pp. 251-71.

Gross, U., Brandes, J., Strunz, V., Bab, I. & Sela, J. (1981) 'The ultrastructure of the interface between a glass ceramic and bone', *J Biomed Mater Res*, Vol. 15, No. 3, pp. 291-305.

Gross, U., Kinne, R., Schmitz, H.J. & Strunz, V. (1988) 'The response of bone to surface active glass/glass-ceramics', *CRC Critical Reviews on Biocompatibility*, Vol. 4, p. 2.

Gross, U., Roggendorf, W., Schmitz, H.J. & Strunz, V. (1986a) 'Testing procedures for surface reactive biomaterials', in Christel, P., Meunier, A. & Lee, A.J.C. (Eds.): *Biological and Biomechanical Performance of Biomaterials*, Elsevier, Amsterdam, Netherlands, p. 367.

Gross, U., Schmitz, H.J., Strunz, V., Schuppan, D. & Termine, J. (1986b) 'Proteins at the interface of bone-bonding and non-bonding glass-ceramics': *Transaction of the Twelfth Annual Meeting of the Society for Biomaterials*, Society for Biomaterials, Algonquin, IL, p. 98.

Gross, U.M. & Strunz, V. (1980) 'The anchoring of glass ceramics of different solubility in the femur of the rat', *J Biomed Mater Res*, Vol. 14, No. 5, pp. 607-18.

Grossman, D.G. (1991). In: *International Symposium on Computer Restorations*, IL: Quintessenz, Chicago, p. 103.

Guarino, V., Causa, F. & Ambrosio, L. (2007) 'Bioactive scaffolds for bone and ligament tissue', *Expert Review of Medical Devices*, Vol. 4, pp. 405-418.

Haimi, S., Gorianc, G., Moimas, L., Lindroos, B., Huhtala, H., Räty, S., Kuokkanen, H., Sándor, G.K., Schmid, C., Miettinen, S. & Suuronen, R. (2009) 'Characterization of zinc-releasing three-dimensional bioactive glass scaffolds and their effect on human adipose stem cell proliferation and osteogenic differentiation', *Acta Biomaterialia*, Vol. 5, No. 8, pp. 3122-3131.

Hamadouche, M., Meunier, A., Greenspan, DC., Blanchat, C., Zhong, JP., La Torre, GP. & Sedel, L. (2000). Bioactivity of sol-gel bioactive glass coated alumina implants. *J. Biomed. Mater. Res.* 52(2): 422-9.

Han, J., Meng, H. & Xu, L. (2002). Clinical evaluation of bioactive glass in the treatment of periodontal intrabony defects. *Zhonghua kou qiang yi xue za zhi = Zhonghua kouqiang yixue zazhi = Chinese journal of stomatology*, 37(3):225-227.

Hardouin, P., Anselme, K., Flautre, B., Bianchi, F., Bascoulenguet, G. & Bouxin, B. (2000). Tissue engineering and skeletal diseases. *Joint Bone Spine*, 67(5): 419-424.

Hedia, H.S., El-Midany, T.T., Shabara, M.A. & Fouda, N. (2006). Design optimization of cementless metal-backed cup prostheses using the concept of functionally graded material. *Biomed. Mater.*, 1(3):127-33.

Heikkila, J.T., Aho, H.J., Yli-Urpo, A., Happonen, R.P. & Aho, A.J. (1995). Bone formation in rabbit cancellous bone defects filled with bioactive glass granules. *Acta orthopaedica Scandinavica*, 66(5):463-467.

Heikkila, J.T., Mattila, K.T., Andersson, O.H., Yli-Urpo, A. & Aho, A.J. (1995). Behaviour of bioactive glass in human bone, In: *Bioceramics 8*, Hench, L.L. & Wilson, J., pp. 35-41, Elsevier Science, Oxford, U. K.

Helen, W. & Gough, JE. (2008). Cell viability, proliferation and extracellular matrix production of human annulus fibrosus cells cultured within PDLLA/Bioglass composite foam scaffolds in vitro. *Acta. Biomater.*, 4(2): 230-43.

Hench, L. (2006) 'The story of Bioglass', *Journal of Materials Science: Materials in Medicine*, Vol. 17, No. 11, pp. 967-978.

Hench, L.L. (1987) 'Cementless fixation', in Pizzoferrato, A., Marchetti, P.G., Ravaglioli, A. & Lee, A.J.C. (Eds.): *Biomaterials and Clinical Applications*, Elsevier, Amsterdam, Netherl&s, p. 23.

Hench, L.L. (1988) 'Bioactive ceramics', in Ducheyne, P. & Lemons, J. (Eds.): *Bioceramics: Materials Characteristics Versus In Vivo Behaviour*, Annals of New York Academy of Sciences, New York, p. 54.

Hench, L.L. (1991) 'Bioceramics: From Concept to Clinic', *Journal of the American Ceramic Society*, Vol. 74, No. 7, pp. 1487-1510.

Hench, L.L. (1996) 'Biomaterials Science: An Introduction to Materials in Medicine', in Ratner, B.D., Hoffman, A.S., Schoen, F.J. & Lemons, J.E. (Eds.), Academic Press, San Diego, p. 73.

Hench, L.L. (1998) 'Bioceramics', *Journal of the American Ceramic Society*, Vol. 81, No. 7, pp. 1705-1728.

Development and Applications of Varieties of Bioactive Glass Compositions in Dental Surgery, Third Generation
Tissue Engineering, Orthopaedic Surgery and as Drug Delivery System

101

Hench, L.L. & Andersson, Ö.H. (1993) 'Bioactive glasses', in Hench, L.L. & Wilson, J. (Eds.): *An Introduction to Bioceramics Vol. 1*, World Scientific Publishing, Singapore, pp. 41-62.

Hench, L.L. & Clark, A.E. (1982) 'Chapter 6: Adhesion to bone', in Williams, D.F. (Ed.): *Biocompatibility of Orthopaedic Implants*, CRC Press, Boca Raton, FL.

Hench, L.L. & Ethridge, E.C. (1982) *Biomaterials: An interfacial approach*. Academic Press, New York.

Hench, L.L. & Paschall, H.A. (1973) 'Direct chemical bond of bioactive glass-ceramic materials to bone and muscle', *J Biomed Mater Res*, Vol. 7, No. 3, pp. 25-42.

Hench, L.L. & Paschall, H.A. (1974) 'Histochemical responses at a biomaterial's interface', *J Biomed Mater Res*, Vol. 8, No. 3, pp. 49-64.

Hench, L.L., Paschall, H.A., Allen, W.C. & Piotrowski, G. (1975) 'Interfacial behavior of ceramic implants', *National Bureau of Standards Special Publication*, Vol. 415, pp. 19-35.

Hench, L.L. & Polak, J.M. (2002) 'Third-generation biomedical materials', *Science*, Vol. 295, No. 5557, pp. 1014-1017.

Hench, L.L. & Wilson, J. (1984) 'Surface-active biomaterials', *Science*, Vol. 226, No. 4675, pp. 630-6.

Hench, L.L., Spilman, D.B. and Nolletti, D. (1986) 'Fluoride Bioglasses (R)', in Christel, P., Meunier, A. & Lee, A.J.C. (Eds.): *Biological and Biomechanical Performance of Biomaterials*, Elsevier, Amsterdam, Netherlands, pp. 99-104.

Hench, L.L., Splinter, R.J., Allen, W.C. & Greenlee, T.K. (1971) 'Bonding mechanisms at the interface of ceramic prosthetic materials', *Journal of Biomedical Materials Research*, Vol. 5, No. 6, pp. 117-141.

Hench, LL. (1993). Bioactive glasses. In: Hench, LL. & Wilson, J., *An Introduction to Bioceramics*, World Scientific, London.

Heybeli, N., Oktar, FN., Ozyazgan, S., Akkan, G. & Ozsoy, S. (2003). Low-cost antibiotic loaded systems for developing countries. *Technol. Health Care.*, 11(3): 207-16.

Hill, R. (1996) 'An alternative view of the degradation of bioglass', *Journal of Materials Science Letters*, Vol. 15, No. 13, pp. 1122-1125.

Hing, K.A. (2004). Bone repair in the twenty-first century: biology, chemistry or engineering? *Philos. Transact. A Math. Phys. Eng. Sci.*, 362: 2821-50.

Hodgson, AWE., Mueller, Y., Forster, D. & Virtanen, S. (2002). Electrochemical characterisation of passive films on Ti alloys under simulated biological conditions. *Electrochimica Acta.*, 47(12):1913-1923.

Holand, W., Rheinberger, V., Apel, E., Van 't Hoen, C., Holand, M., Dommann, A., Marcel, O., Corinna, M. & Ursula, GH. (2006). Clinical applications of glass-ceramics in dentistry. *Journal of materials science*, 17(11): 1037-1042.

Holand, W., Vogel, W., Naumann, K. & Gummel, J. (1985) 'Interface reactions between machinable bioactive glass-ceramics and bone', *J Biomed Mater Res*, Vol. 19, No. 3, pp. 303-12.

Hsi, C.-S., Cheng, H.-Z., Hsu, H.-J., Chen, Y.-S. & Wang, M.-C. (2007) 'Crystallization kinetics and magnetic properties of iron oxide contained $25Li_2O-8MnO_2-20CaO-$

2P$_2$O$_5$-45SiO$_2$ glasses', *Journal of the European Ceramic Society*, Vol. 27, No. 10, pp. 3171-3176.

Hsiong, SX. & Mooney, DJ. (2006). Regeneration of vascularized bone. *Periodontol*, 41: 109–122.

Hsu, FY., Chueh, SC. & Wang, YJ. (1999). Microspheres of hydroxyapatite/reconstituted collagen as supports for osteoblast cell growth. *Biomaterials*, 20(20): 1931-1936.

Huang, YC., Kaigler, D., Rice, KG., Krebsbach, PH. & Mooney, DJ. (2005). Combined angiogenic and osteogenic factor delivery enhances bone marrow stromal cell-driven bone regeneration. *J. Bone Miner. Res.*, 20: 848–857.

Hulbert, S.F., Bokros, J.C., Hench, L.L., Wilson, J. & Heimke, G. (1987) 'Ceramics in clinical applications: Past, present and future', in Vincenzini, P. (Ed.): *High Tech Ceramics*, Elsevier, Amsterdam, Netherlands, pp. 189-213.

Hutmacher, D., Hürzeler, MB. & Schliephake, H. (1996). A review of material properties of biodegradable and bioresorbable polymers and devices for GTR and GBR applications. *International Journal of Oral and Maxillofacial Implants*, 11(5): 667-678.

Hutmacher, D.W., Schantz, J.T., Lam, C.X.F., Tan, K.C. & Lim, T.C. (2007) 'State of the art and future directions of scaffold-based bone engineering from a biomaterials perspective', *Journal of Tissue Engineering and Regenerative Medicine*, Vol. 1, No. 4, pp. 245-260.

Ido, K., Asada, Y., Sakamoto, T., Hayashi, R. & Kuriyama, S. (2000). Radiographic evaluation of bioactive glass-ceramic grafts in postero-lateral lumbar fusion. *Spinal Cord*, 38(5):315-318.

Itala, A., Koort, J., Ylanen, H.O., Hupa, M. & Aro, H.T. (2003). Biologic significance of surface microroughing in bone incorporation of porous bioactive glass implants. *J. Biomed. Mater. Res. A.*, 67(2): 496-503.

Jackson, I.T. & Yavuzer, R. (2000). Hydroxyapatite cement: an alternative for craniofacial skeletal contour refinements. *British journal of plastic surgery*, 53(1):24-29.

Jackson, I.T., Pellett, C. & Smith, J.M. (1983). The skull as a bone graft donor site. *Annals of plastic surgery*, 11(6):527-532.

Jana, C., Nisch, W. & Grimm, G. (1995). Production and characterization of thin films of Bioverit-type glasses deposited by RF magnetron sputtering, In: Vincenzini, P., *Advances in Science and Technology, Vol12 (Materials in Clinical applications)*. p. 257-262, Faenza: Techna

Jansen, JA., Vehof, JWM., Ruhé, PQ., Kroeze-Deutman, H., Kuboki, Y., Takita, H., Hedberg E.L. & Mikos, AG. (2005). Growth factor-loaded scaffolds for bone engineering. *J. Control. Release*, 101: 127–136.

Jarcho, M. (1981) 'Calcium phosphate ceramics as hard tissue prosthetics', *Clin Orthop Relat Res*, No. 157, pp. 259-78.

Jell, G., Notingher, I., Tsigkou, O., Notingher, P., Polak, JM., Hench, LL. & Stevens, MM. (2008). Bioactive glass-induced osteoblast differentiation: a noninvasive spectroscopic study. J. Biomed. Mater. Res., 86(1): 31–40.

Johnson, M.W., Sullivan, S.M., Rohrer, M. & Collier, M. (1997). Regeneration of peri-implant infrabony defects using PerioGlas: a pilot study in rabbits. *Int. J. Oral Maxillofac. Implants.*, 12(6):835-9.

Development and Applications of Varieties of Bioactive Glass Compositions in Dental Surgery, Third Generation
Tissue Engineering, Orthopaedic Surgery and as Drug Delivery System

103

Jones, J.R. (2007) 'Bioactive ceramics and glasses', in Boccaccini, A.R. & Gough, J.E. (Eds.): *Tissue Engineering Using Ceramics and Polymers Vol. 1*, Woodhead Publishing Limited CRC Press, Cambridge, U. K., pp. 52-71.

Jones, J.R. (2009) 'New trends in bioactive scaffolds: The importance of nanostructure', *Journal of the European Ceramic Society*, Vol. 29, No. 7, pp. 1275-1281.

Jones, J.R., Gentleman, E. & Polak, J. (2007). Bioactive glass scaffolds for bone regeneration. *Elements*, 3(6):393–9.

Jones, JR., Tsigkou, O., Coates, EE., Stevens, MM., Polak, JM. & Hench, LL. (2007). Extracellular matrix formation and mineralization on a phosphate-free porous bioactive glass scaffold using primary human osteoblast (HOB) cells. *Biomaterials*, 28(9): 1653-63.

Kanczler, J.M. & Oreffo, R.O. (2008) 'Osteogenesis and angiogenesis: the potential for engineering bone', *Eur Cell Mater*, Vol. 15, pp. 100-14.

Kanellakopoulou, K. & Giamarellos-Bourboulis, EJ. (2000). Carrier systems for the local delivery of antibiotics in bone infections. *Drugs*, 59(6): 1223–32.

Kangasniemi, K. & Yti-Urpo, A. (1990) 'Biological response of glasses in the SiO_2-Na_2O-CaO-P_2O_5-B_2O_3 system', in Yamamuro, T., Hench, L.L. & Wilson, J. (Eds.): *Handbook of Bioactive Ceramics Vol. I*, CRC Press, Boca Raton, FL, pp. 97-108.

Karageorgiou, V. & Kaplan, D. (2005). Porosity of 3D biomaterial scaffolds and osteogenesis, *Biomaterials*, 26: 5474–5491.

Karatzas, S., Zavras, A., Greenspan, D. & Amar, S. (1999). Histologic observations of periodontal wound healing after treatment with PerioGlas in nonhuman primates. *Int. J. Periodontics Restorative Dent.*, 19(5):489-99.

Karlsson, K.H., Ylänen, H. & Aro, H. (2000) 'Porous bone implants', *Ceramics International*, Vol. 26, No. 8, pp. 897-900.

Kawanabe, K., Okada, Y., Matsusue, Y., Iida, H. & Nakamura, T. (1998). Treatment of osteomyelitis with antibiotic-soaked porous glass ceramic. *The Journal of bone and joint surgery* 80(3): 527-530.

Kaysinger, KK. & Ramp, WK. (1998). Extracellular pH modulates the activity of cultured human osteoblasts. *Cell Biochem.*, 68: 83-89

Keshaw, H., Forbes, A. & Day, Richard M. (2005). Release of angiogenic growth factors from cells encapsulated in alginate beads with bioactive glass. *Biomaterials*, 26(19): 4171-4179

Kinnunen, I., Aitasalo, K., Pollonen, M. & Varpula, M. (2000). Reconstruction of orbital floor fractures using bioactive glass. *J. Craniomaxillofac. Surg.*, 28(4):229-234.

Kitsugi, T., Yamamuro, T. & Kokubo, T. (1989) 'Bonding behavior of a glass-ceramic containing apatite and wollastonite in segmental replacement of the rabbit tibia under load-bearing conditions', *J Bone Joint Surg Am*, Vol. 71, No. 2, pp. 264-72.

Klein, M., Goetz, H., Pazen, S., Al-Nawas, B., Wagner, W. & Duschner, H. (2009) 'Pore characteristics of bone substitute materials assessed by microcomputed tomography', *Clinical Oral Implants Research*, Vol. 20, No. 1, pp. 67-74.

Klongnoi, B., Rupprecht, S., Kessler, P., Thorwarth, M., Wiltfang, J. & Schlegel, KA. (2006). Influence of platelet-rich plasma on a bioglass and autogenous bone in sinus augmentation. An explorative study. *Clin. Oral. Implants Res.*, 17(3):312-20.

Knapp, C.I., Feuille, F., Cochran, D.L. & Mellonig, J.T. (2003). Clinical and histologic evaluation of bone-replacement grafts in the treatment of localized alveolar ridge defects. Part 2: bioactive glass particulate. *Int. J. Periodontics Restorative Dent.*, 23(2):129-37.

Kohlhauser, C., Hellmich, C., Vitale-Brovarone, C., Boccaccini, A.R., Rota, A. & Eberhardsteiner, J. (2009) 'Ultrasonic Characterisation of Porous Biomaterials Across Different Frequencies', *Strain*, Vol. 45, No. 1, pp. 34-44.

Kokubo, T., Ito, S., Sakka, S. & Yamamuro, T. (1986) 'Formation of a high-strength bioactive glass-ceramic in the system $MgO-CaO-SiO_2-P_2O_5$', *Journal of Materials Science*, Vol. 21, No. 2, pp. 536-540.

Kokubo, T., Shigematsu, M., Nagashima, Y., Tashiro, M., Nakamura, T., Yamamuro, T. & Higashi, S. (1982) 'Apatite- and wollastonite-containg glass-ceramics for prosthetic application', *Bulletin of the Institute for Chemical Research, Kyoto University*, Vol. 60, No. 3-4, pp. 260-268.

Kundu, B., Nandi, SK., Dasgupta, S., Datta, S., Mukherjee, P., Roy, S., Singh, AK., Mandal, TK., Das, P., Bhattacharya, R. & Basu, D. (2011). Macro-to-micro porous special bioactive glass and ceftriaxone-sulbactam composite drug delivery system for treatment of chronic osteomyelitis: an investigation through in vitro and in vivo animal trial. *J. Mater. Sci. Mater. Med.*, 22(3):705-20.

Lacefield, WR. & Hench, LL. (1986). The bonding of Bioglass to a cobalt-chromium surgical implant alloy. *Biomaterials*, 7(2): 104-8.

Langer, R. (1980). Polymeric delivery systems for controlled drug release. *Chemical Engineering Communications*, 6(1-3): 1-48.

Langer, R. (1990). New methods of drug delivery. *Science*, 249(4976): 1527-1533.

Langer, R. & Vacanti, JP. (1993). Tissue Engineering. Science, 260(5110): 920-926

Larsson, C., Thomsen, P., Aronsson, BO., Rodahl, M., Lausmaa, J., Kasemo, B. & Ericson, LE. (1996). Bone response to surface-modified titanium implants: studies on the early tissue response to machined and electropolished implants with different oxide thicknesses. *Biomaterials*, 17: 605-616.

Lasserre, A. & Bajpai, PK. (1998). Ceramic drug-delivery devices. *Critical reviews in therapeutic drug carrier systems*, 15(1): 1-56.

Leach, JK., Kaigler, D., Wang, Z., Krebsbach, PH. & Mooney, DJ. (2006). Coating of VEGF-releasing scaffolds with bioactive glass for angiogenesis and bone regeneration, *Biomaterials*, 27: 3249–3255.

Leonetti, J.A, Rambo, H.M. & Throndson, R.R. (2000). Osteotome sinus elevation and implant placement with narrow size bioactive glass. *Implant dentistry*, 9(2):177-182.

Leu, A., Stieger, S.M., Dayton, P., Ferrara, K.W. & Leach. J.K. (2009). Angiogenic response to bioactive glass promotes bone healing in an irradiated calvarial defect. *Tissue Eng. Part A*, 15(4):877-85.

Li, M., Zhang, R., Wang, J. & Yang, S. (2007). Study of different biocomposite coatings on Ti alloy by a subsonic thermal spraying technique. *Biomed. Mater.*, 2(1): 1-5.

Lin, F.-H., Huang, Y.-Y., Hon, M.-H. & Wu, S.-C. (1991) 'Fabrication and biocompatibility of a porous bioglass ceramic in a $Na_2O-CaO-SiO_2-P_2O_5$ system', *Journal of Biomedical Engineering*, Vol. 13, No. 4, pp. 328-334.

Development and Applications of Varieties of Bioactive Glass Compositions in Dental Surgery, Third Generation
Tissue Engineering, Orthopaedic Surgery and as Drug Delivery System
105

Linati, L., Lusvardi, G., Malavasi, G., Menabue, L., Menziani, M.C., Mustarelli, P. & Segre, U. (2005) 'Qualitative and quantitative structure-property relationships analysis of multicomponent potential bioglasses', *The Journal of Physical Chemistry B*, Vol. 109, No. 11, pp. 4989-4998

Liu, A., Hong, Z., Zhuang, X., Chen, X., Cui, Y., Liu, Y. & Jing, X. (2008) 'Surface modification of bioactive glass nanoparticles and the mechanical and biological properties of poly(l-lactide) composites', *Acta Biomaterialia*, Vol. 4, No. 4, pp. 1005-1015.

Liu, X., Huang, W., Fu, H., Yao, A., Wang, D., Pan, H. & Lu, W. (2009a) 'Bioactive borosilicate glass scaffolds: improvement on the strength of glass-based scaffolds for tissue engineering', *Journal of Materials Science: Materials in Medicine*, Vol. 20, No. 1, pp. 365-372.

Liu, X., Huang, W., Fu, H., Yao, A., Wang, D., Pan, H., Lu, W., Jiang, X. & Zhang, X. (2009b) 'Bioactive borosilicate glass scaffolds: in vitro degradation and bioactivity behaviors', *Journal of Materials Science: Materials in Medicine*, Vol. 20, No. 6, pp. 1237-1243.

Livingston, T., Ducheyne, P. & Garino, J. (2002). In vivo evaluation of a bioactive scaffold for bone tissue engineering. *J. Biomed. Mater. Res.*, 62(1): 1-13.

Lockyer, M.W.G., Holland, D. & Dupree, R. (1995) 'NMR investigation of the structure of some bioactive and related glasses', *Journal of Non-Crystalline Solids*, Vol. 188, No. 3, pp. 207-219.

Lopez-Esteban, S., Saiz, E., Fujino, S., Oku, T., Suganuma, K. & Tomsia, AP. (2003). Bioactive glass coatings for orthopedic metallic implants. *J. Eur. Ceram. Soc.*, 23(15): 2921-2930.

Loty, C., Sautier, J.M., Tan, M.T., Oboeuf, M., Jallot, E., Boulekbache, H., Greenspan, D. & Forest, N. (2001) 'Bioactive glass stimulates *in vitro* osteoblast differentiation and creates a favorable template for bone tissue formation', *Journal of Bone and Mineral Research*, Vol. 16, No. 2, pp. 231-239.

Lovelace, T.B., Mellonig, J.T., Meffert, R.M., Jones, A.A., Nummikoski, P.V. & Cochran, D.L. (1998). Clinical evaluation of bioactive glass in the treatment of periodontal osseous defects in humans. *Journal of periodontology*, 69(9):1027-1035.

Low, S.B., King, C.J. & Krieger, J. (1997). An evaluation of bioactive ceramic in the treatment of periodontal osseous defects. *The International journal of periodontics and restorative dentistry*, 17(4):358-367.

Lu, H.H., El-Amin, S.F., Scott, K.D. & Laurencin, C.T. (2003) 'Three-dimensional, bioactive, biodegradable, polymer-bioactive glass composite scaffolds with improved mechanical properties support collagen synthesis and mineralization of human osteoblast-like cells in vitro', *Journal of Biomedical Materials Research Part A*, Vol. 64A, No. 3, pp. 465-474.

Lu, HH., Tang, A., Oh, SC, Spalazzi, JP. & Dionisio, K. (2005). Compositional effects on the formation of a calcium phosphate layer and the response of osteoblast-like cells on polymer-bioactive glass composites. *Biomaterials*, 26(32): 6323-34.

Luciani, A., Coccoli, V., Orsi, S., Ambrosio, L. & Netti, PA. (2008). PCL microspheres based functional scaffolds by bottom-up approach with predefined microstructural properties and release profiles. *Biomaterials*, 29(36):4800-4807.

Mader, JT., Landon, GC. & Calhoun, J. (1993). Antimicrobial treatment of osteomyelitis. *Clin. Orthop. Relat. Res.*, 295: 87–95.

Mahmood, J., Takita, H., Ojima, Y., Kobayashi, M., Kohgo, T. & Kuboki, Y. (2001) 'Geometric Effect of Matrix upon Cell Differentiation: BMP-Induced Osteogenesis Using a New Bioglass with a Feasible Structure', *Journal of Biochemistry*, Vol. 129, No. 1, pp. 163-171.

Malafaya, PB., Santos, TC., Van Griensven, M. & Reis, RL. (2008). Morphology, mechanical characterization and in vivo neo-vascularization of chitosan particle aggregated scaffolds architectures. *Biomaterials*, 29(29): 3914-3926.

Mankin, H.J., Fogelson, F.S., Thrasher, Z.A. & Jaffer, F. (1976). Massive resection and allograft transplantation in the treatment of malignant bone tumours. *N. Engl. J. Med.*, 294: 1247-1250.

Manson, P.N., Crawley, W.A. & Hoopes, J.E. (1986). Frontal cranioplasty: risk factors and choice of cranial vault reconstructive material. *Plastic and reconstructive surgery*, 77(6):888-904.

Mantsos, T., Chatzistavrou, X., Roether, J.A., Hupa, L., Arstila, H. & Boccaccini, A.R. (2009) 'Non-crystalline composite tissue engineering scaffolds using boron-containing bioactive glass and poly(D,L-lactic acid) coatings', *Biomed Mater*, Vol. 4, No. 5, p. 055002.

Marciani, R.D., Gonty, A.A., Giansanti, J.S. & Avila, J. (1977). Autogenous cancellous marrow bone graft in irradiated (i) long mandibles. *Oral. Surg.*, 43: 365-368.

Mardare, CC., Mardare, AI., Fernandes, JR. & Joanni, ED. (2003). Imposition of bioactive glass-ceramic thin-films by RF magnetron sputtering. *J. European. Ceram. Soc.*, 23:1027–1030.

Marelli, B., Ghezzi, C.E., Barralet, J.E., Boccaccini, A.R. & Nazhat, S.N. (2010). Three-dimensional mineralization of dense nanofibrillar collagen-bioglass hybrid scaffolds. *Biomacromolecules*, 11(6):1470-9.

McCarthy, R.E., Peek, R.D., Morrissy, R.T. & Hough, Jr A.J. (1986). Allograft bone in spinal fusion for paralytic scoliosis. *J. Bone Joint Surg. Am.*, 68: 370−5.

Meffert, R.M., Thomas, J.R., Hamilton, K.M. & Brownstein, C.N. (1985). Hydroxylapatite as an alloplastic graft in the treatment of human periodontal osseous defects. *Journal of periodontology*, 56(2):63-73.

Meinert, K., Uerpmann, C., Matschullat, J. & Wolf, GK. (1998). Corrosion and leaching of silver doped ceramic IBAD coatings on SS 316L under simulated physiological conditions. *Surface and Coatings Technology*, 103-104: 58-65.

Mengel, R., Schreiber, D. & Flores-de-Jacoby, L. (2006). Bioabsorbable membrane and bioactive glass in the treatment of intrabony defects in patients with generalized aggressive periodontitis: results of a 5-year clinical & radiological study. *J. Periodontol.*, 77(10):1781-7.

Meseguer-Olmo, L., Ros-Nicolás, M., Vicente-Ortega, V., Alcaraz-Baños, M., Clavel-Sainz, M., Arcos, D., Ragel, C., Vallet-Regí, M. & Meseguer-Ortiz, C. (2006). A bioactive sol-gel glass implant for in vivo gentamicin release. Experimental model in Rabbit. *Journal of Orthopaedic Research,* 24: 454–460.

Middleton, E.T., Rajaraman, C.J., O'Brien, D.P., Doherty, S.M. & Taylor, A.D. (2008). The safety and efficacy of vertebroplasty using Cortoss cement in a newly established vertebroplasty service. *Br. J. Neurosurg.,* 22:252–6.

Miguel, B.S., Kriauciunas, R., Tosatti, S., Ehrbar, M., Ghayor, C., Textor, M. & Weber, F.E. (2010) 'Enhanced osteoblastic activity and bone regeneration using surface-modified porous bioactive glass scaffolds', *Journal of Biomedical Materials Research Part A,* Vol. 94A, No. 4, pp. 1023-1033.

Miliauskaite, A., Selimovic, D. & Hannig, M. (2007). Successful management of aggressive periodontitis by regenerative therapy: a 3-year follow-up case report. *J. Periodontol.,* 78(10):2043-50.

Milosev, I., Metikos-Hukovic, M. & Strehblow, HH. (2000). Passive film on orthopaedic TiAlV alloy formed in physiological solution investigated by X-ray photoelectron spectroscopy. *Biomaterials,* 21(20): 2103-2113.

Misra, S.K., Ansari, T., Mohn, D., Valappil, S.P., Brunner, T.J., Stark, W.J., Roy, I., Knowles, J.C., Sibbons, P.D., Jones, E.V., Boccaccini, A.R. & Salih, V. (2010a) 'Effect of nanoparticulate bioactive glass particles on bioactivity and cytocompatibility of poly(3-hydroxybutyrate) composites', *Journal of The Royal Society Interface,* Vol. 7, No. 44, pp. 453-465.

Misra, S.K., Ansari, T.I., Valappil, S.P., Mohn, D., Philip, S.E., Stark, W.J., Roy, I., Knowles, J.C., Salih, V. & Boccaccini, A.R. (2010b) 'Poly(3-hydroxybutyrate) multifunctional composite scaffolds for tissue engineering applications', *Biomaterials,* Vol. 31, No. 10, pp. 2806-2815.

Misra, S.K., Mohn, D., Brunner, T.J., Stark, W.J., Philip, S.E., Roy, I., Salih, V., Knowles, J.C. & Boccaccini, A.R. (2008) 'Comparison of nanoscale and microscale bioactive glass on the properties of P(3HB)/Bioglass® composites', *Biomaterials,* Vol. 29, No. 12, pp. 1750-1761.

Misra, S.K., Valappil, S.P., Roy, I. & Boccaccini, A.R. (2006) 'Polyhydroxyalkanoate (PHA)/Inorganic Phase Composites for Tissue Engineering Applications', *Biomacromolecules,* Vol. 7, No. 8, pp. 2249-2258.

Mistry, S., Kundu, D., Datta, S. & Basu, D. (2011). Comparison of bioactive glass coated and hydroxyapatite coated titanium dental implants in the human jaw bone. *Australian Dental Journal,* 56: 68–75.

Mohamad Yunos, D., Bretcanu, O. & Boccaccini, A. (2008) 'Polymer-bioceramic composites for tissue engineering scaffolds', *Journal of Materials Science,* Vol. 43, No. 13, pp. 4433-4442.

Mohn, D., Zehnder, M., Imfeld, T. & Stark, W.J. (2010). Radio-opaque nanosized bioactive glass for potential root canal application: evaluation of radiopacity, bioactivity and alkaline capacity. *Int. Endod. J.,* 43(3):210-7.

Moimas, L., Biasotto, M., Di Lenarda, R., Olivo, A. & Schmid, C. (2006). Rabbit pilot study on the resorbability of three-dimensional bioactive glass fibre scaffolds. *Acta biomaterialia Mar.,* 2(2):191-199.

Moimas, L., Biasotto, M., Lenarda, R.D., Olivo, A. & Schmid, C. (2006) 'Rabbit pilot study on the resorbability of three-dimensional bioactive glass fibre scaffolds', *Acta Biomaterialia*, Vol. 2, No. 2, pp. 191-199.

Moreira-Gonzalez, A., Lobocki, C., Barakat, K., Andrus, L., Bradford, M., Gilsdorf, M. & Jackson, IT. (2005). Evaluation of 45S5 bioactive glass combined as a bone substitute in the reconstruction of critical size calvarial defects in rabbits. *J. Craniofac. Surg.* 16(1): 63-70.

Muller, W. (1890). Zur frage der tempoaren schadelresektion an stele der trepanation. *Zentralbl. Chir.*, 4:65.

Munukka, E., Leppäranta, O., Korkeamäki, M., Vaahtio, M., Peltola, T., Zhang, D., Hupa, L., Ylänen, H., Salonen, J., Viljanen, M. & Eerola, E. (2008) 'Bactericidal effects of bioactive glasses on clinically important aerobic bacteria', *Journal of Materials Science: Materials in Medicine*, Vol. 19, No. 1, pp. 27-32.

Mylonas, D., Vidal, M.D., De Kok, I.J., Moriarity, J.D. & Cooper, L.F. (2007). Investigation of a thermoplastic polymeric carrier for bone tissue engineering using allogeneic mesenchymal stem cells in granular scaffolds. *J. Prosthodont.*, 16(6):421-30.

Naber, C.L., Reid, O.M. & Hammer, J.E. III. (1972). Gross and histologic evaluation of an autogenous bone graft. 57th month post operatively. *J. Periodontal.*, 43: 702.

Nakamura, T., Yamamuro, T., Higashi, S., Kokubo, T. & Itoo, S. (1985) 'A new glass-ceramic for bone replacement: evaluation of its bonding to bone tissue', *J Biomed Mater Res*, Vol. 19, No. 6, pp. 685-98.

Nandi, S.K., Kundu, B., Datta, S., De, D.K. & Basu, D. (2009) 'The repair of segmental bone defects with porous bioglass: An experimental study in goat', *Research in Veterinary Science*, Vol. 86, No. 1, pp. 162-173.

Nandi, SK., Kundu, B., Mukherjee, P., Mandal, TK., Datta, S., De, DK. & Basu, D. (2009). In vitro and in vivo release of cefuroxime axetil from bioactive glass as an implantable delivery system in experimental osteomyelitis. *Ceram. Int.*, 35(8): 3207-3216.

Neo, M., Nakamura, T., Ohtsuki, C., Kasai, R., Kokubo, T. & Yamamuro, T. (1994). Ultrastructural study of the A-W GC-bone interface after long-term implantation in rat and human bone. *Journal of biomedical materials research*, 28(3):365-372.

Neo, M., Nakamura, T., Ohtsuki, C., Kokubo, T. & Yamamuro, T. (1993). Apatite formation on three kinds of bioactive material at an early stage in vivo: a comparative study by transmission electron microscopy. *Journal of biomedical materials research*, 27(8):999-1006.

Nickell, W.B., Jurkiewicz, M.J. & Salyer, K.E. (1972). Repair of skull defects with autogenous bone. *Arch. Surg.*, 105(3):431-433.

Nicoll Steven, B., Radin, S., Santos, EM., Tuan, RS. & Ducheyne, P. (1997). *In vitro* release kinetics of biologically active transforming growth factor -β1 from a novel porous glass carrier. *Biomaterials*, 18 (12): 853-859

Norton, M.R. & Wilson, J. (2002). Dental implants placed in extraction sites implanted with bioactive glass: human histology and clinical outcome. *The International journal of oral and maxillofacial implants*, 17(2):249-257.

Development and Applications of Varieties of Bioactive Glass Compositions in Dental Surgery, Third Generation
Tissue Engineering, Orthopaedic Surgery and as Drug Delivery System

109

Ochoa, I., Sanz-Herrera, J.A., GarcÃa-Aznar, J.M., DoblarÃ©, M., Yunos, D.M. & Boccaccini, A.R. (2009) 'Permeability evaluation of 45S5 BioglassÂ®-based scaffolds for bone tissue engineering', *Journal of Biomechanics*, Vol. 42, No. 3, pp. 257-260.

O'Donnell, M.D. & Hill, R.G. (2010) 'Influence of strontium and the importance of glass chemistry and structure when designing bioactive glasses for bone regeneration', *Acta Biomaterialia*, Vol. 6, No. 7, pp. 2382-2385.

Ohtsuki, C., Kushitani, H., Kokubo, T., Kotani, S. & Yamamuro, T. (1991). Apatite formation on the surface of Ceravital-type glass-ceramic in the body. *Journal of biomedical materials research*, 25(11):1363-1370.

Olding, T., Sayer, M. & Barrow, D. (2001) 'Ceramic sol-gel composite coatings for electrical insulation', *Thin Solid Films*, Vol. 398-399, pp. 581-586.

Oliveira, A.L., Mano, J.F. & Reis, R.L. (2003) 'Nature-inspired calcium phosphate coatings: present status and novel advances in the science of mimicry', *Current Opinion in Solid State and Materials Science*, Vol. 7, No. 4-5, pp. 309-318.

Pajamaki, K.J., Andersson, O.H., Lindholm, T.S., Karlsson, K.H. & Yli-Urpo, A. (1993). Induction of new bone by allogeneic demineralized bone matrix combined to bioactive glass composite in the rat. *Annales chirurgiae et gynaecologiae*, 207:137-143.

Pajamaki, K.J., Andersson, O.H., Lindholm, T.S., Karlsson, K.H., Yli-Urpo, A. & Happonen, R.P. (1993). Effect of bovine bone morphogenetic protein and bioactive glass on demineralized bone matrix grafts in the rat muscular pouch. *Annales chirurgiae et gynaecologiae*, 207:155-161.

Palussiere, J., Berge, J., Gangi, A., Cotton, A., Pasco, A., Bertagnoli, R., Hans, J., Paolo, C. & Hervé, D. (2005). Clinical results of an open prospective study of a bis-GMA composite in percutaneous vertebral augmentation. *Eur. Spine J.*, 14: 982–91.

Pan, H.B., Zhao, X.L., Zhang, X., Zhang, K.B., Li, L.C., Li, Z.Y., Lam, W.M., Lu, W.W., Wang, D.P., Huang, W.H., Lin, K.L. & Chang, J. (2010) 'Strontium borate glass: potential biomaterial for bone regeneration', *Journal of The Royal Society Interface*, Vol. 7, No. 48, pp. 1025-1031.

Patka, P., Haarman, H.J. & Bakker, F.C. (1998). Bone transplantation and bone replacement materials. *Ned. Tijdschr. Geneeskd.*,142: 893–6.

Peltola, M., Suonpaa, J., Aitasalo, K., Maattanen, H., Andersson, O., Yli-Urpo, A. & Laippala, P. (2000). Experimental follow-up model for clinical frontal sinus obliteration with bioactive glass (S53P4). *Acta. Otolaryngol Suppl* 543: 167-169.

Peltola, MJ., Suonpaa, JT., Andersson, H., Maattanen, HS., Aitasalo, KM., Yli-Urpo, A. & Laippala, PJ. (2000). In vitro model for frontal sinus obliteration with bioactive glass S53P4. *Journal of Biomedical Materials Research*, 53(2): 161-166.

Phan, PV., Grzanna, M., Chu, J., Polotsky, A., El-Ghannam, A., Van Heerden, D., Hungerford, DS. & Frondoza, CG. (2003). The effect of silica-containing calcium-phosphate particles on human osteoblasts in vitro. *J. Biomed Mater. Res, A.* 67(3): 1001-8

Queiroz, AC., Santos, JD., Monteiro, FJ., Gibson, IR. & Knowles, JC. (2001). Adsorption and release studies of sodium ampicillin from hydroxyapatite and glass-reinforced hydroxyapatite composites. *Biomaterials*, 22 (11): 1393-1400

Quinones, C.R. & Lovelace, T.B. (1997). Utilization of a bioactive synthetic particulate for periodontal therapy & bone augmentation techniques. *Pract. Periodont. Aesthet. Dent.*, 9:1-7.

Radha, G. & Ashok, K. (2008) 'Bioactive materials for biomedical applications using sol-gel technology', *Biomedical Materials*, Vol. 3, No. 3, p. 034005.

Radice, S., Kern, P., Bürki, G., Michler, J. & Textor, M. (2007). Electrophoretic deposition of zirconia-Bioglass composite coatings for biomedical implants. *J. Biomed. Mater. Res. A*, 82(2): 436-44.

Rainer, A., Giannitelli, S.M., Abbruzzese, F., Traversa, E., Licoccia, S. & Trombetta, M. (2008) 'Fabrication of bioactive glass-ceramic foams mimicking human bone portions for regenerative medicine', *Acta Biomaterialia*, Vol. 4, No. 2, pp. 362-369.

Ramp, WK., Lenz, LG. & Kaysinger, KK. (1994). Medium pH modulates matrix, mineral, and energy metabolism in cultured chick bones and osteoblast-like cells. *Bone Miner.*, 24(1): 59-73.

Ray, N.H. (1978) *Inorganic Polymers*. Academic Press, London.

Reck, R. (1981). Tissue reactions to glass ceramics in the middle ear. *Clin. Otolaryngol. Allied Sci.*, 6:63–5.

Reck, R. (1983). Bioactive glass ceramic: a new material in tympanoplasty. *The Laryngoscope*, 93(2):196-199.

Renghini, C., Komlev, V., Fiori, F., Verné, E., Baino, F. & Vitale-Brovarone, C. (2009) 'Micro-CT studies on 3-D bioactive glass-ceramic scaffolds for bone regeneration', *Acta Biomaterialia*, Vol. 5, No. 4, pp. 1328-1337.

Rezwan, K., Chen, Q.Z., Blaker, J.J. & Boccaccini, A.R. (2006) 'Biodegradable and bioactive porous polymer/inorganic composite scaffolds for bone tissue engineering', *Biomaterials*, Vol. 27, No. 18, pp. 3413-3431.

Rivero, DP., Fox, J., Skipor, AK., Urban, RN. & Galante, JO. (1988). Calcium phosphate-coated porous titanium implants for enhanced skeletal fixation, *Journal of Biomedical Materials Research* 22: 191-201.

Roessler, S., Zimmermann, R., Scharnweber, D., Werner, C. & Worch, H. (2002). Characterization of oxide layers on Ti6Al4V and titanium by streaming potential and streaming current measurements. *Colloids and Surfaces B: Biointerfaces*, 26(4): 387-395.

Roether, JA., Gough, JE., Boccaccini, AR., Hench, LL., Maquet, V. & Jérôme, R. (2002). Novel bioresorbable and bioactive composites based on bioactive glass and polylactide foams for bone tissue engineering. *J. Mater. Sci. Mater. Med.*, 13(12): 1207-14.

Ross, N., Tacconi, L. & Miles, J.B. (2000). Heterotopic bone formation causing recurrent donor site pain following iliac crest bone harvesting. *Br. J. Neurosurg.*, 14: 476–9.

Ryu, H.S., Seo, J.H., Kim, H., Hong, K.S., Park, H.J., Kim, D.J., Lee, J.H., Lee, D.H., Chang, B.S. & Lee, C.K. (2003) 'Bioceramics 15', Trans Tech Publications Limited, Zurich-Uotikon, p 261

Saino, E., Maliardi, V., Quartarone, E., Fassina, L., Benedetti, L., De Angelis, MG., Mustarelli, P., Facchini, A. & Visai, L. (2010). In vitro enhancement of SAOS-2 cell calcified matrix deposition onto radio frequency magnetron sputtered bioglass-coated titanium scaffolds. *Tissue Eng. Part A.*, 16(3): 995-1008.

Development and Applications of Varieties of Bioactive Glass Compositions in Dental Surgery, Third Generation
Tissue Engineering, Orthopaedic Surgery and as Drug Delivery System
111

Saravanapavan, P., Gough, J.E., Jones, J.R. & Hench, L.L. (2003) 'Antimicrobial macroporous gel-glasses: Dissolution and cytotoxicity', *Key Engineering Materials*, Vol. 254-256, pp. 1087-1090.

Scala, M., Gipponi, M., Pasetti, S., Dellachá, E., Ligorio, M., Villa, G., Margarino, G., Giannini, G. & Strada, P. (2007). Clinical applications of autologous cryoplatelet gel for the reconstruction of the maxillary sinus. A new approach for the treatment of chronic oro-sinusal fistula. *In Vivo.*, 21(3):541-7.

Schepers, E., de Clercq, M., Ducheyne, P. & Kempeneers, R. (1991). Bioactive glass particulate material as a filler for bone lesions. *Journal of oral rehabilitation*, 18(5):439-452.

Schnettler, R. (1997). Markgraf E. Knochenersatzmaterialen und Wachstumsfaktoren. Thieme: Stuttgart

Scotchford, C.A., Shataheri, M., Chen, P.S., Evans, M., Parsons, A.J., Aitchison, G.A., Efeoglu, C., Burke, J.L., Vikram, A., Fisher, S.E. & Rudd, C.D. (2011). Repair of calvarial defects in rats by prefabricated, degradable, long fibre composite implants. *J. Biomed. Mater. Res. A*, 96(1):230-8.

Seeherman, H. & Wozney, JM. (2005). Delivery of bone morphogenic proteins for orthopedic tissue regeneration. *Cytokine Growth Factor Rev.*, 16: 329–345.

Seiler, J.G. & Johnson, J. (2000). Iliac crest autogenous bone grafting: donor site complications. *J. South Orthop. Assoc.*, 9: 91 — 7.

Sepulveda, P., Jones, J.R. & Hench, L.L. (2001) 'Characterization of melt-derived 45S5 and sol-gel-derived 58S bioactive glasses', *Journal of Biomedical Materials Research*, Vol. 58, No. 6, pp. 734-740.

Shapoff, C.A., Alexander, D.C. & Clark, A.E. (1997). Clinical use of a bioactive glass particulate in the treatment of human osseous defects. *Compend. Contin. Educ. Dent.*, 18(4):352-4.

Skaggs, DL., Samuelson, MA., Hale, JM., Kay, RM. & Tolo, VT. (2000). Complications of posterior iliac crest bone grafting in spine surgery in children. *Spine*, 25: 2400 — 2

Smit, R.S., van der Velde, D. & Hegeman, J.H. (2008). Augmented pin fixation with Cortoss for an unstable AO-A3 type distal radius fracture in a patient with a manifest osteoporosis. *Arch. Orthop. Trauma. Surg.*, 128:989–93.

Smith, A.W., Yousefi, J. & Jackson, I.T. (1999). Screw fixation of methylmethacrylate in the craniofacial area. *Eur J Plast Surg.*, 22:17-21.

Sooksaen, P., Suttiruengwong, S., Oniem, K., Ngamlamiad, K. & Atireklapwarodom, J. (2008) 'Fabrication of porous bioactive glass-ceramics via decomposition of natural fibres', *Journal of Metals, Materials and Minerals*, Vol. 18, No. 2, pp. 85-91.

Spaans, CJ., Belgraver, VW., Rienstra, O., de Groot, JH., Veth, RP. & Pennings, AJ. (2000). Solvent-free fabrication of micro-porous polyurethane amide and polyurethane-urea scaffolds for repair and replacement of the knee-joint meniscus. *Biomaterials*, 21(23): 2453-2460.

Stanley, H.R., Clark, A.E., Pameijer, C.H. & Louw. N.P. (2001). Pulp capping with a modified bioglass formula (#A68-modified). *Am. J. Dent.*, 14(4):227-32.

Stevens, M.M. & George, J.H. (2005) 'Exploring and Engineering the Cell Surface Interface', *Science*, Vol. 310, No. 5751, pp. 1135-1138.

Stevenson, S. & Horowitz, M. (1992). The response to bone allografts. *J. Bone Joint Surg. Am.*, 74:939–50.

Strnad, Z. (1992) 'Role of the glass phase in bioactive glass-ceramics', *Biomaterials*, Vol. 13, No. 5, pp. 317-321.

Summers, B.N. & Eisenstein, S.M. (1989). Donor site pain from the ilium: a complication of lumbar spine fusion. *J. Bone Joint Surg. Br.*, 71-B: 677 – 80.

Suominen, E. & Kinnunen, J. (1996). Bioactive glass granules and plates in the reconstruction of defects of the facial bones. Scandinavian journal of plastic and reconstructive surgery. *Nordisk plastikkirurgisk forening and Nordisk klubb for handkirurgi*, 30(4):281-289.

Suonpaa. J., Sipila, J., Aitasalo, K., Antila, J. & Wide, K. (1997). Operative treatment of frontal sinusitis. *Acta Otolaryngol. Suppl.*, 529:181-183.

Sy, I.P. (2002). Alveolar ridge preservation using a bioactive glass particulate graft in extraction site defects. *General dentistry*, 50(1):66-68.

Taboas, J.M., Maddox, R.D., Krebsbach, P.H. & Hollister, S.J. (2003) 'Indirect solid free form fabrication of local and global porous, biomimetic and composite 3D polymer-ceramic scaffolds', *Biomaterials*, Vol. 24, No. 1, pp. 181-194.

Tadjoedin, E.S., de Lange, G.L., Lyaruu, D.M., Kuiper, L. & Burger, E.H. (2002). High concentrations of bioactive glass material (BioGran) vs. autogenous bone for sinus floor elevation. *Clinical oral implants research*, 13(4):428-436.

Temenoff, JS. & Mikos, AG.(2000). Review: tissue engineering for regeneration of articular cartilage. *Biomaterials*, 21(5): 431-440.

Thomas, KA., Kay, JF., Cook, SD. & Jarcho, M. (1987). The effect of surface macrotexture & hydroxylapatite coating on the mechanical strengths and histologic profiles of titanium implant materials. *Journal of Biomedical Materials Research*, 21: 1395-414.

Thomas, MV., Puleo, DA. & Al-Sabbagh, M. (2005). Bioactive glass three decades on, *J. Long-Term Eff. Med. Implants*, 15 (6): 585–597.

Thompson, I. & Hench, L. (1998) 'Mechanical properties of bioactive glasses, glass-ceramics and composites', *Proceedings of the Institution of Mechanical Engineers, Part H: Journal of Engineering in Medicine*, Vol. 212, No. 2, pp. 127-136.

Thompson, I.D. (2005) 'Biocomposites', in Hench, L.L. and Jones, J.R. (Eds.): *Biomaterials, Artificial Organs and Tissue Engineering*, Woodhead Publishing Limited CRC Press, Cambridge, U. K., pp. 48-58.

Throndson, R.R. & Sexton, S.B. (2002). Grafting mandibular third molar extraction sites: a comparison of bioactive glass to a nongrafted site. *Oral surgery, oral medicine, oral pathology, oral radiology, and endodontics*, 94(4):413-419.

Tsigkou, O., Hench, L.L., Boccaccini, A.R., Polak, J.M. & Stevens, M.M. (2007). Enhanced differentiation and mineralization of human fetal osteoblasts on PDLLA containing bioglass composite films in the absence of osteogenic supplements. *J. Biomed. Mater. Res. A.*, 80(4):837–51

Tsigkou, O., Jones, J.R., Polak, J.M. & Stevens, M.M. (2009). Differentiation of fetal osteoblasts and formation of mineralized bone nodules by 45S5 bioglass conditioned medium in the absence of osteogenic supplements. *Biomaterials*, 30(21): 3542–50.

Development and Applications of Varieties of Bioactive Glass Compositions in Dental Surgery, Third Generation
Tissue Engineering, Orthopaedic Surgery and as Drug Delivery System
113

Urist, M.R. (1965). Bone: formation by autoinduction. *Science*,150: 893–9.

Valimaki, V.V. & Aro, H.T. (2006). Molecular basis for action of bioactive glasses as bone graft substitute. *Scand. J. Surg.*, 95:95–102.

Vallet-Regí, M., Ragel, C.V. & Salinas, Antonio J. (2003) 'Glasses with Medical Applications', *European Journal of Inorganic Chemistry*, Vol. 2003, No. 6, pp. 1029-1042.

Vargas, G.E., Mesones, R.V., Bretcanu, O., López, J.M.P., Boccaccini, A.R. & Gorustovich, A. (2009) 'Biocompatibility and bone mineralization potential of 45S5 Bioglass®-derived glass-ceramic scaffolds in chick embryos', *Acta Biomaterialia*, Vol. 5, No. 1, pp. 374-380.

Verné, E., Fernández, Vallés C., Vitale Brovarone, C., Spriano, S. & Moisescu, C. (2004). Double-layer glass-ceramic coatings on Ti6Al4V for dental implants. *J. Eur. Ceram. Soc.* 24(9): 2699-2705.

Verné, E., Ferraris, M., Jana, C. & Paracchini, L. (2000). Bioverit® I base glass/Ti particulate biocomposite: "In situ" vacuum plasma spray deposition. *J. Eur. Ceram. Soc.*, 20(4): 473-479.

Verné, E., Ferraris, M., Ventrella, A., Paracchini, L., Krajewski, A. & Ravaglioli, A. (1998). Sintering and plasma spray deposition of bioactive glass-matrix composites for biomedical applications. *J. Eur. Ceram. Soc.*, 18(4): 363-372.

Villacam J,H., Novaes, A.B. Jr., Souza, S.L., Taba, M. Jr., Molina, G.O. & Carvalho, T.L. (2005). Bioactive glass efficacy in the periodontal healing of intrabony defects in monkeys. *Brazilian dental journal*, 16(1):67-74.

Vitale Brovarone, C., Verné, E. & Appendino, P. (2006) 'Macroporous bioactive glass-ceramic scaffolds for tissue engineering', *Journal of Materials Science: Materials in Medicine*, Vol. 17, No. 11, pp. 1069-1078.

Vitale-Brovarone, C., Baino, F. & Verné, E. (2010) 'Feasibility and Tailoring of Bioactive Glass-ceramic Scaffolds with Gradient of Porosity for Bone Grafting', *Journal of Biomaterials Applications*, Vol. 24, No. 8, pp. 693-712.

Vitale-Brovarone, C., Baino, F. & Verné, E. (2009b) 'High strength bioactive glass-ceramic scaffolds for bone regeneration', *Journal of Materials Science: Materials in Medicine*, Vol. 20, No. 2, pp. 643-653.

Vitale-Brovarone, C., Baino, F., Bretcanu, O. & Verné, E. (2009a) 'Foam-like scaffolds for bone tissue engineering based on a novel couple of silicate-phosphate specular glasses: synthesis and properties', *Journal of Materials Science: Materials in Medicine*, Vol. 20, No. 11, pp. 2197-2205.

Vitale-Brovarone, C., Miola, M., Balagna, C. & Verné, E. (2008) '3D-glass-ceramic scaffolds with antibacterial properties for bone grafting', *Chemical Engineering Journal*, Vol. 137, No. 1, pp. 129-136.

Vitale-Brovarone, C., Nunzio, S.D., Bretcanu, O. & Verné, E. (2004) 'Macroporous glass-ceramic materials with bioactive properties', *Journal of Materials Science: Materials in Medicine*, Vol. 15, No. 3, pp. 209-217.

Vitale-Brovarone, C., Vernè, E., Bosetti, M., Appendino, P. & Cannas, M. (2005) 'Microstructural and *in vitro* characterization of SiO_2-Na_2O-CaO-MgO glass-ceramic bioactive scaffolds for bone substitutes', *Journal of Materials Science: Materials in Medicine*, Vol. 16, No. 10, pp. 909-917.

Vitale-Brovarone, C., Verné, E., Robiglio, L., Appendino, P., Bassi, F., Martinasso, G., Muzio, G. & Canuto, R. (2007) 'Development of glass-ceramic scaffolds for bone tissue engineering: Characterisation, proliferation of human osteoblasts and nodule formation', *Acta Biomaterialia*, Vol. 3, No. 2, pp. 199-208.

Vogel, W., Hohland, W., Naumann, K., Vogel, J., Carl, G., Gotz, W. & Wange, P. (1990) 'Glass-ceramics for medicine and dentistry', in Yamamuro, T., Hench, L.L. & Wilson, J. (Eds.): *Handbook of Bioactive Ceramics Vol. I*, CRC Press, Boca Raton, FL, p. 353.

Vollenweider, M., Brunner, T.J., Knecht, S., Grass, R.N., Zehnder, M., Imfeld, T. & Stark, W.J. (2007) 'Remineralization of human dentin using ultrafine bioactive glass particles', *Acta Biomaterialia*, Vol. 3, No. 6, pp. 936-943.

Walenkamp, GHIM. (1997). Chronic osteomyelitis. *Acta. Orthop. Scand.*, 68(5): 497–506.

Wallace, K.E., Hill, R.G., Pembroke, J.T., Brown, C.J. & Hatton, P.V. (1999) 'Influence of sodium oxide content on bioactive glass properties', *Journal of Materials Science: Materials in Medicine*, Vol. 10, No. 12, pp. 697-701.

Weber, R.S., Kearns, D.B. & Smith, R.J. (1987). Split calvarium cranioplasty. *Archives of otolaryngology--head and neck surgery*,113(1):84-89.

Webster, T.J. & Ahn, E.S. (2007) 'Nanostructured biomaterials for tissue engineering bone': *Tissue Engineering II Vol. 103*, Springer, Berlin, Germany, pp. 275-308.

Weiner, S. (1986). Organization of extracellularly mineralized tissues: A comparative study of biological crystal growth. *CRC Crit. Rev. Biochem.*, 20: 365-408.

Wei-Tao, J., Xin, Z., Chang-Qing, Z., Xin, L., Wen-Hai, H., Mohamed, NR. & Day, DE. (2010). Elution characteristics of teicoplanin-loaded biodegradable borate glass/chitosan composite. *International Journal of Pharmaceutics*, 387(1-2): 184-186

Wei-Tao, J., Xin, Z., Shi-Hua, L., Xin, L., Wen-Hai, H., Mohamed, NR., Day, DE., Chang-Qing, Z., Zong-Ping, X. & Jian-Qiang, W. (2010). Novel borate glass/chitosan composite as a delivery vehicle for teicoplanin in the treatment of chronic osteomyelitis. Acta Biomaterialia 6: 812–819

Wen, H.B., Moradian-Oldak, J. & Fincham, A.G. (1999). Modulation of apatite crystal growth on Bioglass by recombinant amelogenin. *Biomaterials*, 20(18):1717-25.

Wennerberg, A., Albrektsson, T. & Andersson, B. (1996). Bone tissue response to commercially pure titanium implants blasted with fine and coarse particles of aluminum oxide. *Int. J. Oral Maxillofac. Implants*, 11: 38-45.

Wheeler, DL., Montfort, MJ. & McLoughlin, SW. (2001). Differential healing response of bone adjacent to porous implants coated with hydroxyapatite and 45S5 bioactive glass. *J. Biomed. Mater. Res.*, 55(4): 603-12.

Whitaker, L.A., Munro, I.R., Salyer, K.E., Jackson, I.T., Ortiz-Monasterio, F. & Marchac, D. (1979).   Combined report of problems and complications in 793 craniofacial operations. *Plastic and reconstructive surgery*, 64(2):198-203.

Wilda, H. & Gough. JE. (2006). In vitro studies of annulus fibrosus disc cell attachment, differentiation and matrix production on PDLLA/45S5 Bioglass composite films. *Biomaterials*, 27(30): 5220-9.

Development and Applications of Varieties of Bioactive Glass Compositions in Dental Surgery, Third Generation
Tissue Engineering, Orthopaedic Surgery and as Drug Delivery System

115

Wilson, J. & Nolletti, D. (1990) 'Bonding of soft tissues of Bioglass (R)', in Yamamuro, T., Hench, L.L. & Wilson, J. (Eds.): *Handbook of Bioactive Ceramics Vol. I, Bioactive Glasses and Glass-Ceramics*, CRC Press, Boca Raton, FL, pp. 283-302.

Wilson, J., Pigott, G.H., Schoen, F.J. & Hench, L.L. (1981) 'Toxicology and biocompatibility of bioglasses', *J Biomed Mater Res*, Vol. 15, No. 6, pp. 805-17.

Wu, C. (2009) 'Methods of improving mechanical and biomedical properties of CaSi-based ceramics and scaffolds', *Expert Review of Medical Devices*, Vol. 6, No. 3, pp. 237-241.

Wu, S.C., Hsu, H.C., Hsiao, S.H. & Ho, W.F. (2009). Preparation of porous 45S5 Bioglass-derived glass-ceramic scaffolds by using rice husk as a porogen additive. *J. Mater. Sci. Mater. Med.,* 20(6):1229-36.

Wu, TJ., Huang, HH., Lan, CW., Lin, CH., Hsu, FY. & Wang, YJ. (2004). Studies on the microspheres comprised of reconstituted collagen and hydroxyapatite. *Biomaterials,* 25(4): 651-658.

Xia, W. & Chang, J. (2006). Well-ordered mesoporous bioactive glasses (MBG): A promising bioactive drug delivery system. *Journal of Controlled Release,* 110(3): 522-530

Xie, XH., Yu, XW., Zeng, SX., Du, RL., Hu, YH., Yuan, Z., Lu, EY., Dai, KR. & Tang, TT. (2010). Enhanced osteointegration of orthopaedic implant gradient coating composed of bioactive glass and nanohydroxyapatite. *J. Mater. Sci. Mater. Med.,* 21(7): 2165-73.

Xin, Z., WeiTao, J., YiFei, G., Wei, X., Xin, L., DePing, W., ChangQing, Z., WenHai, H., Mohamed, NR., Day, DE. & Nai, Z. (2010). Teicoplanin-loaded borate bioactive glass implants for treating chronic bone infection in a rabbit tibia osteomyelitis model. *Biomaterials* 31(22): 5865-5874

Xu, C., Su, P., Chen, X., Meng, Y., Yu, W., Xiang, A.P. & Wang, Y. (2011). Biocompatibility and osteogenesis of biomimetic Bioglass-Collagen-Phosphatidylserine composite scaffolds for bone tissue engineering. *Biomaterials,* 32(4):1051-8.

Xu, C., Su, P., Wang, Y., Chen, X., Meng, Y., Liu, C., Yu, X., Yang, X., Yu, W., Zhang, X. & Xiang, A.P. (2010). A novel biomimetic composite scaffold hybridized with mesenchymal stem cells in repair of rat bone defects models. *J. Biomed. Mater. Res. A.,* 95(2):495-503.

Xynos, ID., Hukkanen, MV., Batten, JJ., Buttery, LD., Hench, LL. & Polak, JM. (2000). Bioglass 45S5 stimulates osteoblast turnover and enhances bone formation In vitro: implications and applications for bone tissue engineering. *Calcif. Tissue Int.,* 67(4): 321-9.

Yamamuro, T., Hench, L.L. & Wilson, J. (1990a) *Bioactive glasses and glass-ceramics Vol. I.* CRC Press, Boca Raton, FL.

Yamamuro, T., Hench, L.L. & Wilson, J. (1990b) *Calcium phosphate and hydroxylapatite ceramics Vol. II.* CRC Press, Boca Raton, FL.

Yamamuro, T., Shikata, J., Kakutani, Y., Yoshii, S., Kitsugi, T. & Ono, K. (1988) 'Novel methods for clinical applications of bioactive ceramics', in Ducheyne, P. and Lemons, J.E. (Eds.): *Bioceramics: Material Characteristics Versus In Vivo Behaviour,* Annals of New York Academy of Sciences, New York, p. 107.

Yang, S., Leong, K.-F., Du, Z. & Chua, C.-K. (2001) 'The Design of Scaffolds for Use in Tissue Engineering. Part I. Traditional Factors', *Tissue Engineering*, Vol. 7, No. 6, pp. 679-689.

Yang, S., Leong, K.-F., Du, Z. & Chua, C.-K. (2002) 'The Design of Scaffolds for Use in Tissue Engineering. Part II. Rapid Prototyping Techniques', *Tissue Engineering*, Vol. 8, No. 1, pp. 1-11.

Yang, XB., Webb, D., Blaker, J., Boccaccini, AR., Maquet, V., Cooper, C. & Oreffo, RO. (2006). Evaluation of human bone marrow stromal cell growth on biodegradable polymer/bioglass composites. *Biochem. Biophys. Res. Commun.*, 342(4): 1098-107.

Yılmaz, S., Ipek, M., Celebi, GF. & Bindal, C. (2005). The effect of bond coat on mechanical properties of plasma-sprayed Al2O3 and Al2O3-13 wt% TiO2 coatings on AISI 316L stainless steel. *Vacuum*, 77(3): 315-321.

Yoshii, S., Kakutani, Y., Yamamuro, T., Nakamura, T., Kitsugi, T., Oka, M., Kokubo, T. & Takagi, M. (1988) 'Strength of bonding between A-W glass-ceramic and the surface of bone cortex', *J Biomed Mater Res*, Vol. 22, No. 3 Suppl, pp. 327-38.

Younger, E.M. & Chapman, M.W. (1989). Morbidity at bone graft donor sites. *J. Orthop. Trauma.*, 3: 192-5.

Yue, TM., Yu, JK., Mei, Z. & Man, HC. (2002). Excimer laser surface treatment of Ti-6Al-4V alloy for corrosion resistance enhancement. *Materials Letters*, 52(3): 206-212.

Yukna, R.A., Evans, G.H., Aichelmann-Reidy, M.B. & Mayer, E.T. (2001). Clinical comparison of bioactive glass bone replacement graft material and expanded polytetrafluoroethylene barrier membrane in treating human mandibular molar class II furcations. *J. Periodontol.*, 72(2):125-33.

Yun, H.-s., Kim, S.-e. & Hyeon, Y.-t. (2007) 'Design and preparation of bioactive glasses with hierarchical pore networks', *Chemical Communications*, No. 21, pp. 2139-2141.

Zaffe, D., Bertoldi, C. & Consolo, U. (2003). Element release from titanium devices used in oral and maxillofacial surgery. *Biomaterials*, 24(6): 1093-1099.

Zamet, J.S., Darbar, U.R., Griffiths, G.S., Bulman, J.S., Brägger, U., Bürgin, W. & Newman, H.N. (1997). Particulate bioglass as a grafting material in the treatment of periodontal intrabony defects. *J. Clin. Periodontol.*, 24(6):410-8.

Zhang, J., Wang, M., Cha, JM. & Mantalaris, A. (2009). The incorporation of 70s bioactive glass to the osteogenic differentiation of murine embryonic stems cells in 3D bioreactors. *J. Tissue Eng. Regen. Med.* 3(1): 63-71.

Zhao, L., Yan, X., Zhou, X., Zhou, L., Wang, H., Tang, J. & Yu, C. (2008). Mesoporous bioactive glasses for controlled drug release. *Microporous and Mesoporous Materials*, 109(1-3): 210-215

Zhu Yufang & Kaskel Stefan. 2009. Comparison of the in vitro bioactivity and drug release property of mesoporous bioactive glasses (MBGs) and bioactive glasses (BGs) scaffolds. Microporous and Mesoporous Materials. 118 (1-3): 176-182

Zietek, M., Radwan-Oczko, M., Konopka, T. & Kozlowski, Z. (1998). Use of the BIOGRAN preparation in surgical treatment of periodontal disease. *Polim. Med.*, 28(3-4):63-9.

Zongping, Xie., Xin, Liu., Weitao, Jia., Changqing, Z., Wenhai, H. & Jianqiang, W. 2009. Treatment of osteomyelitis and repair of bone defect by degradable bioactive borate glass releasing vancomycin. *Journal of Controlled Release*, 139(2): 118-126

5

Application of Low-Temperature Plasma Processes for Biomaterials

Uwe Walschus[1], Karsten Schröder[2], Birgit Finke[2],
Barbara Nebe[3], Jürgen Meichsner[1], Rainer Hippler[1],
Rainer Bader[3], Andreas Podbielski[3] and Michael Schlosser[1]

[1]*University of Greifswald, Greifswald*
[2]*Leibniz Institute for Plasma Science and Technology, Greifswald*
[3]*University of Rostock, Rostock*
Germany

1. Introduction

Physical plasma is defined as a gas in which part of the particles that make up the matter are present in ionized form. This is achieved by heating a gas leading to dissociation of the molecular bonds and subsequently ionization of the free atoms. Thereby, plasma consists of positively and negatively charged ions and negatively charged electrons as well as radicals, neutral and excited atoms and molecules (Raizer, 1997; Conrads and Schmidt, 2000). On the one hand, plasma is a natural phenomenon as more than 90 % of the universe is in the plasma state, for example in fire, in the polar aurora borealis and perhaps most importantly in the nuclear fusion reactions of the sun. On the other hand, plasma can be created artificially and has found applications in technology like plasma screens or light sources. The use of high temperature plasma for energy production is still the focus of ongoing research.

For the modification of biomaterial surfaces, low temperature plasma which is sometimes also called cold plasma is used. It is characterized by a low degree of ionization at low or atmospheric pressure (Roth, 1995; Roth 2001; Hippler et al., 2008). To create low temperature plasmas, a compound is first transformed into a gas and then ionized by applying energy in the form of heat, direct or alternating electric current, radiation or laser light. Commonly used plasma gas sources are oxygen, nitrogen, hydrogen or argon. Two typical research plasma reactors for different applications are shown in Fig. 1. Depending on the nature and amount of energy, low temperature plasmas are characterized by a non-equilibrium between electron temperature and gas temperature. Thus the main parameters which define the characteristics of a plasma and thereby its applicability are its temperatures, types and densities of radicals and its level of ionization. In material science, possible applications of low-temperature plasmas include the modification of surface properties like electrochemical charge or amount of oxidation as well as attachment or modification of surface-bound chemical groups. Consequently, properties like hardness, resistance to chemical corrosion or physical abrasion, wettability, the water absorption capacity as well as the affinity toward specific molecules can be modulated specifically and precisely by the use of low-temperature plasmas (Meichsner et al., 2011).

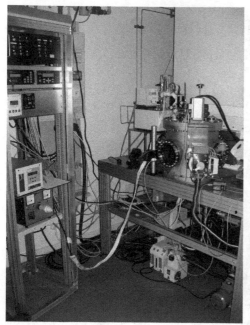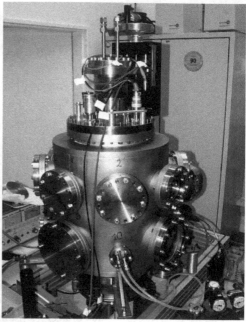

Fig. 1. Laboratory-size low-temperature plasma reactors for argon / ethylenediamine plasma (left) and pulsed magnetron sputtering (right)

Plasma treatments can be used to improve different aspects of the therapeutic characteristics of medical implants (Ohl & Schröder, 2008; Schröder et al., 2011). Possible applications include the incorporation of therapeutic agents into implants or the attachment of drug molecules onto the material surface. This includes for example plasma processes used for surface coupling of antibiotic substances or for integration of metal ions into biomaterial surfaces to create implants which exhibit long-lasting antibacterial properties after implantation. By creating such implants with antibacterial properties, the often devastating effects of implant-related infections could be markedly reduced. Therapeutic agents for other applications can be loaded onto implant surfaces via plasma treatment as well to achieve their controlled release over time. Possible applications are drug-eluting stents and vascular prostheses which release drugs to reduce blood coagulation and thombosis as well as to prevent intima hyperplasia and restenosis.

Low-temperature plasma-modified surfaces were furthermore found to possess specific bioactive properties in vitro and in vivo. For example, such surfaces influence the attachment and growth of osteoblasts, fibroblasts and inflammatory cells which provides the possibility to enhance implant ingrowth and tissue regeneration as well as to reduce implant-related inflammation, thereby improving the biocompatibility. Another field of application is plasma sterilization of prosthetic materials which is a gentle approach that can be adapted for many different materials and which is especially advantageous over conventional methods regarding the required time. From a process technology point of view, sterilization would also be a beneficial concomitant effect of other plasma treatments aimed at modulating specific material properties. The range of materials which can be treated with low-temperature plasma processes includes many materials with an established track record in regenerative medicine, for example ceramics like hydroxyapatite, polymeric materials like polyester, polypropylene, silicone and polytetrafluoroethylene, and metals like titanium, titanium-based alloys and steel. Consequently, the possible utilization of plasma treatments in the field of biomaterials includes a wide range of applications in cardiovascular and reconstructive surgery, orthopaedics and dentistry. Therefore, low-temperature plasma processes have great potential for improvement of medical implants. In the following, a concise overview of the respective applications and the underlying plasma processes is presented, putting an emphasis on recent developments. The main directions of research in this developing field are reviewed in terms of the respective aims, the relevant materials and the potential clinical applications.

2. Plasma-assisted creation of implants containing therapeutic compounds

The coating of implant surfaces with therapeutic agents is an interesting approach to improve the clinical outcome of implantation. In this field, the treatment with plasma can be used to either facilitate the surface attachment of the respective drug itself or to create a layer on top of a coating with a therapeutic compound to modulate the kinetics of its release. Among the multitude of possible applications, recent research activities are focused on two main directions: the equipment of implants with antibiotics and other compounds with antibacterial properties to prevent implant-related infections and the coating with anti-thrombogenic agents to prevent the formation of blood clots and thrombosis for implants with blood contact like vascular prostheses and stents. In principle, most of the plasma-based approaches used in these areas could also be applied with other drugs which have already been examined for drug-eluting implants, for example paclitaxel and everolimus (Butt et al., 2009), dexamethasone (Radke et al., 2004) or trapidil, probucol and cilostazol (Douglas, 2007) all aimed at reducing restenosis after implantation of vascular stents which is an emerging and clinically promising field for controlled drug release in biomaterials research.

2.1 Implant surfaces with antibacterial properties

The equipment of implants with antibacterial properties can be achieved either by attaching antibiotic substances or by creating surfaces which release metal ions which are known to have anti-infective effects. Polyvinylchloride, a polymer which is used for endotracheal tubes and catheters, was equipped with triclosan and bronopol, compounds with immediate and persistent broad-spectrum antimicrobial effects, after the surface was activated with oxygen plasma to produce more hydrophilic groups for effective coating (Zhang et al., 2006). Experiments using *Staphylococcus aureus* and *Escherichia coli* demonstrated the effectiveness of these surfaces. Similarly, polyvinylidenfluoride used for hernia meshes was modified by plasma-induced graft polymerization of acrylic acid with subsequent binding of the antibiotic gentamycin (Junge et al., 2005). In addition to the microbiological examination of the gentamycin-releasing material, the in vitro and in vivo biocompatibility was examined by cytotoxicity testing and implantation into Sprague-Dawley rats for up to 90 days, and no side effects on biocompatibility were observed. The fact that an implant coating with a sustained release of gentamycin is effective against bacteria with no adverse effects on cellular proliferation was also confirmed by the evaluation of titanium implants with gentamycin grafted onto the surface of a plasma sprayed wollastonite coating (Li et al., 2008). Wollastonite was previously found to be a promising material for bone tissue repair due to its high bonding strength to titanium substrates, its mechanical properties and its bioactivity and biocompatibility (Liu et al., 2008).

Due to their well-known antibacterial effects, metals like silver, copper or tin are possible alternatives to classical antibiotic compounds as an effective and sustained release from coatings is possibly easier to achieve due to their small size. Similarly to gentamycin as mentioned before, silver has been used as a powder added to a plasma-sprayed wollastonite coating on titanium implants (Li et al., 2009). In comparison to a coating without silver, tests with *Escherichia coli* confirmed the antibacterial activity of the silver while an examination of osteoblast morphology revealed no obvious difference between both coatings. Furthermore, the release of silver was also examined for amino-hydrocarbon plasma polymer coatings (Lischer et al., 2011), after plasma immersion ion implantation into polyethylene (Zhang et al., 2008) and for silver nanoparticles bound to an allylamine plasma polymer thin film (Vasilev et al., 2010b). Similarly, the use of copper for antibacterial implant coatings has also been studied by plasma implantation into polyethylene (Zhang et al., 2007). The use of plasma immersion ion implantation is however not restricted to polymer materials as demonstrated by recent work on the application of this process for equipment of titantium surfaces with copper ions (Polak el al., 2010). Compared to controls, the implants created by this Plasma immersion ion implantation of copper reduced the number of methicillin-resistant *Staphylococcus aureus* cultivated on the respective surfaces (Schröder et al., 2010a). Ion implantation can also be used for non-metals like fluorine which is of particular relevance for dental applications. This was examined with titanium, stainless steel and polymethyl methacrylate for fluorine alone (Nurhaerani et al., 2006) or with stainless steel for a combination of fluorine with silver (Shinonaga & Arita, 2009).

2.2 Implant surfaces with reduced thrombogenicity

Another field of interest for plasma applications is the coating of implants with anti-thrombogenic agents. This is of special importance for vascular prostheses and stents which are in constant contact with blood. For these implants, thrombosis and blood clot formation are severe and potentially life-threatening complications. Classical anti-coagulants used for thrombosis prophylaxis and treatment include coumarin derivates like phenprocoumon for oral application as well as heparin which is physiologically found in the body and extracted for medicinal use from mucosal tissues of slaughtered meat animals and hirudin, originally from the European medical leech *Hirudo medicinalis*, for parenteral use. The Plasma-based attachment of heparin has for example been examined for stainless steel which is used in stents (Yang et al., 2010). For this application, a pulsed-plasma polymeric allylamine film with a high amino group density was created to subsequently immobilize heparin via its carboxylic groups and established coupling chemistry using 1-Ethyl-3-(3-dimethylaminopropyl) carbodiimide and N-Hydroxysuccinimide. In a similar way, a heparin coating of polystyrene surfaces was achieved by preadsorption with undecylenic acid, a FDA-approved natural fungicide for skin disorders, followed by treatment with argon plasma and covalent immobilization of an albumin-heparin conjugate (van Delden et al., 1997). Another example is the heparinization of polyurethane by low temperature plasma and grafting of poly(acrylic acid), water-soluble chitosan and heparin (Lin et al., 2005). In addition to well-established anti-coagulants, the endothelial membrane protein thrombomodulin, a co-factor in the thrombin-activated anticoagulant pathway, has also been examined regarding plasma-based attachment on biomaterial surfaces. This application was studied for polytetrafluoroethylene, a common material for vascular prostheses, via CO_2 plasma activation and subsequent vapour phase graft polymerization of acrylic acid (Vasilets et al., 1997; Sperling et al., 1997). Another surface modification which was examined for reduced thrombogenicity was plasma-induced graft polymerization of 2-methacryloyloxyethyl phosphorylcholine on titanium alloy surfaces which resulted in reduced deposition and activation of platelets in subsequent in vitro experiments with ovine blood (Ye et al., 2009).

2.3 Regulation of drug release by barrier layers

In addition to plasma-assisted surface attachment of therapeutic compounds, plasma processes can also be used to create an over-coating which acts as a barrier to regulate the drug release. This application has for example been examined using daunomycin, an antibiotic substance, and rapamycin, a compound with immunosuppressive and anti-proliferative effects which is used for example in stents to prevent excessive tissue growth, in combination with a plasma polymerized tetramethylcyclo-tetrasiloxane coating (Osaki et al., 2011). Changing the deposition time length resulted in different coating thickness which, like the molecular weight of the drug, was found to influence the drug-release rate. A comparable approach was used on polyetherurethane onto which a plasma-deposited poly(butyl methyacrylate) membrane with controlled porosity was applied to control the release of ciprofloxacin (Hendricks et al., 2000). Adhesion and colonization of *Pseudomonas aeruginosa* was evaluated to assess the antimicriobial effectiveness.

Furthermore, an over-coating can also be applied to surfaces which release metal ions. For instance, the antibacterial surfaces created by plasma immersion ion implantation of copper as mentioned before were also treated with an additional layer of plasma-polymerized allylamine to regulate the Cu release and to modulate cellular adhesion and spreading. This combination reduced the antibacterial effects of the surface to some extent but did not completely disable it (Schröder et al., 2010a). On the other hand, the combined treatment also led to lower local inflammatory reactions after implantation into rats (Schlosser, unpublished data), highlighting the need to find an optimal balance between in vivo biocompatibility and sufficient antibacterial effects. Another study demonstrated that creation of thin films by plasma polymerization for controlled release of silver ions and traditional antibiotics is applicable to the surface of many different medical devices (Vasilev et al., 2010a).

The use of an over-coating to regulate the release rate is not only possible for antibiotics but also for antithrombogenic agents. This has for example been studied for hirudin for which an additional layer of 2-hydroxyethyl methacrylate created by glow discharge plasma deposition on drug-loaded polyurethane matrices served as a diffusional barrier controlling the hirudin release kinetics depending on the plasma coating conditions (Kim et al., 1998).

Of more general interest for the field of drug-releasing implants is a recent study which describes the use of liposomes, artificial vesicles enclosed by a lipid bilayer. Liposomes can be used as drug containers by encapsulation of therapeutic compounds, in some cases additionally targeted to their site of action by antibodies, and potentially offer a wide range of applications. Covalent coating of liposomes onto stainless steel was achieved via radiofrequency glow plasma assisted creation of a thin film of acrylic acid characterized by surface carboxylic groups to which the liposomes were attached via formation of amide bonds (Mourtas et al., 2011). While the study was considered by the authors to be a proof of principle, the presented method seems to be a versatile approach due to possible changes of process parameters for the liposome immobilization procedure as well as regarding the choice of different drugs for encapsulation.

3. Plasma-based surface functionalization

Medical implants interact with their surrounding tissue in a complex manner. For example, a so called neointima layer is formed over time at the inner surface of vascular prostheses. Bone implants based on calcium phosphate possess osteoconductive and osteoinductive properties. Most importantly, all biomaterials are foreign to the body and the aim of acute and chronic inflammatory reactions which can persist for as long as the implant remains in the body. While short-term temporary implants which are removed some time after implantation should rather be inert, long-term implants intended for permanent presence in the recipient's body should ideally possess bioactive properties to facilitate proper tissue integration. A multitude of different approaches has been examined with the aim to influence the interactions between biomaterials and the host tissue, for example by regulation of protein and cell attachment to improve the implant ingrowth and to reduce implant-related inflammation. Possible methods include for example the coating with different proteins, with biomembrane-derived phospholipids, with diamond-like carbon or ceramics or the attachment of chemical groups to create surfaces with a specific electric charge. Low-temperature plasmas have extensively been examined in vitro and in vivo for these applications.

3.1 Creation of bioactive surfaces
The cell-material and tissue-material interactions can be influenced by modifying the surface charge via chemical groups. For example, an enhanced osteoblast growth in vitro was observed for surfaces modified with plasma-polymerized 1-aminoheptane (Zhao et al., 2011). The plasma-based deposition of acetaldehyde and allylamine polymer coatings on silicon and perfluorinated poly(ethylene-co-propylene) was found to influence the outgrowth of bovine corneal epithelial tissue for up to 21 days (Thissen et al., 2006). A treatment of Titanium samples with a comparable process called plasma-polymerized allylamine, based on the polymerization of allylamine after activation with a continuous wave oxygen-plasma, creates a positively charged amino group rich surface aimed at improving attachment of the negatively charged matrix substance hyaluronan. This coating was found to be advantageous concerning initial osteoblast adhesion and spreading (Nebe et al., 2007) and to have beneficial effects in vitro on the formation of focal adhesions as well as on cell morphology and spreading (Finke et al., 2007) and vinculin mobility (Rebl et al., 2010) of osteoblasts. An in vivo examination in rats revealed no negative influence on the number of total and tissue macrophages, T cells and MHC class II antigen-presenting cells in the peri-implant tissue (Hoene et al., 2010). Furthermore, it was demonstrated that the

plasma parameters influence the surface properties and thereby the host response. Samples with a lower plasma duty cycle (ratio of plasma on-time t_{on} divided by the overall pulse duration t_{on} + t_{off}) resulted in a higher layer thickness and protein absorption as well as a lower oxygen uptake due to sonication in distilled water. Consequently, the hydrogel-like character of the plasma-polymerized allylamine films was probably more developed for the high duty cycle samples, resulting in an overall lower inflammatory response in vivo than for the implants created with a low duty cycle (Hoene et al., 2010). Similar results regarding enhanced cell adhesion were also obtained for a plasma consisting of a mixture of argon and ethylenediamine (Finke et al., 2011). A treatment of a hip prosthesis with this plasma process is exemplarily shown in Fig. 2.

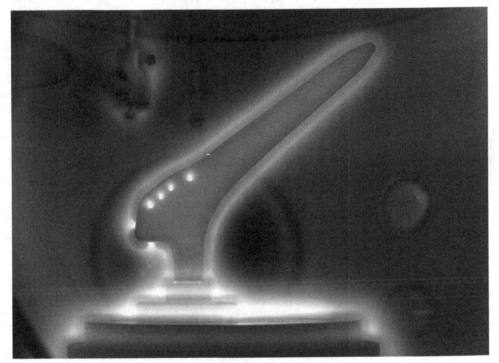

Fig. 2. Hip joint implant in low pressure plasma using a mixture of argon and ethylenediamine for cell adhesive coating

In contrast to these positively charged NH_2 films, a coating of Titanium implants with acrylic acid after similar plasma activation, called plasma-polymerized acrylic acid, results in a negatively charged COOH-group rich surface which was found to facilitate osteogenic differentiation by stimulation of mRNA expression of early (ALP, COL, Runx2) as well as late (BSP, OCN) bone differentiation markers (Schröder et al., 2010b). However, the long-term inflammatory response in vivo caused by this coating were increased compared to uncoated controls (Schröder et al., 2010b), highlighting the difficult balance that improving one specific aspect of implant characteristics is often accompanied by adverse changes in other parameters. Furthermore, it illustrates the problem that the results of in vitro experiments on the one hand and in vivo studies on the other are often inconsistent due to the complex nature of reactions in a living organism which can only partially and often inadequately be modelled using in vitro approaches.

Similar to metals and metal alloys, cell attachment on polymers can also be modulated by plasma treatment. The application of glow-discharge plasma of mixed ammonia and oxygen on polytetrafluoroethylene surfaces reduced the hydrophobicity and increased the attachment of aorta endothelial cells (Chen et al., 2003). Furthermore, an oxygen plasma has been shown to improve surface attachment of mouse fibroblasts L-929 on thermoplastic polyetherurethane used for gastric implants (Schlicht et al., 2010).

Low-temperature plasma can also be used to achieve immobilization of bioactive molecules. This was demonstrated for example by an oxygen plasma treatment to enhance the immobilization of simvastatin, which stimulates bone formation, onto Ti surfaces (Yoshinari et al., 2006). The deposition of thin film from ethylene plasma on Ti surfaces allows the chemical attachment of hydroxyethylmethacrylate onto Ti to improve the in vitro adhesion of mouse fibroblasts L-929 (Morra & Cassinelli, 1997). Albumin nanoparticles conjugated with a truncated fragment of fibronectin were directly patterned onto polymers to elicit adhesion and spreading of human mesenchymal stem cells and fibroblasts (Rossi et al., 2010). Stable coating of collagen type I onto two different metal alloys (Ti6Al4V, X2CrNiMo18) was achieved using a argon-hydrogen plasma and found to increase the viability and attachment of human osteoblast-like osteosarcoma cells SAOS-2 (Hauser et al., 2010), and coating of collagen onto silicone performed with an argon-oxygen plasma led to increased adhesion and viability of mouse fibroblasts 3T3 (Hauser et al., 2009). Poly(lactide-co-glycolide), a biodegradable polymer widely used as scaffold material for tissue engineering, was modified by oxygen plasma treatment followed by anchorage of cationized gelatine for improved attachment and growth of mouse fibroblasts 3T3 (Shen et al, 2007).

A popular material for bioactive coatings on implants for bone replacement is calcium phosphate which is the main natural component in the bone matrix where it accounts for more than half of the bone weight. It exists in a variety of different chemical preparations differing in their atomic and ionic lattice configuration, their Ca:P ratio, the number and size of pores, and their surface area. One calcium phosphate preparation commonly used for biomaterials is hydroxyapatite ($Ca_{10}(PO_4)_6(OH)_2$) which is generally considered to be osteoconductive and osteoinductive (Walschus et al., 2009). Using a process called plasma spraying, it is possible to deposit thin and dense layers of hydroxyapatite onto metal implant surfaces (de Groot et al., 1987). Due to the well-established bioactive properties and good biocompatibility of hydroxyapatite, these coatings have been clinically used in dentistry and orthopedics since the mid 1980s (Tang et al., 2010). Furthermore, plasma spraying can also be used to create other layers like Ca-Si-Ti-based sphene ceramics (Wu et al., 2009), hydroxyapatite/ silica ceramics (Morks 2008), zirconia (Morks & Kobayashi 2008; Wang et al., 2010), yttria-stabilized zirconia (Wang et al., 2009) or hydroxyapatite/ yttria/ zirconia composites (Chang et al., 1997; Gu et al., 2004). One important advantage of plasma-sprayed coatings for biomaterials is the ability to precisely modify the microstructure by modulating the parameters of the plasma process (Khor et al., 2004; Huang et al., 2010) to study and improve microstructure-related tissue growth stimulation.

3.2 Plasma-assisted vapour deposition of inert diamond-like carbon layers

Another field of increasing interest which should be mentioned briefly in this chapter is the plasma-based coating of implants with diamond-like carbon for which plasma-assisted chemical vapour deposition is the most commonly used deposition method. Diamond-like carbon layers can exhibit the typical diamond crystalline structure, an amorphous structure or a mixture of both (Schlosser & Ziegler, 1997). Furthermore, depending on the coating procedure, they can consist of pure carbon or contain other elements. Overall, diamond-like carbon films are characterized by an excellent mechanical stability and hardness, a high corrosion resistance as well as reduced tissue-material interactions and no detectable cytotoxicity (Schlosser & Ziegler, 1997). Particularly for implants where inertness of the surface is required, they are therefore an attractive option for coating of medical implants in a number of applications in reconstructive surgery and dentistry (Roy & Lee, 2007). Diamond-like carbon coatings have for example been examined for ureteral stents (Laube et al., 2007), orthodontic archwires (Kobayashi et al., 2007), joint implants (Thorwarth et al., 2010) or cardiovascular stents (De Scheerder et al., 2000).

4. Plasma sterilization

Sterilization as the elimination of living microorganisms like bacteria, viruses and fungi, especially pathogenic agents, is an important aspect in biomaterials applications to prevent implant-related infections. Commonly used methods to achieve sterility include the treatment with heat, chemicals and irradiation. Each of those methods has its specific disadvantages and not all are equally usable for the sterilization of medical implants. For example, a heat treatment can lead to irreversible modifications of heat-labile materials and to denaturation of protein coatings. Irradiation with UV or gamma rays requires cost-intensive equipment with high safety requirements and can also cause irreversible modifications of proteins such as albumin and collagen used as sealing impregnation of vascular prostheses, as well as biomaterials like polymers. Chemical sterilization using for example ethylene oxide could result in residuals on the treated surface. Therefore, the application of low-temperature plasma processes as an alternative sterilization technique which is a gentle process from a physico-chemical point of view has been the focus of ongoing research since several years. It is known that exposure to plasma effectively and irreversibly damages cells from different bacteria species like for example *Escherichia coli, Staphylococcus aureus, Pseudomonas aeruginosa, Bacillus cereus* or *Bacillus subtilis* (Bazaka et al., 2011). Especially for modified or functionalized biomaterials, sterilization with low-temperature plasma would therefore be an attractive option as it could be achieved as a secondary effect of plasma treatment aimed at other surface modification purposes (Bazaka et al., 2011).

The application of plasma sterilization of heat-sensitive silicone implants has recently been demonstrated (Hauser et al., 2011). Similarly, sterilization of poly-L-lactide electrospun microfibers which can be used to repair tissue defects can effectively be achieved by hydrogen peroxide gas plasma which ensures sterility of the scaffolds and does not affect their chemical and morphological features (Rainer et al., 2010). Biodegradable polyester three-dimensional tissue engineering scaffolds which are particularly prone to morphological degeneration by high temperature and pressure were successfully sterilized with an argon-based radio-frequency glow discharge plasma (Holy et al., 2001), demonstrating the usefulness of plasma sterilization for damageable materials. Similar results were also obtained for starch based biomaterials for which a recent study found that treatment with oxygen plasma resulted in more hydrophilic surfaces compared to UV-irradiation (Pashkuleva et al., 2010). Furthermore, both methods gave comparable results regarding osteoblast adherence, from which the authors concluded that plasma sterilization as well as UV-irradiation improved the biocompatibility and can be used as cost-effective methods for sterilization.

For metal implants, it was found that rapid and efficient sterilization of different alloys like X2CrNiMo18-15-3, Ti6Al7Nb und Ti6Al4V is possible with plasmas based on different gas mixtures such as argon/oxygen, argon/hydrogen and argon/nitrogen (Hauser et al., 2008). Sterilization of non-woven polyethylene terephthalate fiber structures for vascular grafts with either ethylene oxide or low temperature plasma resulted in comparable fibroblastic viability but a significantly higher TNF-α release, indicating activation of macrophages, for macrophages incubated on the fibres which were treated with ethylene oxide (Dimitrievska et al., 2011). Subcutaneous implantation into mice demonstrated inflammation accompanied by a foreign body reaction with no difference after 30 days between the samples treated with the two sterilization methods. A comparison of the effects of sterilization with gamma irradiation, ethylene oxide treatment, electron beam irradiation and plasma sterilization on the in vitro behaviour of polylactide fibres revealed that sterilization with both gamma and electron beam irradiation caused a decrease of the intrinsic viscosity while treatment with ethylene oxide and plasma sterilization had no pronounced effects on the sample properties (Nuutinen et al., 2002). These results also highlight the potential of plasma sterilization as a gentle alternative to other commonly used sterilization methods. However, it is not equally suitable for all materials as it might have adverse effects on relevant material properties. For example, demineralized bone matrix which was sterilized with low-temperature gas-plasma sterilization lost its osteoinductive capacity (Ferreira et al., 2001).

Another application related to sterilization is the removal of surface contaminations. This is particularly important for residues like prion proteins which have contagious and pathogenic properties. The usefulness of plasma treatment for molecular-level removal of proteinaceous contamination was recently demonstrated for silicon and surgical stainless steel surfaces (Banerjee et al., 2010).

5. Conclusions and outlook

Low temperature plasmas offer a wide range of applications in biomaterials research to improve the clinical performance of medical implants by modifying their surface characteristics. In many cases, the use of plasmas facilitates modifications which are difficult or unable to achieve by conventional physical or chemical methods, like for example the stable attachment of molecules onto noble metal surfaces. The concise overview presented in this chapter demonstrates the potential of low temperature plasma processes for the precise modification of specific implant surface properties while retaining the overall characteristics of the material. The main aims of research in this field are to reduce implant-related complications like infections, thrombus formation and inflammation as well as to modulate the cell-material and tissue-material interactions for improved implant ingrowth. Another equally important area of research is the use of plasmas for sterilization. The studies which were presented here indicate that plasma processes are applicable for practically all commonly used biomaterials including metals, polymers, ceramics and composites, offering a wide range of clinical applications in all fields of reconstructive medicine.

Given the versatility of low temperature plasma processes and the diverse nature of materials and clinical applications, it is difficult to predict future developments in this field. If there is any specific trend, then it is an increase in the number of studies which deal with biodegradable materials, reflecting an overall surge of interest in biomaterials research for this kind of materials. Another development is the use of increasingly sophisticated methods for surface analysis, making it possible to draw precise conclusions regarding relationships between process parameters, surface characteristics and the biological response. Two important aspects in need of more research are on the one hand the aging-related surface changes of plasma-modified biomaterials and on the other hand their in vivo behaviour. Most of the studies discussed here used only in vitro methods to assess the biocompatibility. However, for the step from the lab into clinical practice it is essential to examine the in vivo biocompatibility by using appropriate animal models. There are several aspects of biocompatibility, both short- and long-term, which can not be adequately examined with in vitro methods like cell culture techniques. More detailed in vivo testing together with a better understanding of the influence of the plasma parameters on the physico-chemical material properties and on the response of cells, tissues and living organisms will ultimately turn currently promising research projects into clinical applications for improved implants. The increasing interest in the application of low-temperature plasmas in biomaterials science is illustrated by the formation of long-term and large-scale research projects, scientific centers and institutional networks in recent years, for example the Plasma Physics and Radiation Technology Cluster at the Eindhoven University of Technology in the Netherlands, the Center for Advanced Plasma Surface Technology (CAPST) in Korea, and the Campus PlasmaMed at the Leibniz Institute of Plasma Science and Technology Greifswald, the University of Greifswald and the University of Rostock in Germany.

6. References

Banerjee K.K., Kumar S., Bremmell K.E. & Griesser H.J. (2010). Molecular-level removal of proteinaceous contamination from model surfaces and biomedical device materials by air plasma treatment. *Journal of Hospital Infection*, Vol. 76, No. 3, pp. 234-242.

Bazaka K., Jacob M.V., Crawford R.J. & Ivanova E.P. (2011). Plasma-assisted surface modification of organic biopolymers to prevent bacterial attachment. *Acta Biomaterialia*, Vol. 7, No. 5, pp. 2015-2028.

Butt M., Connolly D. & Lip G.Y. (2009). Drug-eluting stents: a comprehensive appraisal. *Future Cardiology*, Vol. 5, No. 2, pp. 141-157.

Chang E., Chang W.J., Wang B.C. & Yang C.Y. (1997). Plasma spraying of zirconia-reinforced hydroxyapatite composite coatings on titanium. Part I: phase, microstructure and bonding strength. *Journal of Materials Science: Materials in Medicine*, Vol. 8, No. 4, pp. 193-200.

Chen M., Zamora P.O., Som P., Peña L.A. & Osaki S. (2003). Cell attachment and biocompatibility of polytetrafluoroethylene (PTFE) treated with glow-discharge plasma of mixed ammonia and oxygen. *Journal of Biomaterials Science: Polymer Edition*, Vol. 14, No. 9, pp. 917-935.

Conrads H. & Schmidt M. (2000). Plasma generation and plasma sources. *Plasma Sources Science and Technology*, Vol. 9, No. 4, pp. 441-454.

de Groot K., Geesink R., Klein C.P. & Serekian P. (1987). Plasma sprayed coatings of hydroxylapatite. *Journal of Biomedical Materials Research*, Vol. 21, No. 12, pp. 1375-1381.

De Scheerder I., Szilard M., Yanming H., Ping X.B., Verbeken E., Neerinck D., Demeyere E., Coppens W. & Van de Werf F. (2000). Evaluation of the biocompatibility of two new diamond-like stent coatings (Dylyn) in a porcine coronary stent model. *Journal of Invasive Cardiology*, Vol. 12, No. 8, pp. 389-394.

Dimitrievska S., Petit A., Doillon C.J., Epure L., Ajji A., Yahia L. & Bureau M.N. (2011). Effect of sterilization on non-woven polyethylene terephthalate fiber structures for vascular grafts. *Macromolecular Bioscience*, Vol. 11, No. 1, pp. 13-21.

Douglas J.S. Jr. (2007). Pharmacologic approaches to restenosis prevention. *American Journal of Cardiology*, Vol. 100, No. 5 Suppl. 1, pp. S10-S16.

Ferreira S.D., Dernell W.S., Powers B.E., Schochet R.A., Kuntz C.A., Withrow S.J. & Wilkins R.M. (2001). Effect of gas-plasma sterilization on the osteoinductive capacity of demineralized bone matrix. *Clinical Orthopaedics and Related Research*, Vol. 388, pp. 233-239.

Finke B., Lüthen F., Schröder K, Mueller P.D., Bergemann C., Frant M., Ohl A. & Nebe B.J. (2007). The effect of positively charged plasma polymerization on initial osteoblastic focal adhesion on titanium surfaces. *Biomaterials*, Vol. 28, No. 30, pp. 4521-4534.

Finke B., Hempel F., Testrich H., Artemenko A., Rebl H., Kylián O., Meichsner J., Biederman H., Nebe B., Weltmann K.-D., Schröder K. (2011). Plasma processes for cell-adhesive titanium surfaces based on nitrogen-containing coatings. *Surface & Coatings Technology*, Vol. 205, Suppl. 2, pp. S520-S524

Gu Y.W., Khor K.A., Pan D. & Cheang P. (2004). Activity of plasma sprayed yttria stabilized zirconia reinforced hydroxyapatite/Ti-6Al-4V composite coatings in simulated body fluid. *Biomaterials*, Vol. 25, No. 16, pp. 3177-3185.

Hauser J., Halfmann H., Awakowicz P., Köller M. & Esenwein S.A. (2008). A double inductively coupled low-pressure plasma for sterilization of medical implant materials. *Biomedical Engineering*, Vol. 53, No. 4, pp. 199-203.

Hauser J., Zietlow J., Köller M., Esenwein S.A., Halfmann H., Awakowicz P. & Steinau H.U. (2009). Enhanced cell adhesion to silicone implant material through plasma surface modification. *Journal of Materials Science: Materials in Medicine*, Vol. 20, No. 12, pp. 2541-2548.

Hauser J., Köller M., Bensch S., Halfmann H., Awakowicz P., Steinau H.U. & Esenwein S. (2010). Plasma mediated collagen-I-coating of metal implant materials to improve biocompatibility. *Journal of Biomedical Materials Research Part A*, Vol. 94, No. 1, pp. 19-26.

Hauser J., Esenwein S.A., Awakowicz P., Steinau H.U., Köller M. & Halfmann H. (2011). Sterilization of heat-sensitive silicone implant material by low-pressure gas plasma. *Biomedical Instrumentation & Technology*, Vol. 45, No. 1, pp. 75-79.

Hendricks S.K., Kwok C., Shen M., Horbett T.A., Ratner B.D. & Bryers J.D. (2000). Plasma-deposited membranes for controlled release of antibiotic to prevent bacterial adhesion and biofilm formation. *Journal of Biomedical Materials Research*, Vol. 50, No. 2, pp. 160-170.

Hippler R., Kersten H., Schmidt M. & Schoenbach K.H. (2008). Low temperature plasma physics: Fundamental aspects and applications. Wiley-VCH, Weinheim, Germany.

Hoene A., Walschus U., Patrzyk M., Finke B., Lucke S., Nebe B., Schröder K., Ohl A. & Schlosser M. (2010). In vivo investigation of the inflammatory response against allylamine plasma polymer coated titanium implants in a rat model. *Acta Biomaterialia*, Vol. 6, No. 2, pp. 676-683.

Holy C.E., Cheng C., Davies J.E. & Shoichet M.S. (2001). Optimizing the sterilization of PLGA scaffolds for use in tissue engineering. *Biomaterials*, Vol. 22, No. 1, pp. 25-31.

Huang Y., Song L., Liu X., Xiao Y., Wu Y., Chen J., Wu F. & Gu Z. (2010). Hydroxyapatite coatings deposited by liquid precursor plasma spraying: controlled dense and porous microstructures and osteoblastic cell responses. *Biofabrication*, Vol. 2, No. 2, paper 045003.

Junge K., Rosch R., Klinge U., Krones C., Klosterhalfen B., Mertens P.R., Lynen P., Kunz D., Preiss A., Peltroche-Llacsahuanga H. & Schumpelick V. (2005). Gentamicin supplementation of polyvinylidenfluoride mesh materials for infection prophylaxis. *Biomaterials*, Vol. 26, No. 7, pp. 787-793.

Khor K.A., Gu Y.W., Pan D. & Cheang P. (2004). Microstructure and mechanical properties of plasma sprayed HA/YSZ/Ti-6Al-4V composite coatings. *Biomaterials*, Vol. 25, No. 18, pp. 4009-4017.

Kim D.D., Takeno M.M., Ratner B.D. & Horbett T.A. (1998). Glow discharge plasma deposition (GDPD) technique for the local controlled delivery of hirudin from biomaterials. *Pharmaceutical Research*, Vol. 15, No. 5, pp. 783-786.

Kobayashi S., Ohgoe Y., Ozeki K., Hirakuri K. & Aoki H. (2007). Dissolution effect and cytotoxicity of diamond-like carbon coatings on orthodontic archwires. *Journal of Materials Science: Materials in Medicine*, Vol. 18, No. 12, pp. 2263-2268.

Laube N., Kleinen L., Bradenahl J. & Meissner A. (2007). Diamond-like carbon coatings on ureteral stents--a new strategy for decreasing the formation of crystalline bacterial biofilms? *Journal of Urology*, Vol. 177, No. 5, pp. 1923-1927.

Li B., Liu X., Cao C., Dong Y., Wang Z. & Ding C. (2008). Biological and antibacterial properties of plasma sprayed wollastonite coatings grafting gentamicin loaded collagen. *Journal of Biomedical Materials Research Part A*, Vol. 87, No. 1, pp. 84-90.

Li B., Liu X., Cao C., Dong Y. & Ding C. (2009). Biological and antibacterial properties of plasma sprayed wollastonite/silver coatings. *Journal of Biomedical Materials Research Part B: Applied Biomaterials*, Vol. 91, No. 2, pp. 596-603.

Lin W.C., Tseng C.H. & Yang M.C. (2005). In-vitro hemocompatibility evaluation of a thermoplastic polyurethane membrane with surface-immobilized water-soluble chitosan and heparin. *Macromolecular Bioscience*, Vol. 5, No. 10, pp. 1013-1021.

Lischer S., Körner E., Balazs D.J., Shen D., Wick P., Grieder K., Haas D., Heuberger M. & Hegemann D. (2011). Antibacterial burst-release from minimal Ag-containing plasma polymer coatings. *Journal of the Royal Society Interface*, Vol. 8, No. 60, pp. 1019-1030.

Liu X., Morra M., Carpi A. & Li B. (2008). Bioactive calcium silicate ceramics and coatings. *Biomedicine & Pharmacotherapy*, Vol. 62, No. 8, pp. 526-529.

Meichsner J., Schmidt M., Wagner H.E. (2011). Non-thermal Plasma Chemistry and Physics. Taylor & Francis, London, UK.

Morks M.F. (2008). Fabrication and characterization of plasma-sprayed HA/SiO(2) coatings for biomedical application. *Journal of the Mechanical Behavior of Biomedical Materials*, Vol. 1, No. 1, pp. 105-111.

Morks M.F. & Kobayashi A. (2008). Development of ZrO2/SiO2 bioinert ceramic coatings for biomedical application. *Journal of the Mechanical Behavior of Biomedical Materials*, Vol. 1, No. 2, pp. 165-171.

Morra M. & Cassinelli C. (1997). Organic surface chemistry on titanium surfaces via thin film deposition. *Journal of Biomedical Materials Research*, Vol. 37, No. 2, pp. 198-206.

Mourtas S., Kastellorizios M., Klepetsanis P., Farsari E., Amanatides E., Mataras D., Pistillo B.R., Favia P., Sardella E., d'Agostino R. & Antimisiaris S.G. (2011). Covalent immobilization of liposomes on plasma functionalized metallic surfaces. *Colloids and Surfaces B: Biointerfaces*, Vol. 84, No. 1, pp. 214-220.

Nebe B., Finke B., Lüthen F., Bergemann C., Schröder K., Rychly J., Liefeith K. & Ohl A. (2007). Improved initial osteoblast functions on amino-functionalized titanium surfaces. *Biomolecular Engineering*, Vol. 24, No. 5, pp. 447-54.

Nurhaerani, Arita K., Shinonaga Y. & Nishino M. (2006). Plasma-based fluorine ion implantation into dental materials for inhibition of bacterial adhesion. *Dental Materials Journal*, Vol. 25, No. 4, pp. 684-692.

Nuutinen J.P., Clerc C., Virta T. & Törmälä P. (2002). Effect of gamma, ethylene oxide, electron beam, and plasma sterilization on the behaviour of SR-PLLA fibres in vitro. *Journal of Biomaterials Science: Polymer Edition*, Vol. 13, No. 12, pp. 1325-1336.

Ohl A., Schröder K. (2008). Plasma assisted surface modification of biointerfaces. In: Hippler R., Kersten H., Schmidt M. & Schoenbach K.H. Low temperature plasma physics: Fundamental aspects and applications. Wiley-VCH, Weinheim, Germany, pp. 803-819.

Osaki S.G., Chen M. & Zamora P.O. (2011). Controlled Drug Release through a Plasma Polymerized Tetramethylcyclo-tetrasiloxane Coating Barrier. *Journal of Biomaterials Science: Polymer Edition*, published online before print January 28, 2011, doi: 10.1163/092050610X552753.

Pashkuleva I., Marques A.P., Vaz F. & Reis R.L. (2010). Surface modification of starch based biomaterials by oxygen plasma or UV-irradiation. *Journal of Materials Science: Materials in Medicine*, Vol. 21, No. 1, pp. 21-32.

Polak M., Ohl A., Quaas M., Lukowski G., Lüthen F., Weltmann K.-D. & Schröder K. (2010). Oxygen and Water Plasma-Immersion Ion Implantation of Copper into Titanium for Antibacterial Surfaces of Medical Implants. *Advanced Engineering Materials*, Vol. 12, No. 9, pp. B511-B518.

Radke P.W., Weber C., Kaiser A., Schober A. & Hoffmann R. (2004). Dexamethasone and restenosis after coronary stent implantation: new indication for an old drug? *Current Pharmaceutical Design*, Vol. 10, No. 4, pp. 349-355.

Rainer A., Centola M., Spadaccio C., Gherardi G., Genovese J.A., Licoccia S. & Trombetta M. (2010). Comparative study of different techniques for the sterilization of poly-L-lactide electrospun microfibers: effectiveness vs. material degradation. *International Journal of Artificial Organs*, Vol. 33, No. 2, pp. 76-85.

Raizer Y.P. (1997). Gas Discharge Physics. Springer, Berlin, Germany.

Rebl H., Finke B., Ihrke R., Rothe H., Rychly J., Schröder K. & Nebe B.J. (2010). Positively Charged Material Surfaces Generated by Plasma Polymerized Allylamine Enhance Vinculin Mobility in Vital Human Osteoblasts. *Advanced Engineering Materials*, Vol. 12, No. 8, pp. B356-B364.

Rossi M.P., Xu J., Schwarzbauer J. & Moghe P.V. (2010). Plasma-micropatterning of albumin nanoparticles: Substrates for enhanced cell-interactive display of ligands. *Biointerphases*, Vol. 5, No. 4, pp. 105-113.

Roth J.R. (1995). Industrial Plasma Engineering. Volume 1: Principles. Institute of Physics Publishing, Bristol, UK.

Roth J.R. (2001). Industrial Plasma Engineering. Volume 2: Applications to Nonthermal Plasma Processing. Institute of Physics Publishing, Bristol, UK.

Roy R.K. & Lee K.R. (2007). Biomedical applications of diamond-like carbon coatings: a review. *Journal of Biomedical Materials Research Part B: Applied Biomaterials*, Vol. 83, No. 1, pp. 72-84.

Schlicht H., Haugen H.J., Sabetrasekh R. & Wintermantel E. (2010). Fibroblastic response and surface characterization of O(2)-plasma-treated thermoplastic polyetherurethane. *Biomedical Materials*, Vol. 5, No. 2, paper 25002

Schlosser M. & Ziegler M. (1997). Biocompatibility of Active Implantable Devices. In: Fraser, D.M. (Ed.). Biosensors in the Body. Continuous In Vivo Monitoring. John Wiley & Sons, Chicester, UK, pp. 140-170.

Schröder K., Finke B., Polak M., Lüthen F., Nebe J.B., Rychly J., Bader R., Lukowski G., Walschus U., Schlosser M., Ohl A. & Weltmann K.-D. (2010a). Gas-Discharge Plasma-Assisted Functionalization of Titanium Implant Surfaces. *Materials Science Forum*, Vols. 638-642, pp. 700-705.

Schröder K., Finke B., Ohl A., Lüthen F., Bergemann C., Nebe B., Rychly J., Walschus U., Schlosser M. Liefeith K., Neumann H.-G. & Weltmann K.-D. (2010b). Capability of Differently Charged Plasma Polymer Coatings for Control of Tissue Interactions with Titanium Surfaces. *Journal of Adhesion Science and Technology*, Vol. 24, No. 7, pp. 1191-1205.

Schröder K., Foest R., Ohl A. (2011). Biomedical applications of plasmachemical surface functionalization. In: Meichsner J., Schmidt M., Wagner H.E. Non-thermal Plasma Chemistry and Physics. Taylor & Francis, London, UK, in press

Shen H., Hu X., Yang F., Bei J. & Wang S. (2007). Combining oxygen plasma treatment with anchorage of cationized gelatin for enhancing cell affinity of poly(lactide-co-glycolide). *Biomaterials*, Vol. 28, No. 29, pp. 4219-4230.

Shinonaga Y. & Arita K. (2009). Surface modification of stainless steel by plasma-based fluorine and silver dual ion implantation and deposition. *Dental Materials Journal*, Vol. 28, No. 6, pp. 735-742.

Sperling C., König U., Hermel G., Werner C., Müller M., Simon F., Grundke K., Jacobasch H.J., Vasilets V.N. & Ikada Y. (1997). Immobilization of human thrombomodulin onto PTFE. *Journal of Materials Science: Materials in Medicine*, Vol. 8, No. 12, pp. 789-791.

Tang Q., Brooks R., Rushton N. & Best S. (2010). Production and characterization of HA and SiHA coatings. *Journal of Materials Science: Materials in Medicine*, Vol. 21, No. 1, pp. 173-181.

Thissen H., Johnson G., Hartley P.G., Kingshott P. & Griesser H.J. (2006). Two-dimensional patterning of thin coatings for the control of tissue outgrowth. *Biomaterials*, Vol. 27, No. 1, pp. 35-43.

Thorwarth G., Falub C.V., Müller U., Weisse B., Voisard C., Tobler M. & Hauert R. (2010). Tribological behavior of DLC-coated articulating joint implants. *Acta Biomaterialia*, Vol. 6, No. 6, pp. 2335-2341.

van Delden C.J., Lens J.P., Kooyman R.P., Engbers G.H. & Feijen J. (1997). Heparinization of gas plasma-modified polystyrene surfaces and the interactions of these surfaces with proteins studied with surface plasmon resonance. *Biomaterials*, Vol. 18, No. 12, pp. 845-852.

Vasilets V.N., Hermel G., König U., Werner C., Müller M., Simon F., Grundke K., Ikada Y. & Jacobasch H.J. (1997). Microwave CO2 plasma-initiated vapour phase graft polymerization of acrylic acid onto polytetrafluoroethylene for immobilization of human thrombomodulin. *Biomaterials*, Vol. 18, No. 17, pp. 1139-1145.

Vasilev K., Simovic S., Losic D., Griesser H.J., Griesser S., Anselme K. & Ploux L. (2010a). Platforms for controlled release of antibacterial agents facilitated by plasma polymerization. *Conference Proceedings of the IEEE Engineering in Medicine and Biology Society*, pp. 811-814.

Vasilev K., Sah V.R., Goreham R.V., Ndi C., Short R.D. & Griesser H.J. (2010). Antibacterial surfaces by adsorptive binding of polyvinyl-sulphonate-stabilized silver nanoparticles. *Nanotechnology*, Vol. 21, No. 21, paper 215102.

Walschus U., Hoene A., Neumann H.-G., Wilhelm L., Lucke S., Lüthen F., Rychly J. & Schlosser M. (2009). Morphometric immunohistochemical examination of the inflammatory tissue reaction after implantation of calcium phosphate-coated titanium plates in rats. *Acta Biomaterialia*, Vol. 5, No. 2, pp. 776-784.

Wang G., Liu X., Gao J. & Ding C. (2009). In vitro bioactivity and phase stability of plasma-sprayed nanostructured 3Y-TZP coatings. *Acta Biomaterialia*, Vol. 5, No. 6, pp. 2270-2278.

Wang G., Meng F., Ding C., Chu P.K. & Liu X. (2010). Microstructure, bioactivity and osteoblast behavior of monoclinic zirconia coating with nanostructured surface. *Acta Biomaterialia*, Vol. 6, No. 3, pp. 990-1000.

Wu C., Ramaswamy Y., Liu X., Wang G. & Zreiqat H. (2009). Plasma-sprayed CaTiSiO5 ceramic coating on Ti-6Al-4V with excellent bonding strength, stability and cellular bioactivity. *Journal of the Royal Society Interface*, Vol. 6, No. 31, pp. 159-168.

Yang Z., Wang J., Luo R., Maitz M.F., Jing F., Sun H. & Huang N. (2010). The covalent immobilization of heparin to pulsed-plasma polymeric allylamine films on 316L stainless steel and the resulting effects on hemocompatibility. *Biomaterials*, Vol. 31, No. 8, pp. 2072-2083.

Ye S.H., Johnson C.A. Jr., Woolley J.R., Oh H.I., Gamble L.J., Ishihara K. & Wagner W.R. (2009). Surface modification of a titanium alloy with a phospholipid polymer prepared by a plasma-induced grafting technique to improve surface thromboresistance. *Colloids and Surfaces B: Biointerfaces*, Vol. 74, No. 1, pp. 96-102.

Yoshinari M., Hayakawa T., Matsuzaka K., Inoue T., Oda Y., Shimono M., Ide T. & Tanaka T. (2006). Oxygen plasma surface modification enhances immobilization of simvastatin acid. *Biomedical Research*, Vol. 27, No. 1, pp. 29-36.

Zhang W., Chu P.K., Ji J., Zhang Y., Liu X., Fu R.K., Ha P.C. & Yan Q. (2006). Plasma surface modification of poly vinyl chloride for improvement of antibacterial properties. *Biomaterials*, Vol. 27, No. 1, pp. 44-51.

Zhang W., Zhang Y., Ji J., Yan Q., Huang A. & Chu PK. (2007). Antimicrobial polyethylene with controlled copper release. *Journal of Biomedical Materials Research Part A*, Vol. 83, No. 3, pp. 838-844.

Zhang W., Luo Y., Wang H., Jiang J., Pu S. & Chu PK. (2008). Ag and Ag/N2 plasma modification of polyethylene for the enhancement of antibacterial properties and cell growth/proliferation. *Acta Biomaterialia*, Vol. 4, No. 6, pp. 2028-2036.

Zhao J.H., Michalski W.P., Williams C., Li L., Xu H.S., Lamb P.R., Jones S., Zhou Y.M. & Dai X.J. (2011). Controlling cell growth on titanium by surface functionalization of heptylamine using a novel combined plasma polymerization mode. *Journal of Biomedical Materials Research Part A*, Vol. 87, No. 2, pp. 127-134.

6

Elasticity of Spider Dragline Silks Viewed as Nematics: Yielding Induced by Isotropic-Nematic Phase Transition

Linying Cui[1], Fei Liu[2] and Zhong-can Ou-Yang[2]
[1]Department of Physics, Tsinghua University, Beijing,
[2]Center for Advanced Study, Tsinghua University, Beijing,
China

1. Introduction

Spider dragline silk (SDS), the main structural web silk regarded as the "spider's lifeline", exhibits a fascinating combination of high tensile strength and high extensibility (1). Its toughness is over 10 times that of Kevlar, the material for making bullet-proof suits (2). In addition, SDS has a unconventional sigmoidal shaped stress-strain curve and shape memory capability after the tension and torsion test (3; 4) (Figure 1). All these intriguing properties have aroused the broad interest of scientists to understand the underlying deformation mechanism of SDS.

Leaving the open question of why SDS is that mechanically superb aside, people have already started to produce artificial SDS for numerous applications. Various methods to spin artificial SDS have been explored. These include conventional wet spinning of regenerated SDS obtained through forced silking (5; 6), solvent spinning of recombinant SDS protein analogue produced via bacteria and yeast cell cultures doped with chemically synthesized artificial genes (6; 7), and spinning of silk monofilaments from aqueous solution of recombinant SDS protein obtained by inserting the silk-producing genes into mammalian cells (6; 8). The applications also cover a broad biomedical range. For example, the silk-silica fusion proteins was used for bone regeneration by combining the self-assembling domains of SDS (*Nephila clavipes*) as scaffolds and the silaffin-derived R5 peptide of *Cylindrotheca fusiformis* that is responsible for silica mineralization (6; 9). Improved cell adhesion and proliferation of mouse osteoblast (MC3T3-E1) cells was achieved with films composed of *B. mori* fibroin and recombinantly produced proteins based upon *N. clavipes* SDS (incorporating the RGD integrin recognition sequence) *in vitro* (6; 10). SDS based antibacteria materials was also demonstrated by incorporating silk proteins with inorganic antibacteria nanoparticles such as silver nanoparticles (11) and titanium dioxide nanoparticles (12). In addition, silk films are promising candidates for biocompatible coatings for biomedical implants. For instance, gold nanoparticles, silver nanoparticles, and transition metal oxides/sulfides were dip-coated by SDS proteins and showed novel electrical, magnetic, optical properties, and at the same time, biocompatibility (6; 13–16).

Going back to the fundamental question of the structure-property relation of SDS, several experimental studies have been carried out to determine the supra-molecular structure of

SDS (17–22). X-ray diffraction patterns showed that there are many well oriented beta-sheet nanocrystals in the silk, with the long axis of the beta-sheet parallel to the silk axis (17–19). And polarized FTIR spectroscopy and Raman spectroscopy revealed more structures beyond the beta-sheet nanocrystal, including beta-coils, beta-turns, alpha-helices or the more compact and left-handed 3(1)-helices, all of which have quite low orientation in un-stressed SDS (1; 23–26). NMR data also suggested that there are two regions in SDS, a highly oriented beta-sheet nanocrystal region and a poorly oriented polypeptide chain region (22; 27; 28).Furthermore, these structural study results were confirmed by the protein sequence analysis (20; 29). Based on all these results, it is generally accepted that SDS is semicrystalline polymer with beta-sheet nanocrystals embedded in the amorphous region, which was a polypeptide chain network (23; 24; 30) (Figure 2(a)). The beta-sheet nanocrystals were always highly oriented to the axis of SDS, while the polypeptide chain network exhibited random orientation under zero external stress (19). When SDS was subjected to external tension stress, the orientation of the components in the polypeptide chain network was observed to increase significantly as the strain increased (17; 25; 28).

A few models were proposed (18; 23; 30; 31) to understand the structure-property relation of SDS based upon deformation theories of polymers and composite materials. For example, the model by Termonia (23) treated SDS as a hydrogen-bonded amorphous matrix embedded with stiff crystals as cross-links. In the interfacial region, an extremely high modulus is required to get SDS's overall behavior on deformation. While in the model of Porter and Vollrath (30; 31), parameters linking to chemical compositions and morphological order were used to interpret thermo-mechanical properties of SDS. But some parameters such as ordered/disordered fractions are difficult to be obtained from experiments. A recent model (18) connecting deformations on the macroscopic and molecular length scales still did not consider the change of the orientation of nanocomposites during deformation. Especially, as pointed out by Vehoff *at al.* recently (32), basic polymer theories such as the freely jointed chain, the freely rotating chain and the worm-like chain, as well as a hierarchical chain model of the spider capture silk (33) could not reproduce the sigmoidal shape or even the steep initial regime of SDS (Fig. 2(a)) (32). While nonlinear polymer theories can give a general description of the entire deformation process of the silk, some special conditions are invoked (30; 31) and the uniqueness in SDS is not taken into account. In one word, a more natural and unified description for the extraordinary properties of SDS as a model biomaterial still seems to be lacking.

Quite a few works (4; 17; 19; 22; 34–37) have pointed out that SDS is liquid crystalline material and liquid crystal (LC) phase plays a vital role in both its spinning process and mechanical properties. In the spinning process, the spider's 'spinning dope' is liquid crystalline, which make it possible to efficiently spin a thread from large silk protein molecules (4; 38–40). Specifically, in the spider's gland and duct the molecules form a nematic phase (4; 38) — a phase that makes the silk solution flow as a liquid but maintain some of the orientational order characteristic of a crystal, with the long axes of neighboring molecules aligned approximately parallel to one another. In the final extrusion stage of the spinning process, the liquid crystal phase is even more enhanced and frozen into the beta-sheet structure of the silk: The forming thread stretches, narrows and pulls away from the walls of the duct, which bring the dope molecules into better alignment and into a more extended conformation to facilitate hydrogen bonds formation to give the anti-parallel beta conformation of the final thread (4; 38). The final silk contains 40 vol % anti-parallel beta-nanocrystals highly aligned to the silk axis as a frozen LC phase from the spinning process (31).

For the solid SDS, the LC phase transition is an important feature in SDS's deformation process and contributes a lot to the silk's combination of high strength and high extensibility, as well as the shape memory property. In the unstressed state of SDS, the polypeptide chain network has random orientation (25) with many components present, such as beta-coils, beta-turns, alpha-helices or the more compact and left-handed 3(1)-helices (1; 22–24; 26). All of these structures have elongated shapes and the tendency to form LC phase (41). Under increasing tensile stress, the orientations of the elongated components increase substantially as revealed by polarized FTIR spectroscopy and DECODER (direction exchange with correlation for orientation distribution evaluation and reconstruction) NMR (25; 28). The sigmoidal shape of the stress-strain curve (Figure 1(a)) indicates that a LC phase transition takes place at the yield point, resulting in the huge extensibility of SDS after the yield point.

Although some work proposed SDS to be a biological LC elastomer together with the silkworm's silk (37), a detailed description of the deformation mechanism of SDS from the LC point of view is lacking. We constructed an analytical LC model. The polypeptide chain network is set to be in the isotropic state at the beginning with the tendency to transit into the LC phase. Under external stress, the Maier-Saupe theory (42) of nematic LC is employed to monitor the change of the orientation of the polypeptide chain network. We show that during deformation SDS undergoes significant increase of the orientation of the chain network, with a force-induced isotropic-nematic phase transition at the yield point which especially facilitates the extension of the SDS after the yield point. The comprehensive agreement between theory and experiments on the stress-strain curve strongly indicates SDS to belong to LC materials. Especially, the remarkable yielding elasticity of SDS is understood for the first time as the force-induced isotropic-nematic phase transition of the chain network. The present theory also predicts a drop of the stress in supercontracted SDS, an early found effect of humidity on the mechanical properties in many silks (30; 32; 43).

2. Model

Because the beta-sheet nanocrystal has high orientation along the silk axis as spun and deforms much smaller than that of the bulk (17), we will neglect the deformation and rotation of the beta-sheet nanocrystal under external stress and focus on the deformation change of the amorphous polypeptide chain network in the current work. This assumption is also supported by the observations that SDS's high extensibility results primarily from the disordered region (18; 20; 21), and that the deformation of the beta-sheet nanocrystal is at least a factor of 10 smaller than that of the bulk (17).

We take the polypeptide chain network in the amorphous region of SDS as a molecular LC field with each chain section corresponding to a mesogenic molecule (i.e. a molecule having the tendency to form liquid crystal phase under specific conditions); see Fig. 2. Following the LC continuum theory in the absence of forces, the potential of a mesogenic molecule takes the Maier-Saupe interaction form (42)

$$V(\cos \theta) = -aS\left(\frac{3}{2}\cos^2 \theta - \frac{1}{2}\right), \tag{1}$$

where θ is the angle between the long axis of the molecule and the silk axis (the z-axis), which is also the direction of $\hat{n}$ (Fig. 2 (b)). a is the strength of the mean field. S is the orientation order parameter of the LC, defined as the average of second Legendre polynomial (41)

$$S = \left\langle \frac{3}{2}\cos^2\theta - \frac{1}{2} \right\rangle. \tag{2}$$

We notice that the Maier-Saupe potential has been used by Pincus and de Gennes when investigating LC phase transition in a polypeptide solution (44). Using the LC potential to describe the interaction between the segments of the polypeptide chain network is a good mean-field approach because a large part of the polypeptide chain network bears alpha helix and beta coil structures (20; 24), which tend to form a LC phase due to their elongated shape (41). When a uniform force field f along z-axis is applied, the potential of a molecule is written as

$$U(\cos\theta) = V - fl\cos\theta, \tag{3}$$

where l denotes the length of the mesogenic molecule.
From the definition of the order parameter S, we get a self-consistency equation

$$S = \int_{-1}^{1}(\frac{3}{2}\cos^2\theta - \frac{1}{2})\exp(\frac{3aS}{2k_BT}\cos^2\theta + \alpha\cos\theta)d\cos\theta \\ \Big/ \int_{-1}^{1}\exp(\frac{3aS}{2k_BT}\cos^2\theta + \alpha\cos\theta)d\cos\theta\,, \tag{4}$$

with $\alpha = fl/k_BT$. The solution of the above equation may not be unique, in order to obtain physically sound solution we need to apply the free energy minimization criterion (41) given by

$$F_{MS} = -k_BT\ln Z + \frac{1}{2}aS^2, \tag{5}$$

where Z is the partition function $Z = \int_{-1}^{1}e^{-U(\cos\theta)/k_BT}d\cos\theta$, and the second term at the right-hand side corrects for the double counting arising from the mean field method (45).
The orientation function S was calculated numerically at different temperatures $T^* = T/T_{ni}$ and forces f, and the results were shown in Fig. 3(b). Here $T_{ni} = a/(4.541k_B)$ is the isotropic-nematic transition temperature in the absence of forces (42). At temperatures below T_{ni} the molecules have spontaneous nematic order, and the force does not induce further order significantly. While for the molecules initially in paranematic state (i.e. an isotropic state close to the nematic state), the applied force field will induce a first-order phase transition — S jumps discontinuously to a higher value at a certain critical force $f_C(T^*)$. At even higher temperatures, nematic field is weaker and the effect of the force is less dramatic.
To compare with experiment data, we give the expressions of stress and strain in our model. Apparently, the stress σ of the bulk is $\sigma \equiv F/A = Nf$: F is the force on the surface of the bulk, A is the area of the surface, and N is the number of molecules per area. The strain ε of the bulk is defined as $\varepsilon = [L(f) - L_0]/L_0$, where $L(f)$ is the length of the bulk along z-axis when the force field f is applied and we can take it as $L(f) = \langle l|\cos\theta|\rangle$, and $L_0 = L(f = 0) = l/2$. Then the strain ε is $\varepsilon = 2\langle|\cos\theta|\rangle - 1$. The curve of ε versus σ at different temperatures is shown in Fig. 3(c). At temperatures below T_{ni}, the strain grows smoothly with the stress. For temperatures just above T_{ni}, the strain grows with the stress in an almost linear way under small forces, then a jump in the strain occurs at the critical force $f_C(T^*)$, after which the strain increases smoothly with the stress again. At higher temperatures, the nematic field is weaker

and the jump is replaced by a smooth increase in strain, with a plateau in a certain range of force.

In our model, the reduced temperature T^* is an essential parameter, which needs to be chosen specifically in order to predict the stress-strain curve of SDS. Because the silk solution is in LC state at ambient temperature (4; 34; 35) while for the solid silk the orientation of the polypeptide chain network is very low (25), it is likely that the solid polypeptide chain network still has a high tendency to form LC state and is in paranematic state under zero loading. Namely, the isotropic-nematic transition temperature T_{ni} of the chain network is slightly lower than the room temperature T_r, i. e. T^* is just above 1. Actually, the curves of $T^* = 1.01$ and 1.02 agree well with the experimental stress-strain curve of SDS, with a steep linear relation at the beginning and more abrupt increase of the strain after the yield point. Due to viscoelasticity (46), defects and polydomain effects (45), the real SDS exhibit a smoother strain increase after the yield point, while the non-viscoelastic and defect-free LC model predicts an abrupt increase of the strain. From the curves of $T^* = 1.01$ and 1.02, we get the estimation of the yield strain $\varepsilon_y \approx 0.04$, the yield stress $\sigma_y = \alpha N k_B T / l \approx 8.4\text{MPa}$, and the Young's modulus at the linear region $E \equiv \sigma_y / \varepsilon_y \approx 210\text{MPa}$, given $\alpha \sim 0.2$, $N/l \sim 10\text{nm}^{-3}$, and $k_B T_r \sim 4.1\text{pNnm}$. These estimations well agree with the experimental results for the low reeling speed SDS, with the yield strain $\varepsilon_y \approx 0.04$, the yield stress $\sigma_y \approx 10\text{MPa}$, and the Young's modulus at the linear region $E \approx 250\text{MPa}$ (Fig. 3(d)) (19).

3. Discussion

The stress-strain curve of paranematic state in the LC model well explains the main features of the stress-strain curve of SDS: With low loading, entropy is dominating and the polypeptide chain network is isotropic. Mesogenic molecules only respond individually to the external stress field by rotating a little bit to the stress direction on average, so the increase of the strain is small and the Young's modulus is high. As the stress increases, the competition between the entropy and the mesogenic molecule potential (including the LC field and the external force field) in the free energy expression (Eq. 3 and 5) begins to favor the potential field. At the point when the potential begins to dominate over the entropy, the isotropic-nematic phase transition of the mesogenic molecule network (i.e. the polypeptide chain network) occurs. Mesogenic molecules start to rotate collectively to the stress direction to form the nematic LC phase. Since all components in the polypeptide chain network tend to align parallel to the silk axis, the length of the silk increases substantially under a constant stress, resulting in the plateau following the transition initiation point which is called the yield point. Due to viscoelasticity (46), defects and polydomain effects (45), the real SDS has a smoother plateau in the stress-strain curve with the same fact that the majority of the SDS's extensibility results from the softening plateau after the yield point. When the stress increases further, the orientation of the network grows rapidly, as observed by polarized FTIR spectroscopy and DECODER (direction exchange with correlation for orientation distribution evaluation and reconstruction) NMR (25; 28). Finally, the shape memory property of SDS in the tension test can be understood as a reverse phase transition process when the external stress decreases to zero.

In the LC model, we predict an isotropic-nematic phase transition at the yield point. Several experimental observations do support a significant increase of the orientation of the elongated components in the amorphous region with various strain. For example, a polarized FTIR spectroscopy measurement (25) showed that the orientation of some components in the amorphous region increased by 0.3 when the strain reached 24%. A NMR study also suggested the alignment of the components in the amorphous region became poor in the strain relaxation process (28). Further experimental work needs be done to track the orientation change of the polypeptide chain network in the deformation process of SDS in order to better understand its LC character.

We notice that our results agree much better with the mechanical properties of the silks produced by low reeling speed. That is because a high reeling speed will induce a low orientation in the amorphous region, which is not taken into account in the current work.

In addition to describing the stress-strain relation of SDS, our LC model can also qualitatively account for the drop of the stress in wet SDS, i.e. the supercontracted SDS. Take L_0 and R_0 as the initial length and radius of the silk, and L and R as those under stress. Under the assumption of volume conservation we have $\pi R_0^2 L_0 = \pi R^2 L$, so $R/R_0 = \sqrt{1/(1+\varepsilon)}$. The free energy of the bulk can be written as

$$
\begin{aligned}
F &= V - f_{ext}(L - L_0) + 2\pi R L \gamma \\
  &= V - f_{ext}(L - L_0) + 2\pi R_0 L_0 \gamma \sqrt{1+\varepsilon},
\end{aligned}
\tag{6}
$$

where V is the internal energy of the bulk, f_{ext} is the external force on the bulk and γ is the surface energy coefficient. Minimizing F with respect to ε, we get

$$
\sigma = \frac{f_{ext}}{\pi R_0^2} = \frac{1}{\pi R_0^2 L_0}\frac{\partial V}{\partial \varepsilon} + \frac{\gamma}{R_0\sqrt{1+\varepsilon}}.
\tag{7}
$$

When the silk is immersed in water, the surface energy coefficient γ increases, so with the same stress σ we need a bigger strain. Thus our theory can predict the softening of supercontracted silk, an effect observed in many experiments (30; 32; 43; 47; 48).

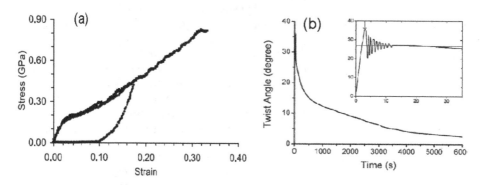

Fig. 1. (a). The stress-strain curves of a spider silk in a deformation cycle and during strain to break. (31) (b). Relaxation dynamics of a torsion pendulum for a spider silk thread. Inset: zoom of the start of the self-relaxation dynamics. The red arrow indicates the end of the excitation and the start of the free relaxation period. Blue line, new equilibrium position. (3)

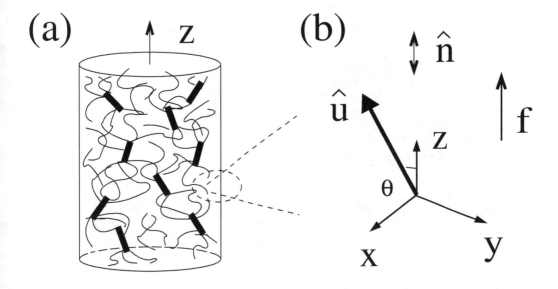

Fig. 2. (a). A schematic diagram of the structure of the dragline silk. The bold lines represent the β-sheet crystals, and the thin lines represent the polypeptide chains in the amorphous region. The z-axis is along the silk axis. (b). The coordinate system of the nematics. n̂ is the director of the nematics, û is the director of the mesogenic molecule, and θ is the angle between the long axis of the molecule and the silk axis z.

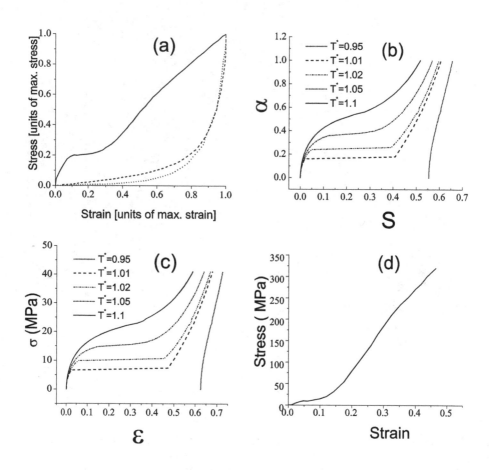

Fig. 3. (Color online.) (a) Comparison of a typical measured dragline silk's stress-strain curve (black solid line) with theoretical curves evaluated by the freely jointed chain (red dash dot line) and the hierarchical chain model (olive dash line) [After T. Vehoff *et al.*]. (b) The orientation order parameter S as a function of $\alpha(= fl/k_BT)$. (c) The stress-strain curves at different temperatures $T^*(= T/T_{ni})$. Calculated with $N/l \sim 10\text{nm}^{-3}$, and $k_BT_r \sim 4.1\text{pNnm}$. (d) The stress-strain curve of the SDS spinned with the speed of 1mms^{-1} (19).

4. Conclusion

In conclusion, we investigate the mechanical properties of SDS from the view point of LC continuum theory. This LC approach is justified by the following considerations: 1) Solid SDS is spined from a polypeptide LC solution and has well aligned beta-sheet nanocrystals as a frozen-in LC phase (36). 2) A large part of the amorphous region (the polypeptide chain network) of the solid SDS has alpha-helix and beta-coils secondary structures, which tend to form LC phase due to their elongated shape (41). 3) By solving a self-consistent equation, both the stress-strain relation and the orientation-reduced temperature relation are obtained from the LC model. These curves agree well with the experimental curves quantitatively and especially help to interpret the high extensibility behavior of SDS at the yield point. 4) The LC model can also describe the shape memory and the supercontraction properties of SDS. 5) The major energy term, the Maier-Saupe potential (41), in the LC model shares the same physical background with the essential energy contributor, the cohesive energy, in polymer theory (31; 49). They both origin from van der Waals forces, although with different emphasis: The LC model focuses on understanding the orientation change and the contribution of LC phase transition to the high extensibility of SDS; while the conventional polymer theories emphasize on either phenomenological descriptions (18) or molecular modelings with high computation requirements (31).

Ongoing work is to develop the model to understand more of the fascinating properties of SDS. More experimental work is highly needed as well to further verify the LC model.

5. References

[1] J. M. Gosline, M. W. Denny, and M. E. Demont, Nature **309**, 551 (1984).

[2] I. Agnarsson, M. Kuntner, T. A. Blackledge, PLoS ONE**5**, e11234 (2010).

[3] O. Emile, A. L. Floch, and F. Vollrath, Nature **440**, 621 (2006).

[4] F. Vollrath and D. P. Knight, Nature **410**, 541 (2001).

[5] M. Kang M, and H. J. Jin, Colloid. Polym. Sci.**285**, 1163 (2007).

[6] J. G. Hardy, and T. R. Scheibel, Prog. Polym. Sci.**35**, 1093 (2010).

[7] C. Fu, Z. Shao, F. Vollrath, Chem. Mater., 6515 (2009).

[8] H. Kim *et al.*, J. Nanosci. Nanotechnol.**8**, 5543 (2008).

[9] A. J. Mieszawska *et al.*, Chem. Mater.**22**, 5780 (2010).

[10] A. W. Morgan *et al.*, Biomaterials**29**, 2556 (2008).

[11] M. Kang *et al.*, J. Nanosci. Nanotechnol.**7**, 3888 (2007).

[12] Y. Xia, G. Gao, and Y. Li, J. Biomed. Mater. Res. Part B**90**, 653 (2009).

[13] A. Singh, S. Hede, and M. Sastry, Small**3**, 466 (2007).

[14] Y. Zhou *et al.*, Chem. Commun.**23**, 2518 (2001).

[15] N. Kukreja *et al.*, Pharmacol Res**57**, 171 (2008).

[16] H. S. Yin, S. Y. Ai, W. J. Shi, and L. S. Zhu, Sens. Actuators B**137**, 747 (2009).

[17] A. Glisąeovic, T. Vehoff, R. J. Davies, and T. Salditt, Macromolecules **41**, 390 (2008).

[18] I. Krasnov *et al.*, Phys. Rev. Lett. **100**, 048104 (2008).

[19] N. Du *et al.*, Biophys. J. **91**, 4528 (2006).

[20] C. Y. Hayashi and R. V. Lewis, J. Mol. Biol. **275**, 773 (1998).

[21] E. Oroudjev *et al.*, Proc. Natl. Acad. Sci. USA **99**, 6460 (2002).

[22] A. H. Simmons, C. A. Michal, and L. W. Jelinski, Science **271**, 84 (1996).

[23] Y. Termonia, Macromolecules **27**, 7378 (1994).

[24] T. Lefevre, M. E. Rousseau, and M. Pezolet, Biophys. J. **92**, 2885 (2007).

[25] P. Papadopoulos, J. Solter, and F. Kremer, Eur. Phys. J. E **24**, 193 (2007).

[26] J. Kummerlen *et al.*, Macromolecules **29**, 2920 (1996).

[27] J. Beek *et al.*, Proc. Natl. Acad. Sci. USA **99**, 10266 (2002).

[28] P. T. Eles and C. A. Michal, Biomacromolecules **5**, 661 (2004).

[29] M. Xu, and R. V. Lewis, Proc. Natl. Acad. Sci. USA **87**, 7120 (1990).

[30] F. Vollrath and D. Porter, Soft Matter **2**, 377 (2006).

[31] D. Porter, F. Vollrath, and Z. Shao, Eur. Phys. J. E **16**, 199 (2005).

[32] T. Vehoff, A. Gliąęsoviąäc, H. Schollmeyer, A. Zippelius, and T. Salditt, Biophys. J. **93**, 4425 (2007).

[33] H. J. Zhou and Y. Zhang, Phys. Rev. Lett. **94**, 028104 (2005).

[34] K. Kerkam, C. Viney, D. Kaplan, and S. Lombardi, Nature **349**, 596 (1991).

[35] P. J. Willcox, S. P. Gido, W. Muller, and D. L. Kaplan, Macromolecules **29**, 5106 (1996).

[36] E. T. Samulski, Liquid Crystalline Order in Polymers, edited by A. Blumstein, (Academic Press, New York, 1978), Chap. 5, p. 186.

[37] D. P. Knight and F. Vollrath, Phil. Trans. R. Soc. Lond. B **357**, 155 (2002).

[38] D. Knight and F. Vollrath, Proc. R. Soc. Lond. B **266**, 519 (1996).

[39] K. Kerkam *et al.*, Nature **349**, 596 (1991).

[40] P. J. Wilcox *et al.*, Macromolecules **29**, 5106 (1996).

[41] P. G. de Gennes, J. Prost, The Physics of Liquid Crystals(2nd edt), (Clarendon Press, Oxford, 1993).

[42] W. Maier and A. Saupe, Z. Naturforsch. A., 14, 882 (1959).

[43] F. I. Bell, I. J. McEwen, and C. Viney, Nature **416**, 37 (2002).

[44] P. Pincus and P. G. de Gennes, J. Polymer Sciences: Polymer Symposium **65**, 85 (1978).

[45] M. Warner, E. M. Terentjev, Liquid Crystal Elastomers, (Clarendon Press, Oxford, 2003).

[46] R. W. Work, J. exp. Biol. **118**, 379 (1985).

[47] R. W. Work, Textile Res. J. **47**, 650 (1977).

[48] R. W. Work, J. Arachnol. **9**, 299 (1981).

[49] D. Porter, Group Interaction Modelling og Polymer Properties, (Marcel Dekker, New York, 1995).

Part 2

Polymer-Based Nanomedicine for Targeted Therapy

7

Nanocrystalline Diamond Films: Applications and Advances in Nanomedicine

Ying-Chieh Chen[1,2], Don-Ching Lee[1] and Ing-Ming Chiu[1,3,4*]

[1]*Institute of Cellular and System Medicine, National Health Research Institutes, Miaoli,*
[2]*Center for Biomedical Engineering, Department of Medicine,*
Brigham and Women's Hospital, Harvard Medical School, Boston,
[3]*Department of Life Sciences, National Chung Hsing University, Taichung*
[4]*Department of Internal Medicine, The Ohio State University, Columbus*
[1,3]*Taiwan*
[2,4]*USA*

1. Introduction

Biomaterials play essential roles in modern strategies in regenerative medicine and tissue engineering by designable biophysical and biochemical cues that direct cellular behavior and function [1-4]. The guidance provided by biomaterials may improve restoration and function of damaged or nonfunctional tissues both in cell-based therapies, such as those where carriers deliver transplanted cells or matrices induce morphogenesis in bioengineered tissues constructed *ex vivo*, and in cellular therapies, such as those where materials induce growth and differentiation of cells from healthy residual tissues *in situ* [3, 5-7].

Stem cells are defined by their ability to self-renew and produce specialized progeny [8, 9]. Consequently, they are the most versatile and promising cell source for the regeneration of aged, injured and diseased tissues. According to their developmental status, stem cells can be classified into two categories: embryonic stem cells and adult stem cells. However, despite the remarkable potential clinical applications of each of these stem-cell populations, their use is currently limited. Thus, a major goal is to develop new culture based approaches, using advanced biomaterials, that more closely mimic what the body already does so well, to promote differentiation of pluripotent cells [3].

Nanomedicine, the application of nanotechnology for medical purpose, is emerging as a new interdisciplinary research field, cutting across biology, chemistry, engineering and medicine. It is expected to lead major advances in disease detection, diagnosis, treatment and further to replacement of damaged tissues and organs. Over the past two decades, there have been significant advances in disease diagnostics, drug delivery, stem cell therapy and tissue engineering. In parallel, nanotechnology has shown great potential for the creation of the next generation of new biomaterials.

Biomaterials that promote regeneration are important in both research and clinical applications [10]. However, current implants have a limited life-expectancy, and younger patients who receive them generally expect to endure revision surgeries to replace worn components. A primary problem with current designs is the generation of wear debris particles at the articulating surface that causes local pain and inflammation. Large debris are normally sequestered by fibrous tissue, while small debris are taken up by macrophages and multinucleated giant cells which may release cytokines that result in inflammation. Thus, the proposed solution for the problem caused by wear debris is to develop durable materials for the articulating surfaces that are more wear resistant, which would reduce the generation of debris particles.

Recently, it was shown that diamond particles (NDs), the diamond structure at a nanometer scale (4-5 nm in size), appear to possess high bioactivity at the molecular level, presenting antioxidant and anticarcinogenic properties. Functionalization of NDs with biological molecules, such as peptides, proteins and nucleic acid, has led to practical significance for biomedical applications, covering their use for single particle imaging in cells, drug delivery and protein separation. For instance, carboxylated nanodiamond has been shown as a useful probe for detecting and labeling the interaction of nanoparticles and bio-objects such as cells and bacteria [11], because NDs can be easily functionalized to conjugate with bio-molecules and can emit bright fluorescence without photobleaching [12-15]. Moreover, the ND particles were phagocytosed into cells by macropinocytosis and clathrin-mediated endocytosis pathways during tracking of cells. However, cell growth ability such as cell division and differentiation were not altered after long-term cell culture for 10 days. Together, NDs are non-cytotoxic and with bright fluorescence, thus has served as a versatile tool in biosensing and bioimaging applications [12, 16].

Diamond has been one of the most desired and investigated materials in the past years. From an extensive list of superlative properties, the ultra-hardness, the chemical inertness, the high thermal conductivity, and the high optical transparency are just a few examples of its remarkable nature. Applications such as cutting tools, abrasives, structural components, heat sinks, bearings, and optical windows (X-ray, IR, and laser windows) are examples that diamond has a wide-ranging impact in many fields.

2. Nanodiamond films

In the late 1980s, polycrystalline diamond films with fine grains were grown for optical coatings [17, 18], wear resistant coatings [19], high-pressure synchrotron X-ray windows [20] and X-ray lithography masks [21]. The first reference to these materials as 'nanocrystalline' was at the Workshop on the Science and Technology of Diamond Films in 1990 [17]. Most of these materials would now be classified as forms of nanocrystalline diamond (NCD) and further characterized the presence of large intrinsic stress and non-diamond phases in these material [22-25]. These NCD materials were all grown in hydrogen-rich chemical vapour deposition (CVD) environments, with typically less than 2% methane (or hydrocarbon) in hydrogen as reactants, exhibiting clusters (cauliflower morphologies), limited surface smoothness, high compressive stress, delamination, and high content of non-diamond phase. NCD was deposited on Si or other substrates which had been 'treated' or 'seeded' to increase the diamond nucleation density [26, 27]. This wet seeding process was in solution containing diamond powder for ultrasonication to create necessary nucleation sites and the process was varied among labs and individuals [28, 29]. By controlling nucleation density and growth conditions, grain sizes were usually 5-150 nm for films less than several μm thick. In 1994, Gruen and coworkers [30-32] developed the growth of nanocrystalline diamond films by CVD under hydrogen-poor and carbon-containing argon gas plasmas conditions. In 1999 [33], this new material was reviewed under the label of 'Nanocrystalline

Diamond Films'. In 2001 [34], the label ultra-nanocrystalline diamond films (UNCD) came to be applied to these materials in order to distinguish them from the more traditional NCD films discussed above [35]. The nanocrystallinity is the result of new growth and nucleation mechanisms, which involve the insertion of C_2, carbon dimer, into carbon-carbon and carbon-hydrogen bonds, resulting in heterogeneous nucleation rates on the order 10^{10} cm^2 s^{-1} [26, 29]. Detailed investigations using synchrotron-based, near-edge X-ray absorption fine-structure spectroscopy (NEXAFS) showed that UNCD films grown using this seeding approach and growth chemistry are of very high quality, with greater than 99% sp^3 bonding [33]. The UNCD films, a form of NCD, has led to applications in micro-electromechanical systems (MEMS) and nano-electromechanical systems (NEMS) [36-38], corrosion resistance [39], biocompatible coatings [40-42], and biosensors [16, 43, 44].

Diamond coatings with nanosized crystallites, NCD, present a great potential in biomedicine and biotechnology. NCD combines surface smoothness with high corrosion resistance and biotolerance, which are ideal features for applications in medicine onto surgical tools and medical implants. For example, joint implants coated with NCD can take benefit of its protective character. The NCD coating acts as a selective protective barrier between the implant and the human environment, preventing the release of metallic ions into the body. NCD presents the highest resistance to bacterial colonization when compared to medical steel and titanium [45]. This property is very important since infection due to microbial colonization of the implant surface may lead to implant rejection. In addition, the high wear resistance and the low coefficient of friction of NCD allow the reduction of the amount of wear debris generated during the joint functioning, thus increasing the life of the prosthesis [46]. Further, the residues formed due to wear in this case are diamond particles, which are completely harmless, initiating little or no adverse reactions from human monocytes and polymorphonuclear leukocytes [47-49]. NCD is also included in this recent group of materials and can be used as a template for the immobilization of active molecules for biological applications or for biosensor applications [44, 50-52]. One example is the functionalization of NCD surface with bone morphogenetic protein-2 (BMP-2) creating a biomimetic coating that results in improved osseointegration, which is a powerful strategy in tissue engineering as well as in bone tissue regeneration [53]. The NCD surface can also be modified with the linking of antibody, human IgG, which provide biomolecular recognition capability and specificity characteristics, proving a biologically sensitive field-effect transistor (Bio-FET) [44].

This paper offers a review of present knowledge of the synthesis and characterization, cell behavior, focused on *in vitro* adhesion, proliferation and differentiation on nanodiamond films. The aim is to highlight nanodiamond films as new generation biomaterials for improving the future development on clinical transplantation and tissue engineering.

3. Surface modifications

Cellular adhesion is of fundamental importance in many biological processes as the adhered cells will sense, interpret, integrate, and then respond to the extracellular signals. Chemical and physical signals from the substrate such as surface energy, topography, electrostatic charge, and wettability play a vital role in stimulating cell adhesion and influencing cell growth behavior. The cellular adhesion properties of as-grown diamond surfaces or functionalized diamond surfaces have been studied recently. The as-grown diamond films were characterized as hydrophobic surfaces with abundance of C-C and C-H bonds [54].

The functionalized surface properties of diamond can be made hydrophobic or hydrophilic with hydrogen or oxygen termination, respectively, which have implications for cellular adhesion. The methods of surface modifications are summarized as following:

1. Hydrogen termination (hydrophobic surface):
2. Diamond films were treated in pure hydrogen plasma treatment at 300-800 W in the microwave plasma CVD system at 5 mTorr for 2-15 min. All freshly prepared hydrogen-terminated diamond samples were used immediately for cell culture.[55-58]
3. Oxygen termination (hydrophilic surface):
    a. Diamond samples were exposed to UV irradiation (18 W, 254 nm) for 18 h in air. After UV functionalization, the samples were rinsed with ultrapure water, tetrahydrofuran, and finally with hexane.[55]
    b. Diamond films were exposed to pure oxygen plasma CVD system at 800 W at 5 mTorr for 10-15 min.[56, 58]
    c. Diamond films were oxidized in concentrated HNO_3 at 60-70° C for 24 hours. This oxidation reaction transformed the face of the film from hydrophobic to hydrophilic surface by adding carboxylate groups to the films. [59, 60]
4. Bio-molecular conjugation [61-64]

4. Nanodiamond-cell interaction: biological performance and response

Cell adhesion is involved in various natural phenomena such as embryogenesis, maintenance of tissue structure, wound healing, immune response, and tissue integration of biomaterial. The biocompatibility of biomaterials is very closely related to cell behavior on contact with them and particularly to cell adhesion to their surface. Surface characteristics of materials, such as their topography, chemistry, or surface energy, play an essential part in cell adhesion on biomaterials. Thus attachment, adhesion and spreading belong to the first phase of cell/material interactions and the quality of this phase will influence the cell's capacity to proliferate or to differentiate itself on contact with the implant. Material/cell interaction depends on the surface aspects of materials which may be described according to their wettability, topography, chemistry and surface energy. These surface characteristics determine how and what kinds of biological molecules will adhere to the surface and more particularly determine the orientation of adhered molecules, and also finally determine the cell behavior while in contact [3, 8, 65]. As previously shown, cells in contact with a surface will firstly attach, adhere and then spread. This first phase depends on specific adhesion proteins such as integrin and cadherin as demonstrated by Chen et al [66]. Thereafter, the quality of this adhesion will influence their morphology, and their capacity for proliferation and differentiation. Early *in vitro* biocompatibility and cytocompatibility studies focused on the morphology and growth capacity of cells on nanodiamond films with various chemical compositions and topographies [15, 53, 56, 58, 67, 68]. Recently, it was found that nanodiamond films further determine the differentiating stage in stem cells, which expands other possibilities for nanodiamond films into organ repair and tissue engineering.

4.1 Biocompatibility tests: morphological aspect and growth capacity of cells on nanodiamond films

NCD films possess numerous valuable physical, chemical and mechanical properties, making NCD an excellent material for implantable biomedical devices. There is still one very important property required for biomaterials, i.e., biocompatibility. The biocompatibility of a material is determined by *in vitro* and *in vivo* tests, involving the interaction of the material with cells.

In vitro studies of biocompatibility of UNCD coatings, produced by MPECVD using Ar/CH_4 as reactive gas, were carried out by Shi et al. [69]. They grew mouse embryonic fibroblasts (MEFs) on UNCD films up to 4 days and found that UNCD film coated substrates can dramatically promote the growth of MEFs, while the quartz substrates inhibit cell attachment. On growing human cervical carcinoma cell line (HeLa), neuronal cell line (PC12) and osteoblastic cells (MC3T3) on UNCD films, no toxicological effects on the cells in culture were observed. It was noted that maximum cell attachment, cell spreading and nuclear coverage were observed on UNCD films compared to two commonly used materials in MEMS platinum and silicon substrates [70]. Amaral et al performed bone marrow cell culture tests on NCD films, prepared by using a hot-filament chemical vapor deposition (HFCVD) technique in $Ar-CH_4-H_2$ gas mixtures, to observe its effects on cellular reaction, osteoblast, and osteoblast activity [71]. The nanometric feature of NCD resulted in increased bone cell proliferation and minimized activity of osteoclast-like cells. Following previous study, Amaral and coworkers cultured primary human gingival fibroblast cell cultures on NCD films for 21 days and no damage to the cells was observed. On performing the cytotoxicity tests using a standard cell line, it was found out that NCD films promotes cell attachment and normal cell growth rates [72]. Several other studies were made on the morphological behavior of mesenchymal stem cells on NCD coating prepared by MPECVD method in hydrogen-rich gas mixtures, which revealed good surface biocompatibility of the coatings [58] . Their investigations indicated that NCD coatings were biocompatible to not only cell lines, but also primary stem cells.

All these *in vitro* studies showed that NCD films tended to promote the growth and adhesion of cells without any toxicological effect. There are other applications where it is desirable that there should not be any cell attachment to a surface, for example, in case of catheters and temporary implants. After getting a primary indication of the biocompatibility of NCD films through *in vitro* tests, several *in vivo* studies were initiated by implants with NCD coating in laboratory animals. An attempt was made to study the osseous healing at the implant sites by inserting implants into 4-year-old female sheep calvaria for 3 days, 1 week and 4 weeks intervals. It was observed that implant surfaces coating with NCD films and then conjugating with BMP-2 enhanced osseointegration *in vivo*. After implanting NCD coated implants in transplantation sites of sheep for different time periods, it has been observed that the NCD-coated implants did not show any significant toxicological effect and are well tolerated in the sheep body. Results further suggest that this technical advancement can be readily applied in clinical therapies with regard to bone healing, since primary human mesenchymal stromal cells strongly activated the expression of osteogenic markers when being cultivated on NCD absorbed with physiological amounts of BMP-2 [73].

The above *in vitro* and *in vivo* studies indicated the biocompatibility of NCD films prepared by a variety of techniques. The general finding so far is that control of cell adhesion and proliferation on NCD can be achieved by altering NCD surface chemistry and surface topography and wettability, probably due to the correlation between these surface properties and the adsorption of endogenous proteins that regulate cell behavior. Adsorbed proteins can be detected on biomaterials within seconds of exposure to the blood, and a monolayer of adsorbed proteins forms in seconds to minutes. Fibronectin, vitronectin and laminin are pro-adhesive proteins, with relatively high concentration in blood, that are recognized by various cellular integrin receptors [74]. It has been observed that fibronectin governs the adhesion and spreading of cells on a material surface [75]. These plasma proteins play an important role in the initial recruitment of cells to the biomaterial surface. The glycoprotein fibronectin consists of multiple specific binding sites and is capable of interacting with a wide variety of other biomaterials, through the formation of fibrilar extracellular matrix or fibrils. So, the specific surface of a biomaterial plays a key role in adsorption of fibronectin or other pro-adhesive proteins and hence better proliferation of cells. The interaction of neural stem cells with UNCD films and the consequent cellular signaling processes are schematized in Figure 1. Some studies revealed that the adhesion and spreading of cells on NCD surfaces is related to the bonding structure present on the surface and the ratio of sp^2/sp^3 [76]. It has also been observed that the microstructure of the NCD films and the kind of treatments seemed to influence the biological effects of cells. However, the correlation between these surface properties (chemistry, topography and wettability) and cell responses is complicated and not clearly understood.

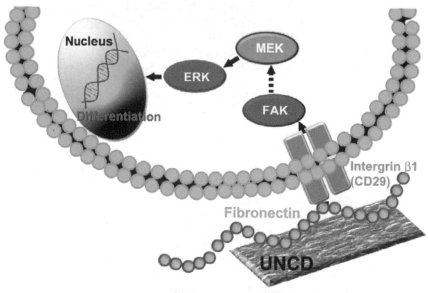

Fig. 1. Schematic drawing summarizes the role of H-UNCD films in mediating differentiation from neural stem cells. Absorbed fibronectin on H-UNCD surface activates integrin β1 (CD29), focal adhesion kinase (FAK) and (extracellular signaling kinase) ERK1/2 pathways and, in turn, leads to an ultimate and specification of neuronal differentiation from NSC.

4.2 Topography effects of nanodiamond films on cells

The comparison of the behavior of different cell types on nanodiamond films shows that they react differently according to surface smoothness [55, 57, 60, 68, 77, 78]. Scanning electron microscopy (SEM) and immunofluorescence staining examinations of osteoblast on nanodiamond films with various surface roughness (nanometer and micrometer) generally demonstrated that enhanced osteoblast functions (including adhesion, proliferation, intracellular protein synthesis, alkaline phosphatase activity and extracellular calcium deposition) on nanocrystalline diamond (RMS~20 nm) compared to submicron diamond grain size films and control for all time periods tested up to 21 days [57, 60]. In addition, an SEM study of osteoblast attachment on NCD films explains the topographical impact diamond had on osteoblast functions by showing complex and longer filopodia extensions.

To investigate the adhesion of normal human dermal fibroblast cells grown on NCD films with various surface smoothnesses, atomic force microscopy were performed. The examination demonstrated that cell viability and adhesion force was better on smooth surfaces (UNCD films) compared to micron diamond grain size films, no matter the terminations of diamond films [55]. Although mesenchymal stem cells and non-differentiated cells adhere similarly on all NCD surfaces with different roughness (20, 270, and 500 nm) and control polystyrene, their metabolic activity on NCD surfaces is increased. On the other hand, osteoblasts adhere on NCD significantly more than on polystyrene, and their metabolic activity is decreased on nano/microrough NCD surfaces in contrast to mesenchymal stem cells. These differences could be attributed to the distinct properties of the two cell types in the human body. Alternatively, the different response of osteoblasts could be attributed to the specific surface topography as well as to the biocompatible properties of diamond. [79]. Hence the controlled topographically structured NCD coatings on various substrates is promising for preparation of better implants, which offer faster colonization by specific cells as well as longer-term stability.

4.3 Surface chemistry effects of nanodiamond films on cells

The bio-compatibility and resistance to chemical corrosion of diamond may increase lifetime of stents, joints, and other implants in the human body. It is also possible to make a chemical functionalization of diamond surface and create bio-passive or bio-active patterns. Kalbacova et al [80] showed that viability and adhesion of human osteoblasts (SAOS-2) cultured on NCD films are predominantly determined by NCD surface termination. Increasing surface nano-roughness plays a secondary yet positive role. Hydrophilic surface of NCD films (O-terminated surface) provides good conditions for osteoblast adhesion and spreading and consequently on their viability (metabolic activity and proliferation). It was shown that hydrophobic H-terminated diamond surfaces are less favorable for osteoblast-like cell adhesion and growth than hydrophilic O-terminated surfaces [80, 81]. This is in agreement with observations on other materials and cells, such as Ti6Al4V titanium alloy [82, 83] and human dermal fibroblast [55]. In addition to cells lines, different kinds of stem cells have also been studied and the results show difference on cell lines and stem cells. Chen et al [56] cultured neural stem cells on different functionalized diamond films in low serum and without any differentiation factors to investigate the biological effects on NSCs. We found that H-terminated UNCD films spontaneously induced cell proliferation and neuronal differentiation and O-terminated UNCD films were also shown to further improve neural differentiation, with a preference to differentiate into oligodendrocytes. Clem [58] reported that H-terminated ultra-smooth nanostructured diamond surfaces supported robust adhesion and survival of mesenchymal stem cells, while oxygen (O)- and fluorine (F)-terminated surfaces resisted cell adhesion. Thalhammer [84] used four different materials (glass, PCD, NCD and Si) coated with monolayers nanodiamonds and displayed promising similarity to the protein-coated materials regarding neuronal cell attachment,

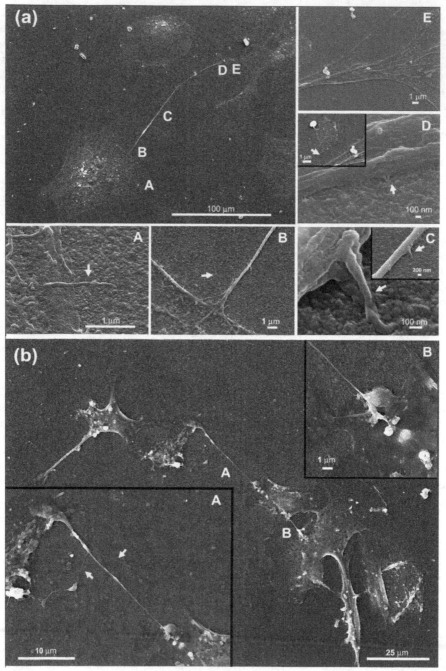

Fig. 2. Scanning electron photomicrographs of neural stem cells cultured on H-UNCD films in regular medium without any differentiating reagents for seven days. Higher

magnification scanning electron microscopy was performed to enlarge different areas (A-E) in graph (a) and (A-B) in graph (b). Yellow arrows show the filopodia at higher magnifications.

neurite outgrowth and functional network formation. Importantly, the neurons were able to grow in direct contact with the NCD-coated material and could be easily maintained in culture for an extended period, equal to those on protein-coated substrates. To further investigate the interaction of cell to NCD film, Chen et al observed the morphology of cells cultured in H-terminated UNCD films and revealed that there were filopodia/nano-diamond interactions (Figure 2). Thus, NCD layering might prove a valuable material for implants on a wide range of substrates. These indicate that diamond films can be easily modified to either promote or prevent cell/biomaterial interactions. This is an interesting feature for tissue engineering and bio-electronics. A question remained though to what kinds of mechanism and key points to affect the degree of the cell adhesion and selectivity.

5. Molecular mechanisms of signaling transduction from UNCD films to nuclei

Cells do not interact with a naked material either *in vitro* or *in vivo*. At the beginning step, the material is conditioned by the biological fluid components. This is a complex process strongly dependent on the cell culture conditions including the underlying substrate and mediating medium/proteins. Surface energy may influence protein adsorption and the structural rearrangement of the proteins on positively and negatively charged substrates (hydrophilic/hydrophobic surface). Protein from serum containing media adsorbed on surfaces forming multiple molecular layers. Hydrophobic H-terminated surfaces were found less favorable for osteoblastic cell adhesion, spreading and viability than hydrophilic O-terminated surfaces [5]. Recently, it was shown that microscopic (30–200 μm) patterns of H- and O-terminated surface can lead to a selective adhesion and arrangement of osteoblasts [85]. This effect also works on human periodontal ligament fibroblast and human cervical carcinoma (HeLa) cells [85-87]. The differential adsorption of "serum proteins" on the negative or positive charged regions from medium with fetal bovine serum (FBS) was studied. It was proposed that the selectivity is due to the serum proteins, which are adsorbed in about the same monolayer thickness (2-4 nm) on both H and O-diamond surfaces, but in different composition and conformations of proteins [88]. When osteoblasts were placed on the diamond surface in McCoy's 5A medium without FBS, cell attachment on H/O-patterned diamond surfaces was not selective [85, 89]. This excluded a direct effect of diamond C-H and C-O surface dipoles on the cell selectivity. FBS adsorption to diamond proceeds in two stages. Formation of monolayer thickness (2-4 nm) FBS layer on both H- and O-diamond was observed within short period of time (<18 h) [86, 88]. AFM nanoshaving showed that this primary FBS layer is less adhesive to H-diamond than to O-diamond. After long time adsorption (6 days), formation of a thick FBS layer was observed on H-diamond (~35 nm) than on O-diamond (~17 nm) [86]. Moreover, it is clear that not only the nature of adsorbed biological molecules but also their conformation and composition will influence consequent cell adhesion. Changes in conformation of pre-adsorbed specific proteins, fibronectin, (not bovine serum albumin or vitronectin, which is abundant in FBS) were observed. These would affected cell binding domain conformations and then affect the affinity with its cell surface receptor [58, 86].

Osteoblast adhesion on materials may also be considered in relation to the expression of the various adhesion proteins and cell receptors. Numerous studies using immunefluorescent staining have shown the presence of vinculin and pY397 focal adhesion kinase (FAK) in cultured human osteoblasts on nanostructured diamond films [60, 78, 79]. The osteoblasts adhered on ultra nano-cones and nano-cones, showing large focal adhesions and relatively strong activation of FAK, are thus more predestined for successful colonization of the entire environment [60, 78]. Hamilton [90] suggested that osteoblast response to substrates with specific topographical features requires FAK-Y397-Src-Y416 complexes for ERK1/2 phosphorylation. Yet on smooth surfaces, Src-independent routes of ERK1/2 activation are present, which finally induce the differentiation of osteoblast further to promote bone formation. The same cell signaling pathway has been studied on other materials, such as titanium alloys [83]. According to published data, the contact of cell to fibronectin could be

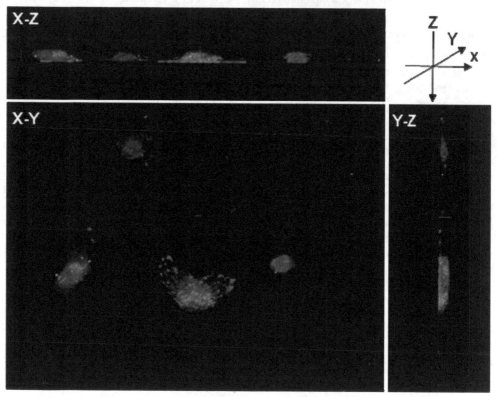

Fig. 3. The confocal immunofluorescence image of neural stem cells grown on the H-UNCD film in the regular medium without any differentiating reagents for 8 hours of culture. Alexafluor 594 labeled phospho-FAK (Red) and DyLight 488 labeled phospho-ERK (Green). The phospho-FAK and phospho-ERK were detected in the cells simultaneously and localized to their proper subcellular positions. In the quadrant of X-Z and Y-Z stacking images, phospho-FAK was observed in basal cell membrane adherent to H-UNCD films, while phosphor-ERK was shown assembled in the cell body.

mediated by integrin β1 [91, 92]. Integrins are transmembrane protein family and composed of α and β subunits as heterodimer. Functions of integrins were involved in the regulation of proliferation, survival, migration and differentiation. The high level of integrin β1 expression has been used to enrich human epidermal and rodent neural stem cells from more restricted progenitor populations [58, 92]. Moreover, Chen et al [66] showed that increased levels of neuronal differentiation in neural stem cells grown on H-UNCD surfaces are due to absorbance of fibronectin from medium to H-terminated UNCD films, resulting in integrin β1-FAK-ERK1/2 signaling (Figure 3) in conditions of low serum-growth factors and free of differentiating reagents.

Number	Function	gi number	Name
1	Extracellular matrix	224863	Fibronectin
2	Blood	78099200	Hemoglobin subunit epsilon
3		126022898	Hemoglobin alpha subunit 1
4		203283896	Apolipoprotein A-I preproprotein
5		3915607	Apolipoprotein A-I
6		77735387	Fetuin B
7		166159174	Angiotensinogen (serpin peptidase inhibitor, clade A, member 8)
8		95147674	Complement factor B
9		2501351	Transferrin
10		27807209	Alpha-2-macroglobulin
11		78369364	Group-specific component (vitamin D binding protein)
12	Epithelium	16303309	Type II keratin 5
13		148747492	Keratin 2
14		73996312	Similar to Keratin, type II cytoskeletal 5 (Cytokeratin 5) (58 kDa cytokeratin) isoform 3
15		9910294	Keratin 71
16		4159806	Type II keratin subunit protein
17	Cytoskeleton	28336	Mutant beta-actin
18	Others	27806907	Clusterin
19		2232299	IgM heavy chain constant region
20		27806809	Regucalcin

Table 1. Differential protein expression profile identified by LC-MS/MS, showing proteins preferentially absorbed on H-UNCD films, but not on Petri dish polystyrene surface.

6. Proteomic analysis of proteins that are adsorbed to UNCD films by using LC-MS/MS

We showed that the abundant fibronectin adsorbed onto the H-UNCD film formed locally dense and conformed layer that allows for the pro-adhesive motifs to be accessible by integrins and further activates the whole signaling pathway [66]. To further investigate what other serum proteins might be bound to UNCD films, we performed proteomic analysis, using LC-MS/MS on serum proteins that are adsorbed to H-UNCD films. We demonstrated that H-UNCD films could adsorb proteins from culture medium more efficient than Petri dish's polystyrene surface could (Table 1). These proteins included not only fibronectin but also proteins that are known to be present in blood, epithelium, cytoskeleton, and others. It would be of interest to further explore the roles of these proteins in shaping the UNCD-cell interaction and the ultimate differentiation into desired cell types.

7. Conclusion

Highly intense research on biocompatibility of NCD films showed that it is a promising material for biomedical applications. NCD films possess easy surface functionalization and nano-topography, offering favorable condition for the growth of fibroblasts, osteoblasts and stem cells without inflammatory response and cytotoxicity. From published *in vitro* studies, NCD films elicited an improved proliferation and differentiation capacity for human osteoblasts and neural stem cells, compared to conventional polystyrene Petri dishes. The relevant mechanism of cellular signaling transduction has been investigated and shown to act through fibronectin-integrin-FAK-ERK pathway. These results suggest the potential usage of NCD films as novel medical devices and implants such as a coating for joint implant and nerve repair in tissue engineering. The delamination and corrosion of the NCD films during its long-term use in medical implants are to be carefully considered for its future biomedical applications. We performed proteomic analysis, using LC-MS/MS, to identify proteins that are adsorbed to UNCD films. We demonstrated proteins such as fibronectin, transferrin, and several keratin proteins that could be adsorbed more efficiently onto UNCD films than to Petri dish's polystyrene surface. It would be of interest to further explore the roles of these proteins in shaping the UNCD-cell interaction and the subsequent differentiation into desired cell types. Finally, more systematic studies *in vivo* are now warranted to confirm its use in biomedical devices for commercial applications.

8. References

[1] Peppas NA, Langer R. New Challenges in Biomaterials. Science 1994 Mar;263(5154):1715-1720.

[2] Hubbell JA. Biomaterials in Tissue Engineering. Bio-Technology 1995 Jun;13(6):565-576.

[3] Lutolf MP, Hubbell JA. Synthetic biomaterials as instructive extracellular microenvironments for morphogenesis in tissue engineering. Nat Biotechnol 2005 Jan;23(1):47-55.

[4] Langer R, Tirrell DA. Designing materials for biology and medicine. Nature 2004 Apr;428(6982):487-492.

[5] Discher DE, Mooney DJ, Zandstra PW. Growth Factors, Matrices, and Forces Combine and Control Stem Cells. Science 2009 Jun;324(5935):1673-1677.

[6] Chai C, Leong KW. Biomaterials approach to expand and direct differentiation of stem cells. Mol Ther 2007 Mar;15(3):467-480.

[7] Hwang NS, Varghese S, Elisseeff J. Controlled differentiation of stem cells. Adv Drug Deliv Rev 2008 Jan;60(2):199-214.

[8] Lutolf MP, Gilbert PM, Blau HM. Designing materials to direct stem-cell fate. Nature 2009 Nov;462(7272):433-441.

[9] Morrison SJ, Spradling AC. Stem cells and niches: Mechanisms that promote stem cell maintenance throughout life. Cell 2008 Feb;132(4):598-611.

[10] Guilak F, Cohen DM, Estes BT, Gimble JM, Liedtke W, Chen CS. Control of Stem Cell Fate by Physical Interactions with the Extracellular Matrix. Cell Stem Cell 2009 Jul;5(1):17-26.

[11] Chao JI, Perevedentseva E, Chung PH, Liu KK, Cheng CY, Chang CC, et al. Nanometer-sized diamond particle as a probe for biolabeling. Biophysical Journal 2007 Sep;93(6):2199-2208.

[12] Liu KK, Wang CC, Cheng CL, Chao JI. Endocytic carboxylated nanodiamond for the labeling and tracking of cell division and differentiation in cancer and stem cells. Biomaterials 2009 Sep;30(26):4249-4259.

[13] Vaijayanthimala V, Tzeng YK, Chang HC, Li CL. The biocompatibility of fluorescent nanodiamonds and their mechanism of cellular uptake. Nanotechnology 2009 Oct;20(42):9.

[14] Ho DA. Beyond the Sparkle: The Impact of Nanodiamonds as Biolabeling and Therapeutic Agents. Acs Nano 2009 Dec;3(12):3825-3829.

[15] Schrand AM, Hens SAC, Shenderova OA. Nanodiamond Particles: Properties and Perspectives for Bioapplications. Critical Reviews in Solid State and Materials Sciences 2009;34(1-2):18-74.

[16] Chan HY, Aslam DM, Wiler JA, Casey B. A Novel Diamond Microprobe for Neuro-Chemical and -Electrical Recording in Neural Prosthesis. Journal of Microelectromechanical Systems 2009 Jun;18(3):511-521.

[17] Ong TP, Chiou WA, Chen FR, Chang RPH. Preparation of Nanocrystalline Diamond Films for Optical Coating Applications Using a Pulsed Microwave Plasma Cvd Method. Carbon 1990;28(6):799-799.

[18] Ong TP, Chang RPH. Low-Temperature Deposition of Diamond Films for Optical Coatings. Applied Physics Letters 1989 Nov;55(20):2063-2065.

[19] Fan WD, Wu H, Jagannadham K, Goral BC. Wear-Resistant Diamond Coatings on Alumina. Surface & Coatings Technology 1995 May;72(1-2):78-87.

[20] Kato M, Fujisawa T. High-pressure solution X-ray scattering of protein using a hydrostatic cell with diamond windows. Journal of Synchrotron Radiation 1998 Sep;5:1282-1286.

[21] Ravet MF, Rousseaux F. Status of diamond as membrane material for X-ray lithography masks. Diamond and Related Materials 1996 May;5(6-8):812-818.

[22] Sharda T, Umeno M, Soga T, Jimbo T. Strong adhesion in nanocrystalline diamond films on silicon substrates. Journal of Applied Physics 2001 May;89(9):4874-4878.

[23] Lifshitz Y, Meng XM, Lee ST, Akhveldiany R, Hoffman A. Visualization of diamond nucleation and growth from energetic species. Physical Review Letters 2004 Jul;93(5):4.

[24] Lee YC, Lin SJ, Chia CT, Cheng HF, Lin IN. Effect of processing parameters on the nucleation behavior of nano-crystalline diamond film. Diamond and Related Materials 2005 Mar-Jul;14(3-7):296-301.

[25] Berry BS, Pritchet WC, Cuomo JJ, Guarnieri CR, Whitehair SJ. INTERNAL-STRESS AND ELASTICITY OF SYNTHETIC DIAMOND FILMS. Applied Physics Letters 1990 Jul;57(3):302-303.

[26] Liu YK, Tso PL, Lin IN, Tzeng Y, Chen YC. Comparative study of nucleation processes for the growth of nanocrystalline diamond. Diamond and Related Materials 2006 Feb-Mar;15(2-3):234-238.

[27] Lee ST, Lin ZD, Jiang X. CVD diamond films: nucleation and growth. Mater Sci Eng R-Rep 1999 Jul;25(4):123-154.

[28] Sumant AV, Gilbert P, Grierson DS, Konicek AR, Abrecht M, Butler JE, et al. Surface composition, bonding, and morphology in the nucleation and growth of ultra-thin, high quality nanocrystalline diamond films. Diam Relat Mat 2007 Apr-Jul;16(4-7):718-724.

[29] Naguib NN, Elam JW, Birrell J, Wang J, Grierson DS, Kabius B, et al. Enhanced nucleation, smoothness and conformality of ultrananocrystalline diamond (UNCD) ultrathin films via tungsten interlayers. Chem Phys Lett 2006 Oct;430(4-6):345-350.

[30] Gruen D, Krauss A. Buckyball precursors produce ultra-smooth diamond films. R&D Magazine 1997 Apr;39(5):57-&.

[31] Gruen DM, Liu SZ, Krauss AR, Luo JS, Pan XZ. FULLERENES AS PRECURSORS FOR DIAMOND FILM GROWTH WITHOUT HYDROGEN OR OXYGEN ADDITIONS. Applied Physics Letters 1994 Mar;64(12):1502-1504.

[32] Gruen DM, Pan XZ, Krauss AR, Liu SZ, Luo JS, Foster CM. DEPOSITION AND CHARACTERIZATION OF NANOCRYSTALLINE DIAMOND FILMS. Journal of Vacuum Science & Technology a-Vacuum Surfaces and Films 1994 Jul-Aug;12(4):1491-1495.

[33] Gruen DM. Nanocrystalline diamond films. Annual Review of Materials Science 1999;29:211-259.

[34] Gruen DM. Ultrananocrystalline diamond in the laboratory and the cosmos. Mrs Bulletin 2001 Oct;26(10):771-776.

[35] Butler JE, Sumant AV. The CVD of nanodiamond materials. Chem Vapor Depos 2008 Jul-Aug;14(7-8):145-160.

[36] Hutchinson AB, Truitt PA, Schwab KC, Sekaric L, Parpia JM, Craighead HG, et al. Dissipation in nanocrystalline-diamond nanomechanical resonators. Applied Physics Letters 2004 Feb;84(6):972-974.

[37] Sekaric L, Parpia JM, Craighead HG, Feygelson T, Houston BH, Butler JE. Nanomechanical resonant structures in nanocrystalline diamond. Applied Physics Letters 2002 Dec;81(23):4455-4457.

[38] Zhang JC, Zimmer JW, Howe RT, Maboudian R. Characterization of boron-doped micro- and nanocrystalline diamond films deposited by wafer-scale hot filament chemical vapor deposition for MEMS applications. Diamond and Related Materials 2008 Jan;17(1):23-28.

[39] Lee CK. Effects of hydrogen and oxygen on the electrochemical corrosion and wear-corrosion behavior of diamond films deposited by hot filament chemical vapor deposition. Applied Surface Science 2008 Apr;254(13):4111-4117.

[40] Yang WS, Auciello O, Butler JE, Cai W, Carlisle JA, Gerbi J, et al. DNA-modified nanocrystalline diamond thin-films as stable, biologically active substrates. Nature Materials 2002 Dec;1(4):253-257.

[41] Yang WS, Auciello O, Butler JE, Cai W, Carlisle JA, Gerbi J, et al. DNA-modified nanocrystalline diamond thin-films as stable, biologically active substrates (vol 1, pg 253, 2002). Nature Materials 2003 Jan;2(1):63-63.

[42] Yang WS, Butler JE, Russell JN, Hamers RJ. Interfacial electrical properties of DNA-modified diamond thin films: Intrinsic response and hybridization-induced field effects. Langmuir 2004 Aug;20(16):6778-6787.

[43] Ariano P, Lo Giudice A, Marcantoni A, Vittone E, Carbone E, Lovisolo D. A diamond-based biosensor for the recording of neuronal activity. Biosensors & Bioelectronics 2009 Mar;24(7):2046-2050.

[44] Yang WS, Hamers RJ. Fabrication and characterization of a biologically sensitive field-effect transistor using a nanocrystalline diamond thin film. Applied Physics Letters 2004 Oct;85(16):3626-3628.

[45] Jakubowski W, Bartosz G, Niedzielski P, Szymanski W, Walkowiak B. Nanocrystalline diamond surface is resistant to bacterial colonization. Diamond and Related Materials 2004 Oct;13(10):1761-1763.

[46] Papo MJ, Catledge SA, Vohra YK. Mechanical wear behavior of nanocrystalline and multilayer diamond coatings on temporomandibular joint implants. J Mater Sci-Mater Med 2004 Jul;15(7):773-777.

[47] Nordsletten L, Hogasen AKM, Konttinen YT, Santavirta S, Aspenberg P, Aasen AO. Human monocytes stimulation by particles of hydroxyapatite, silicon carbide and diamond: In vitro studies of new prosthesis coatings. Biomaterials 1996 Aug;17(15):1521-1527.

[48] Aspenberg P, Anttila A, Konttinen YT, Lappalainen R, Goodman SB, Nordsletten L, et al. Benign response to particles of diamond and SiC: Bone chamber studies of new joint replacement coating materials in rabbits. Biomaterials 1996 Apr;17(8):807-812.

[49] Tang L, Tsai C, Gerberich WW, Kruckeberg L, Kania DR. Biocompatibility of Chemical-Vapor-Deposited Diamond. Biomaterials 1995 Apr;16(6):483-488.

[50] Kulisch W, Popov C, Bliznakov S, Ceccone G, Gilliland D, Sirghi L, et al. Surface and bioproperties of nanocrystalline diamond/amorphous carbon nanocomposite films. Thin Solid Films 2007 Sep;515(23):8407-8411.

[51] Popov C, Kulisch W, Reithmaier JP, Dostalova T, Jelinek M, Anspach N, et al. Bioproperties of nanocrystalline diamond/amorphous carbon composite films. Diamond and Related Materials 2007 Apr-Jul;16(4-7):735-739.

[52] Rubio-Retama J, Hernando J, Lopez-Ruiz B, Hartl A, Steinmuller D, Stutzmann M, et al. Synthetic nanocrystalline diamond as a third-generation biosensor support. Langmuir 2006 Jun;22(13):5837-5842.

[53] Steinmuller-Nethl D, Kloss FR, Najam-U-Haq M, Rainer M, Larsson K, Linsmeier C, et al. Strong binding of bioactive BMP-2 to nanocrystalline diamond by physisorption. Biomaterials 2006 Sep;27(26):4547-4556.

[54] Haensel T, Uhlig J, Koch RJ, Ahmed SIU, Garrido JA, Steinmuller-Nethl D, et al. Influence of hydrogen on nanocrystalline diamond surfaces investigated with HREELS and XPS. Physica Status Solidi a-Applications and Materials Science 2009 Sep;206(9):2022-2027.

[55] Chong KF, Loh KP, Vedula SRK, Lim CT, Sternschulte H, Steinmuller D, et al. Cell adhesion properties on photochemically functionalized diamond. Langmuir 2007 May;23(10):5615-5621.

[56] Chen YC, Lee DC, Hsiao CY, Chung YF, Chen HC, Thomas JP, et al. The effect of ultra-nanocrystalline diamond films on the proliferation and differentiation of neural stem cells. Biomaterials 2009 Jul;30(20):3428-3435.

[57] Yang L, Sheldon BW, Webster TJ. The impact of diamond nanocrystallinity on osteoblast functions. Biomaterials 2009 Jul;30(20):3458-3465.

[58] Clem WC, Chowdhury S, Catledge SA, Weimer JJ, Shaikh FM, Hennessy KM, et al. Mesenchymal stem cell interaction with ultra-smooth nanostructured diamond for wear-resistant orthopaedic implants. Biomaterials 2008 Aug-Sep;29(24-25):3461-3468.

[59] Huang HJ, Chen M, Bruno P, Lam R, Robinson E, Gruen D, et al. Ultrananocrystalline Diamond Thin Films Functionalized with Therapeutically Active Collagen Networks. Journal of Physical Chemistry B 2009 Mar;113(10):2966-2971.

[60] Kalbacova M, Rezek B, Baresova V, Wolf-Brandstetter C, Kromka A. Nanoscale topography of nanocrystalline diamonds promotes differentiation of osteoblasts. Acta Biomaterialia 2009 Oct;5(8):3076-3085.

[61] Popov C, Bliznakov S, Boycheva S, Milinovik N, Apostolova MD, Anspach N, et al. Nanocrystalline diamond/amorphous carbon composite coatings for biomedical applications. Diamond and Related Materials 2008 Apr-May;17(4-5):882-887.

[62] Huang HJ, Pierstorff E, Osawa E, Ho D. Protein-mediated assembly of nanodiamond hydrogels into a biocompatible and biofunctional multilayer nanofilm. Acs Nano 2008 Feb;2(2):203-212.

[63] Jian W, Firestone MA, Auciello O, Carlisle JA. Surface functionalization of ultrananocrystalline diamond films by electrochemical reduction of aryldiazonium salts. Langmuir 2004 Dec;20(26):11450-11456.

[64] Wang J, Carlisle JA. Covalent immobilization of glucose oxidase on conducting ultrananocrystalline diamond thin films. Diamond and Related Materials 2006 Feb-Mar;15(2-3):279-284.

[65] Williams DF. On the nature of biomaterials. Biomaterials 2009 Oct;30(30):5897-5909.

[66] Chen YC, Lee DC, Tsai TY, Hsiao CY, Liu JW, Kao CY, et al. Induction and regulation of differentiation in neural stem cells on ultra-nanocrystalline diamond films. Biomaterials 2010:In press.

[67] Kromka A, Grausova L, Bacakova L, Vacik J, Rezek B, Vanecek M, et al. Semiconducting to metallic-like boron doping of nanocrystalline diamond films and its effect on osteoblastic cells. Diamond and Related Materials Feb-Mar;19(2-3):190-195.

[68] Ariano P, Budnyk O, Dalmazzo S, Lovisolo D, Manfredotti C, Rivolo P, et al. On diamond surface properties and interactions with neurons. European Physical Journal E 2009 Oct;30(2):149-156.

[69] Shi B, Jin QL, Chen LH, Auciello O. Fundamentals of ultrananocrystalline diamond (UNCD) thin films as biomaterials for developmental biology: Embryonic fibroblasts growth on the surface of (UNCD) films. Diamond and Related Materials 2009 Feb-Mar;18(2-3):596-600.

[70] Bajaj P, Akin D, Gupta A, Sherman D, Shi B, Auciello O, et al. Ultrananocrystalline diamond film as an optimal cell interface for biomedical applications. Biomedical Microdevices 2007 Dec;9(6):787-794.

[71] Amaral M, Dias AG, Gomes PS, Lopes MA, Silva RF, Santos JD, et al. Nanocrystalline diamond: In vitro biocompatibility assessment by MG63 and human bone marrow cells cultures. Journal of Biomedical Materials Research Part A 2008 Oct;87A(1):91-99.

[72] Amaral M, Gomes PS, Lopes MA, Santos JD, Silva RF, Fernandes MH. Nanocrystalline diamond as a coating for joint implants: Cytotoxicity and biocompatibility assessment. Journal of Nanomaterials 2008:9.

[73] Kloss FR, Gassner R, Preiner J, Ebner A, Larsson K, Hachl O, et al. The role of oxygen termination of nanocrystalline diamond on immobilisation of BMP-2 and subsequent bone formation. Biomaterials 2008 Jun;29(16):2433-2442.

[74] Tate MC, Garcia AJ, Keselowsky BG, Schumm MA, Archer DR, LaPlaca MC. Specific beta(1) integrins mediate adhesion, migration, and differentiation of neural progenitors derived from the embryonic striatum. Molecular and Cellular Neuroscience 2004 Sep;27(1):22-31.

[75] Hynes RO, Yamada KM. Fibronectins - Multifunctional Modular Glycoproteins. Journal of Cell Biology 1982;95(2):369-377.

[76] Cui FZ, Li DJ. A review of investigations on biocompatibility of diamond-like carbon and carbon nitride films. Surface & Coatings Technology 2000 Sep;131(1-3):481-487.

[77] Yang L, Sheldon BW, Webster TJ. Orthopedic nano diamond coatings: Control of surface properties and their impact on osteoblast adhesion and proliferation. Journal of Biomedical Materials Research Part A 2009 Nov;91A(2):548-556.

[78] Kalbacova M, Broz A, Babchenko O, Kromka A. Study on cellular adhesion of human osteoblasts on nano-structured diamond films. Physica Status Solidi B-Basic Solid State Physics 2009 Dec;246(11-12):2774-2777.

[79] Broz A, Baresova V, Kromka A, Rezek B, Kalbacova M. Strong influence of hierarchically structured diamond nanotopography on adhesion of human osteoblasts and mesenchymal cells. Phys Status Solidi A-Appl Mat 2009 Sep;206(9):2038-2041.

[80] Kalbacova M, Kalbac M, Dunsch L, Kromka A, Vanecek M, Rezek B, et al. The effect of SWCNT and nano-diamond films on human osteoblast cells. Physica Status Solidi B-Basic Solid State Physics 2007 Nov;244(11):4356-4359.

[81] Kalbacova M, Michalikova L, Baresova V, Kromka A, Rezek B, Kmoch S. Adhesion of osteoblasts on chemically patterned nanocrystalline diamonds. Physica Status Solidi B-Basic Solid State Physics 2008 Oct;245(10):2124-2127.

[82] Anselme K, Linez P, Bigerelle M, Le Maguer D, Le Maguer A, Hardouin P, et al. The relative influence of the topography and chemistry of TiAl6V4 surfaces on osteoblastic cell behaviour. Biomaterials 2000 Aug;21(15):1567-1577.

[83] Anselme K. Osteoblast adhesion on biomaterials. Biomaterials 2000 Apr;21(7):667-681.

[84] Thalhammer A, Edgington RJ, Cingolani LA, Schoepfer R, Jackman RB. The use of nanodiamond monolayer coatings to promote the formation of functional neuronal networks. Biomaterials Mar;31(8):2097-2104.

[85] Rezek B, Michalikova L, Ukraintsev E, Kromka A, Kalbacova M. Micro-Pattern Guided Adhesion of Osteoblasts on Diamond Surfaces. Sensors 2009 May;9(5):3549-3562.

[86] Ukraintsev E, Rezek B, Kromka A, Broz A, Kalbacova M. Long-term adsorption of fetal bovine serum on H/O-terminated diamond studied in situ by atomic force microscopy. Physica Status Solidi B-Basic Solid State Physics 2009 Dec;246(11-12):2832-2835.

[87] Michalikova L, Rezek B, Kromka A, Kalbacova M. CVD diamond films with hydrophilic micro-patterns for self-organisation of human osteoblasts. Vacuum 2009 Aug;84(1):61-64.

[88] Rezek B, Ukraintsev E, Michalikova L, Kromka A, Zemek J, Kalbacova M. Adsorption of fetal bovine serum on H/O-terminated diamond studied by atomic force microscopy. Diamond and Related Materials 2009 May-Aug;18(5-8):918-922.

[89] Rezek B, Ukraintsev E, Kromka A, Ledinsky M, Broz A, Noskova L, et al. Assembly of osteoblastic cell micro-arrays on diamond guided by protein pre-adsorption. Diamond and Related Materials Feb-Mar;19(2-3):153-157.

[90] Hamilton DW, Brunette DM. The effect of substratum topography on osteoblast adhesion mediated signal transduction and phosphorylation. Biomaterials 2007 Apr;28(10):1806-1819.

[91] Ivankovic-Dikic I, Gronroos E, Blaukat A, Barth BU, Dikic I. Pyk2 and FAK regulate neurite outgrowth induced by growth factors and integrins. Nature Cell Biology 2000 Sep;2(9):574-581.

[92] Mruthyunjaya S, Manchanda R, Godbole R, Pujari R, Shiras A, Shastry P. Laminin-1 induces neurite outgrowth in human mesenchymal stem cells in serum/differentiation factors-free conditions through activation of FAK-MEK/ERK signaling pathways. Biochemical and Biophysical Research Communications Jan;391(1):43-48.

δ-Free F_oF_1-ATPase, Nanomachine and Biosensor

Jia-Chang Yue[1], Yao-Gen Shu[2], Pei-Rong Wang[1] and Xu Zhang[1]

[1]*Institute of Biophysics, Chinese Academy of Sciences*
[2]*Institute of Theoretical Physics, Chinese Academy of Sciences*
China

1. Introduction

F_oF_1-ATPase is an exquisite nanomachines self-assembled by eight kinds of subunits, and is ubiquitous in the plasma membrane of bacteria, chloroplasts and mitochondria as well as uses the transmembrane electrochemical potential to synthesize ATP. The holoenzyme is a complex of two opposing rotary motors, F_o and F_1, which are mechanically coupled by a common central stalk ("rotor"), $c_n\epsilon\gamma$, and δb_2 subunits connecting two "stator", $\alpha_3\beta_3$ crown in F_1 and a in F_o. The membrane embedded F_o unit converts the proton motive force (p.m.f.) into mechanical rotation of the "rotor", thereby causing cyclic conformational change of $\alpha_3\beta_3$ crown ("stator") in F_1 and driving ATP synthesis. A striking characteristic of this motor is its reversibility. It may rotate in the reverse direction for ATP hydrolysis and utilize the excess energy to pump protons across the membrane(Ballmoos et al., 2009; Boyer, 1997; Feniouk & Yoshida, 2008; Junge, 2004; Saraste, 1999; Weber & Senior, 2003).
The basic hypothesis, "binding change mechanism"(Boyer et al., 1973), however, had not been confirmed until the direct observation of the rotation of F_1-ATPase at single molecule level in 1997(Noji et al., 1997), although it was partly proven by the eccentric structure of γ subunit in 1994(Abrahams et al., 1994). Single molecule technologies have contributed very much to the motor. For example, fluorescence imaging and spectroscopy revealed the physical rotation of isolated F_1(Adachi et al., 2007; Nishizaka et al., 2004; Noji et al., 1997; Yasuda et al., 1998) and F_o(Düser et al., 2009; Zhang et al., 2005), or F_1F_o holoenzyme(Diez et al., 2004; Kaim et al., 2002; Ueno et al., 2005). Magnetic tweezers also be employed to manipulate the ATP synthesis/hydrolysis in F_1(Itoh et al., 2004; Rondelez et al., 2005), and proton translation in F_o(Liu et al., 2006a). Recently, a membrane scaffold protein has been applied to observe the stepping rotation of proton channels (c_n)(Ishmukhametov et al., 2010).
There are three catalytic sites localized three identical β subunits in F_1 respectively. However, the three sites have different affinities for substrate at any given moment in time during catalysis. On the other hand, with different technologies such as AFM, Electron density, and laser-induced liquid bead ion desorption-MS(LILBID-MS) etc., the number of proton channels have been revealed ranging from 10 to 15 for different species(Jiang et al., 2001; Meier et al., 2007; Mitome et al., 2004; Pogoryelov et al., 2005; Seelert et al., 2000; Stock et al., 1999). Thus, it seems reasonable that three ATP molecules will be generated/consumed in F_1 for every cycle, at the same time $n(10 \sim 15)$ protons will be translated transmembrane in F_o because of the tight coupling between the two motors. That is, the H^+/ATP ratio should be $3/n$.
With the development of gene engineering, all subunits of the motor can be expressed in *E. Coli.* such that the motor can be self-assembled *in vitro* into a nanodevice for different

application(Choi & Montemagno, 2005; Liu et al., 2002; Luo et al., 2005; Martin et al, 2007; Soong et al., 2000). For example, if the δ subunit is removed from the motor, the two stators are structurally uncoupled, thereby the F_1 stator only contact with the common rotor. This is named δ-free F_0F_1 motor. Its stator is the a and b_2 subunits, while the rotor is built by c_n, ϵ, γ and $\alpha_3\beta_3$ subunits. Furthermore, this motor can be embedded in a chromatophore which functions as a battery recharged by illumination. Thus, the motor has been reconstructed into a self-driven nanomachine in which the only power is the transmembrane p.m.f. Here, we briefly review our works on the δ-free F_0F_1 motor including reconstituting, direct observation of its rotation, developing as a biosensor and a activator, and so on. However, we begin with the enzymatics of the holoenzyme to investigate the relation between the rotation speed and substrate/product concentrations, transmembrane p.m.f. and damping coefficient etc. which is of benefit to the quantitative analysis.

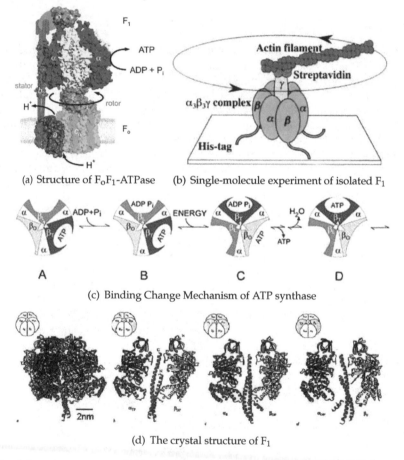

(a) Structure of F_0F_1-ATPase   (b) Single-molecule experiment of isolated F_1

(c) Binding Change Mechanism of ATP synthase

(d) The crystal structure of F_1

Fig. 1. The full-atom structure of the F_0F_1-ATPase(a)(Weber, 2006) and three main breakthroughs including direct observation of rotation of F_1(b)(Noji et al., 1997), basic hypothesis of "binding change mechanism" for ATP synthase(c)(Boyer, 1997) and crystal structure proving of the eccentric rotation of γ subunit(d)(Abrahams et al., 1994).

2. Enzymatics of the holoenzyme

From the viewpoint of enzymatics, conventional theory generally concerned with irreversible reaction on a single substrate which can be described by the Michaelis-Menten kinetics. But ATP can be reversibly synthesized and hydrolyzed in F$_o$F$_1$-ATPase, and the reaction involves several substrates/products. In particular, ATP hydrolysis does spontaneously occur in F$_1$, whereas the thermodynamically unfavorable reaction, ATP synthesis, has to be driven by harnessing the transmembrane proton flow in F$_o$. If it functions as a synthase, the two substrates, ADP and P$_i$, are recombined into one product, ATP. Though it is well established that the mechanical process, chemical reactions in F$_1$ and transmembrane proton transport in F$_o$ are tightly coupled, that is, three ATP molecules will be generated in F$_1$ for every cycle with n protons transmembrane translation in F$_o$, the fundamental relation between the rotation speed and substrate/product concentrations, transmembrane p.m.f. and damping coefficient is still challenging.

2.1 Systematic kinetics of the holoenzyme

A few of theoretical approaches have been proposed aiming for a better understanding of the operating mechanism of this reversible motor. Some work focused on the hydrolysis or synthesis of F$_1$. For example, Oster et al. constructed a 4^3 states model for the couplings among three catalytic sites and provided a physical view of the dynamics(Sun et al., 2004; Wang & Oster, 1998; Xing et al., 2005). However, the model is too sophisticated to be investigated analytically. Some other models studied the mechanism of torque generation of F$_o$ with a turbine or all-atom model(Aksimentiev et al., 2004; Elston et al., 1998; Oster et al., 2000). On the other hand, the kinetics of this motor has been investigated by Pänke et al. with simulations or storage of elastic energy model(Pänke & Rumberg, 1996; 1999). Here, we focus on analytical investigation of the systematic kinetics of the holoenzyme. Furthermore, presumably analytical results could allow for a deeper insight for the working principles of the motor.

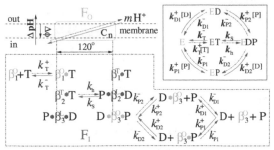

(a) Tri-site filled with random order binding model.

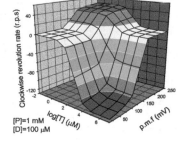

(b) Speed versus ATP concentration and p.m.f.

Fig. 2. (a) Tri-site filled with random order binding model. Synthesis pathway runs from right to left (red solid), whereas hydrolysis one runs from left to right (blue dash dots). (b) Rotational speed of motor versus ATP concentration and p.m.f. Red or blue means that motor works in synthesis or hydrolysis respectively, and yellow represents that motor is near equilibrium(Shu & Lai, 2008).

It is well established that the mechanical process in F_0 and the chemical reactions in F_1 are tightly coupled. Therefore, it is possible to construct a theory which can systematically describe the whole machine. Here, we propose a tri-site filled with random order of ADP and P_i binding model (shown in Fig.2(a)). The kinetics of this reversible reaction may be described by the equations governing the probabilities(denoted by P_E, P_{ET}, P_{EDP}, P_{ED}, and P_{EP}) of these five states:

$$
\left.
\begin{aligned}
\dot{P}_E &= k_T^- P_{ET} + k_{D1}^- P_{ED} + k_{P1}^- P_{EP} - (k_{D1}^+[D] + k_{P1}^+[P] + k_T^+[T])P_E \\
\dot{P}_{ET} &= k_T^+[T]P_E + k_s P_{EDP} - (k_T^- + k_h)P_{ET} \\
\dot{P}_{EDP} &= k_h P_{ET} + k_{P2}^+[P]P_{ED} + k_{D2}^+[D]P_{EP} - (k_{D2}^- + k_{P2}^- + k_s)P_{EDP} \\
\dot{P}_{ED} &= k_{P2}^- P_{EDP} + k_{D1}^+[D]P_E - (k_{D1}^- + k_{P2}^+[P])P_{ED} \\
P_{EP} &= 1 - (P_E + P_{ET} + P_{EDP} + P_{ED})
\end{aligned}
\right\},
\tag{1}
$$

where the square bracket [ ] denotes the concentration, T, D and P represent ATP, ADP and P_i respectively, and $k^+(k^-)$ is the binding(unbinding) constant. The steady-state reaction rate has been derived to be of second degree in ADP and P_i concentrations, and cannot be treated in terms of a Michaelis-Menten form. However, if the bindings and unbindings of ADP and P_i are completely independent and there is no mutual interaction, i.e. $k_{D1}^\pm = k_{D2}^\pm \equiv k_D^\pm$ and $k_{P1}^\pm = k_{P2}^\pm \equiv k_P^\pm$, it can be put into an apparent Michaelis-Menten equation. In addition, clamped ΔpH experiment(Kothen et al., 1995) has shown that binding and unbinding of a substrate (at cosubstrate saturation) are rapid processes as compared to the synthesis/hydrolysis step (mechanical rotation), which means that $k_{s/h} \ll k_L \equiv k_P^+[P] + k_D^+[D] + k_P^- + k_D^-$. Within the framework of steady-state conditions, the clockwise revolution rate of the motor at steady state is given by $\frac{1}{3}(k_s P_{EDP} - k_h P_{ET})$ and can be computed to be

$$
r_c = \frac{\frac{1}{3}v_M^s v_M^h \left\{ [D][P] - \dfrac{[T]}{K_e} \right\}}{(K_M^P[D] + K_M^D[P] + [D][P]) v_M^h + \dfrac{K_M^T + \sigma[T]}{K_e} v_M^s}.
\tag{2}
$$

The definition and meaning of various quantities in the above equation are given below: v_M^s and v_M^h are the saturated rates of synthesis and hydrolysis and are given by

$$
v_M^s \equiv \frac{v_{max}^s k_s}{k_s + k_h + v_{max}^s(1 - k_s/k_L)} \approx \frac{v_{max}^s k_s}{k_s + v_{max}^s + k_h},
\tag{3}
$$

$$
v_M^h \equiv \frac{v_{max}^h k_h}{k_h + v_{max}^h[1 - (k_h - k_s)/k_L]} \approx \frac{v_{max}^h k_h}{k_h + v_{max}^h}
\tag{4}
$$

respectively, where the maximum rates are $v_{max}^s \equiv k_T^-$ and $v_{max}^h \equiv k_P^- k_D^- / (k_P^- + k_D^-)$. The corresponding Michaelis constants are given by

$$
K_M^T \equiv v_M^h \left[\frac{1}{k_T^-} + \frac{1}{k_h} \left(1 + \frac{k_s}{k_T^-} \right) \right] K_d^T \approx \left[1 - v_M^h \left(\frac{1}{v_{max}^h} - \frac{1}{k_T^-} \right) \right] K_d^T,
\tag{5}
$$

$$
K_M^P \equiv v_M^s \left[\frac{1}{k_P^-} + \frac{1}{k_s} \left(1 + \frac{k_h}{k_T^-} \right) \right] K_d^P \approx \left[1 - v_M^s \left(\frac{1}{v_{max}^s} - \frac{1}{k_P^-} \right) \right] K_d^P,
\tag{6}
$$

$$
K_M^D \equiv v_M^s \left[\frac{1}{k_D^-} + \frac{1}{k_s} \left(1 + \frac{k_h}{k_T^-} \right) \right] K_d^D \approx \left[1 - v_M^s \left(\frac{1}{v_{max}^s} - \frac{1}{k_D^-} \right) \right] K_d^D.
\tag{7}
$$

The equilibrium constant is given by $K_e \equiv K_e^b e^{-\Delta G/k_B T}$, where $K_e^b \equiv K_d^T/(K_d^D K_d^P)$ and the dissociations constant are $K_d^I = k_I^-/k_I^+$ with the subscript I=T, D, P respectively. The equilibrium constant varies exponentially with p.m.f.

The inhibitions between substrates and products are complicated because ATP or ADP/P$_i$ binds competitively to the same "open" site no matter the motor functions as a synthase or hydrolase. For convenience, we express the inhibitions in an uncompetitive hydrolysis form with the parameter: $\sigma \equiv 1 + [P]/K_I^{TP} + [D]/K_I^{TD} + [D][P]/K_I^{TDP}$, where $K_I^{TP} \equiv K_d^P \chi k_D^-/k_P^-$, $K_I^{TD} \equiv K_d^D \chi k_P^-/k_D^-$, $K_I^{TDP} \equiv K_d^D K_d^P \chi/[1 + e^{\Delta G/k_B T}]$, and $\chi = e^{\Delta G/k_B T} k_L/v_M^h$.

Eq.(2) implies that the motor is a synthase if $r_c > 0$, a hydrolase if $r_c < 0$, and at equilibrium if $r_c = 0$. Fig.2(b) shows the reversible rotational speed of the motor versus ATP concentration and p.m.f. The motor functions as a synthase only if the ATP concentration is lower than a critical value such as 100μM and p.m.f is higher than 175mV. On the other hand, it becomes a hydrolase when [T]> 100μM and p.m.f< 175mV. The surface in Fig.2(b) also shows the sigmoid kinetics with respect to ΔpH at different Q(Junesch & Gräber, 1987; 1991). The relation between k_h/k_s and ΔpH and damping coefficient of "rotor" can be determined by a stochastic mechanochemical coupling model(Li et al., 2009; Shu & Shi, 2004; Shu & Lai, 2008; Shu et al., 2010)

2.2 Dynamics of system with rotary motor and battery

Recently, F$_o$F$_1$ motor is usually reconstituted in liposomes to investigate the H$^+$/ATP with pH clamp(Steigmiller et al., 2008; Toei et al., 2007; Turina et al., 2003). The dynamics of the system composed of motor and vesicle is urgent. Here we propose a possible experimental situation to study the dynamics of the F$_o$F$_1$ motor and vesicle system. In CF$_o$F$_1$-liposome experiments, a single purified H$^+$-translocating ATP synthase from chloroplast can be reconstituted on a vesicle. If the F$_1$ is extended inside and the vesicle is impermeable except for the proton channel in F$_o$, how long does the system take to achieve equilibrium once the outside pH is disturbed? This question involves the dynamics of the system and seems too complicated to be solved. However, if the diffusions of the substrates and proton in buffer are rapid enough, i.e., the time that the system takes to achieve steady concentrations of substrates and proton inside is much less than the rate-limiting rotational step, the dynamics of this system can be directly derived form Eqs.1 with different initial conditions as shown in Fig.3. Here, we assumed that the rate-limiting rotational step is equal to the rate of ATP hydrolysis/synthesis and may approximately be calculated from Refs(Shu & Lai, 2008; Shu et al., 2010)

Here, we only need to estimate the upper limit of the ATP diffusion time since ATP is the biggest molecule involved with radius $\sim$ 0.7 nm(Ravshan & Yasunobu, 2004). The distance to be covered is, therefore, at most, the radius of the vesicle which has been taken to be $R_v = 350$ nm. With a free diffusion coefficient of $D_A = 0.3 \times 10^9$ nm^2/s, The most diffusion time of ATP may be estimated as $t_A = R_v^2/(6D_A) = 0.06$ ms. This is two orders of magnitude shorter than the time spent for one ATP synthase even at maximum rate. Although this analysis describes a three-dimensional free diffusion, it gives a reasonable estimate for the particular confined geometry when ATP has explored the whole inside of the vesicle and found the corresponding binding site.

Fig.3 shows the dynamics of F$_o$F$_1$ in such a vesicle system calculated from our model. The synthesis/hydrolysis rate achieves a maximum value at 0.1 ms for initial conditions of $P_{EDP} = 1.0$ or $P_{ET} = 1.0$ respectively. After 10 ms, the system enters the steady state. The dynamics is constant with the kinetics values (symbols) and is independent of initial conditions. The rotational rate and inside pH decrease with time, while the ATP concentration

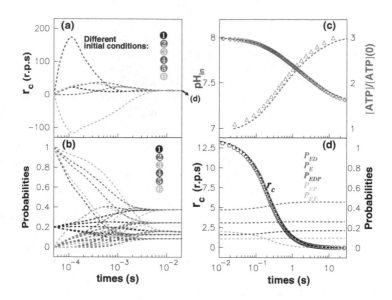

Fig. 3. Dynamics of F_0F_1 motor embedded in a vesicle system. (a) and (b): Evolutions of rotational rates and probabilities with six different initial conditions before 0.02 seconds. (c) Evolutions of pH and ATP concentrations inside. (d) Evolutions of rotational rates and probabilities after 0.01 seconds. The outside pH is constant (=6), while initial inside pH=8, [T]=100 nM, [D]=100 μM, and [P]=1 mM. The diameter of vesicle is 700 nm(Shu & Lai, 2008).

increases monotonically as expected. Here, we do not consider the influence of pH on the activity of F_1. These dynamical predictions can be tested in future experiments.

3. δ-free F_0F_1 rotary motor

An important feature of the two coupled rotary motors is that their stators are rigidly united by b_2 and δ subunits, in which δ subunit connects b_2 and $\alpha_3\beta_3$ crown. Once the δ subunit is deleted, the $\alpha_3\beta_3$ crown stators is no longer constrained, while another stator is still fixed in membrane. Therefore, the $\alpha_3\beta_3$ crown will accompany the "rotor" on rotation, and the transmembrane electrochemical energy is the only power. This is named δ free F_0F_1 rotary motor. On the other hand, chromatophore vesicles are small lipid vesicles that are differentiated to host only the photosynthetic apparatus. These vesicles are closed units, separated from their environment. The the photosynthetic apparatus convert light energy into transmembrane electrochemical energy. The chromatophore vesicle, thus, functions as a rechargeable battery.

We had developed a method to reconstitute the δ free F_0F_1 rotary motor into chromatophore vesicle so that the motor is an ideal self-driven nano-machine(Moriyama et al., 1991; Zhang et al., 2005). Employing a fluorescent actin filament attached to the β-subunits, we have directly observed the light-driven rotation of δ free F_0F_1 rotary motor at single molecule level(Zhang et al., 2005). If the fluorescent actin filament is replaced by a propeller, the motor becomes a self-propelled nano-machine and can serves for nano-submarine in artery to promote thrombolysis. Furthermore, if we exchange an antibody for the fluorescent actin filament, the self-driven nano-machine can detect antigen because it will slowdown due to damp increasing caused by antigen binding. The speed decreasing can be detected by measuring the rate varying of inside pH of chromatophore. Thus, δ free F_oF_1 rotary motor has a great potential to be developed into a biosensor and activator for different applications.

3.1 Reconstitution of δ-free F_oF_1 motor

Purification of the β-subunit, F_1 ($\alpha_3\beta_{(10 \times his\text{-}tag)}3\gamma$), and F_oF_1-ATPase: The F_1-ATPase coding sequence was isolated from thermophilic bacterium PS3, site-directed mutations of a cys193ser and gamaser107cys were introduced, and a 10 *histidine* tag was inserted downstream of the initiation codon.   The mutated construct, pGEMMH, was then cloned into the expression plasmid pQE-30, and the expression plasmid pQE-MH was inserted into *E. coli* JM103(*uncB-UncD*) in which a majority of F_1-ATPase genes have been eliminated. Thermophilic bacterium, *Bacillus* PS3$\beta_{10 \times his\text{-}tag}$ subunit (TF$_1\beta$), and F_1-ATPase ($\alpha_3\beta_{(10 \times his\text{-}tag)}3\gamma$) were expressed and purified as Ref.(Yang et al., 1998), in which the JM103 strain expressing F_1-ATPase was cultured in 2× YT medium (AMP$^+$) for 3-4 h at 37°C. When the A_{660} increased to 0.6-0.8, the expression of the F_1-ATPase was induced by addition of 1 mmol/L isopropylthio-β-D-galactoside for 3 h. Cells were harvested by centrifuging for 15 min at 4000g and cell extractions were prepared using lysozyme (1 mg/mL)/sonication (5 min) in 50 mmol/L Tris-HCl (pH 8.0) buffer containing 0.5 mol/L NaCl and 1 mmol/L phenylmethane sulfonyl fluoride. The extracts were incubated at 60 °C for 30 min, and TF$_1\beta$ was purified using Ni^{2+}-NTA affinity chromatography at 4 °C. F_1-ATPase ($\alpha_3\beta_{(10 \times his\text{-}tag)}3\gamma$) was purified as Ref.(Montemagno & Bachand, 1999) at 25 °C. The F_oF_1-ATP synthase from the *E. coli* JM103(*uncB-UncD*) was purified as Ref.(Yang et al., 1998). The mutant ATP synthase containing the His-tag could be isolated with Ni-NTA column. F_oF_1-ATPase was eluted with buffer B containing 0.05% lysolecithin and 250 mM imidazole at 4 °C, and then further purified by a gel filtration column (Superdex 200 HR 10/30 Pharmacia). The purified protein was analyzed by SDS-PAGE.

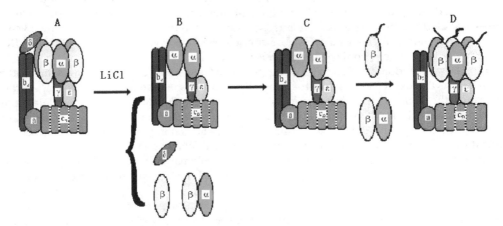

Fig. 4. The procedure of reconstitution of δ-free F_oF_1-ATPase motor. (A) F_oF_1-ATPase; (B) F_oF_1-ATPase is treated by LiCl to remove δ subunit; (C) Rebinding of purified β and α subunits; (D) The reconstituted δ-free F_oF_1-ATPase motor(Zhang et al., 2005).

The procedure of δ-subunit deletion of F_0F_1-ATPase is briefly shown in Fig.4. The proteoliposome containing F_0F_1-ATPase and bacteriorhodopsins (BRs) was incubated with 2 M LiCl, 0.1 mM Tricine-NaOH, 10 mM $MgCl_2$, and 1 mM ATP for 20 min at 4 °C. Then the proteoliposome was washed and isolated by centrifuging. Because some α and β subunits may be removed during δ delation, the LiCl-treated proteoliposome needs incubating with purified $\alpha_3\beta_3\gamma$(or β) subunits at 4 °C for 60 min (for each divided subunit of F_1 with buffer 0.1 mM Tricine-NaOH, 10 mM $MgCl_2$, 50 mM KCl, 0.5 mM NaCl, and 1 mM ATP), and then is cultured at 37 °C for 60 min (for reconstituting of δ-free F_0F_1-ATPase). The proteoliposome needs to be isolated to obtain the reconstituted δ-free F_0F_1-ATPase(Liao et al., 2009; Su et al., 2006; Tao et al., 2008).

3.2 Direct observation of the light-driven rotation of the δ-free F_0F_1 motor

Preparation of motor and liposome: F_0F_1-ATPase from the E. *coli* JM103(*uncB-UncD*) was purified as Ref.(Yang et al., 1998). The purified BR and F_0F_1-ATPase were co-reconstituted into a liposome. The liposome was prepared by reverse-phase evaporation with the mixture of soybean lipid and 1,2-dipalmitoyl-sn-glycero-3 phosphoethanolamine-N-biotinyl (molar ratio: 7:0.001)(Matsui & Yoshida, 1995). The molar ratio of BR and F_0F_1-ATPase was about 100:1, and that of lipids and protein was 30:1(w/w), so that it is possible for one proteoliposome to contain one F_0F_1-ATPase and more than 20 BR molecules.

Preparation of fluorescent actin filaments: The G-actin was co-labeled with FITC and Maleimido-C3-NTA-Ni^{2+} in buffer (50 mM Hepes-KOH, pH 7.6, 4 mM $MgCl_2$, and 0.2 mM ATP) for one night at 4 °C. The free FITC and Maleimido-C3-NTA (Ni-NTA) were removed by a desalting column. Then the labeled G-actin was polymerized in buffer containing 50 mmol/L Hepes-KOH (pH 7.6), 50 mmol/L KCl, 4 mmol/L $MgCl_2$, and 2 mmol/L ATP.

Preparation for immobilization of proteoliposomes in the experimental system for observation. Biotin-AC5-Sulfo-OSu was linked to the polylysine which had previously coated on the bottom of the dishes, and then 100 μl of 10 nM streptavidin was added into the dish bottom. After 5 min, the free streptavidin was washed. The proteoliposomes were conjugated by lipid-biotin-streptavidin-biotin-polylysine to the glass surface. And then the FITC-labeled F-actin filaments were attached to theβ-subunit of F_1 part through the His-tag with Maleimido-C3-NTA, as a marker of orientation for observation under an Olympus IX71 fluorescent microscope equipped with an ICCD camera.

To visualize the rotation of F_0 in proteoliposome, a fluorescent actin filament was attached to β subunits through His-tag, while the proteoliposome was immobilized onto the glass surface through the biotin- streptavidin-biotin complexes(Fig.5A). The sample was exposed under the 570 nm cool light for 30 min to initiate the rotation of the F_0 motor. Before illumination, the buffer containing 2 mM NaN_3 and 2 mM ADP was infused into the chamber. The clockwise rotation of actin filament was traced directly by an Olympus IX71 fluorescent microscope equipped with an ICCD camera (Roper Scientific, Pentamax EEV 512×512 FT) viewing from F_0 side to F_1. Fig.5B shows an example of the sequential clockwise rotation images with 100 ms interval. We have selected six rotational data with different length filaments to show in Fig.5C. The rotation displays occasional pause or even backwards due to Brownian fluctuation. The rotation speed decreases with the length of filament increasing, which is in agreement with the results of single molecule experiments of F_1Noji et al. (1997); Yasuda et al. (1998) as expected. In addition, several control experiments were performed to confirm that the observed rotation is driven by transmembrane proton flow. As shown in Fig.5D, the rotation stopped immediately once 5 μl of 10 μM CCCP was added. It was also found that if the

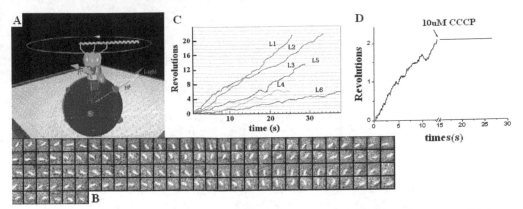

Fig. 5. (A)The system used for observation of the F$_0$ rotation in the proteoliposome which was immobilized on the cover glass with biotin-streptavidin-biotin. (B)The sequential images of a clockwise rotating fluorescent actin filament. Time interval is 100 ms. (C)Time courses of the actin filament rotation with different length. The fluorescent filament was attached to the β subunits through His-tag. The length of filaments denoted L1,L2,L3,L4,L5 and L6 are 1.7, 1.9, 2.0, 2.3, 2.8 and 3.3 μm respectively. (D)The rotation was inhibited by adding CCCP, which verified the motor was indeed driven by transmembrane ΔpH(Zhang et al., 2005).

sample is in dark or is incubated with DCCD before illumination, no rotation has been observed (data are not shown) because CCCP destroyed the transmembrane p.m.f and DCCD blocked the proton channels. Furthermore, if NaN$_3$ and ADP disappeared in the buffer, no rotation of filament was found because NaN$_3$ and ADP prevented the $\alpha_3\beta_3$ crown from sliding to γ subunit(Muneyuki et al., 1993). These results demonstrated that the rotation of filaments depended on the p.m.f produced in proteoliposome. It is interesting that the ΔpH transmembrane of proteoliposome can persist for a long time. After the illumination, some filaments rotated continuously more than 20 min. The proteoliposome function as a recharge battery to supply energy to the rotary motor.

4. Biosensor developed by δ-free F$_o$F$_1$ motor

Light-driven electron transfer causes the proton gradient across the membrane and leads the proton flux through n channels(c$_n$) in F$_0$. The interaction between a subunit and proton flux generates the relative movement between a subunit and c ring. Proton flux will simultaneously alter the inside and outside pH of chromatophore. It is well established that the rotational speed of motor is tightly coupled to the rate of proton transmembrane transport, that is, the changing of speed is equivalent to the altering of proton transfer rate. On the other hand, motor speed can be regulated by changing the load, while the pH altering can be detected by pH-sensitive fluorescent probes such as QDs (quantum dots)(Deng et al., 2007). Thus, the nanomachine can be developed as a sensitive biosensor if the rotor is linked antibody/complementary strand and pH-sensitive probes are labeled outside (or inside) chromatophore.

5. Protein or virus detector

The first type of rotary biosensor was based on the antibody-antigen reaction to capture virus or specific protein. The nanomachine was constructed as shown in Figure6(a): β subunit(1) was linked by its antibody(2), while the antibody(4) of H9 avian influenza virus was connected to β antibody(2) in series by biotin-streptavidin-biotin (3). The chromatophore(6) with F_oF_1 -ATPase was hold on glass surface(7) coated with chitosan. If H9 avian influenza virus(5) exist, they will load to the motor through antibody-antigen reactions. Virus or protein loading, therefore, change motor speed. The speed changing can be detected by monitoring the fluorescent intensity indicated by pH-sensitive dye (or QDs). That is, the fluorescent intensity altering can be used to indirectly detect virus or protein. Its signal-to-noise ratio can be distinguished at single molecular level. Thus, this nanomachine may be a convenient, rapid, and even super-sensitive for detecting virus/protein particles.

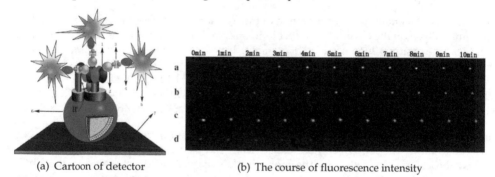

(a) Cartoon of detector　　　　　　(b) The course of fluorescence intensity

Fig. 6. (a) Basic design of biosensor based on δ-free F_oF_1. The fluorescence probe F1300 labeled inside of chromatophores was used as a proton flux indicator. **1** β subunit; **2** antibody of β subunit; **3** the complex of biotin-streptavidin-biotin; **4** the antibody of H9 avian influenza virus; **5** H9 avian influenza virus; **6** chromatophore; **7** glass surface coated with chitosan. (b) Images of intensity change of fluorescence dots caused by pH changing inside chromatophore in the course of 10 min. **a** with virus; **b** without virus; **c** with two antibodies; **d** without ADP(Liu et al., 2006b).

Preparation of H9 avian influenza virus: The avian H9 influenza were propagated in the allantoic cavities of 11-day-old embryonated chicken eggs at 37 °C for 3 days. The allantoic cavities were collected and centrifuged at 4000 rpm for 40 min and then the supernatant was centrifuged again at 100,000g for 2 h. The viruses were resuspended in PBS buffer and used in the experiments.

Labeling of fluorescence probe: The fluorescence probe F1300 was labeled into chromatophore as follows: 3 μl F1300 (0.0015 mol/L, dissolved in ethanol) was added to 150μl chromatophores and then was ultrasonicated in ice for 3 min to make the probe into inner chromatophores. The free fraction was washed by centrifugation at 12,000 rpm for 30 min at 4 °C three times. The precipitate was resuspended in tricine-NaOH buffer.

6. DNA or RNA detector

The second type of rotary biosensor was based on base-pair reaction to capture nucleic acid sequences such as DNA or RNA. Specific RNA/DNA probes, which are the complementary strand of target RNA/DNA, were linked to each β subunits of nanomachine. Once base-pair reaction take places between two strands, the flexible probes will transform into a rigid rods so that motor will slowdown because the damp of rigid rod is much larger than that of flexible single chain. Detection of RNA/DNA was based on the proton flux altering induced by light-driven rotation of δ-free F_0F_1 motor. The base-pair reaction was indicated by changing in the fluorescent intensity of pH-sensitive CdTe quantum dots. Our results showed that the assay was so sensitive (1.2×10^{-18}M) that it can distinguish the target miRNA family members. Moreover, the method could be used to monitor real-time base-pair reaction without any complicated fabrication. The nanomachine has a great potential of clinical application of RNA/DNA.

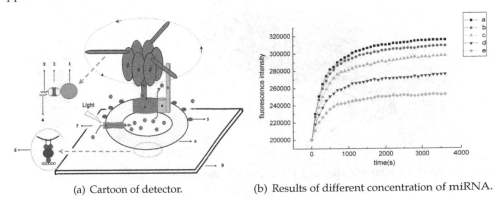

(a) Cartoon of detector.   (b) Results of different concentration of miRNA.

Fig. 7. (a)Schematic diagram of the biosensor based on δ-free F_0F_1-ATPase embedded chromatophore. 1, 2, 3, 4, 5, 6, 7, 8, and 9 represent the antibody against β subunit, the linking complex composed of [biotin-AC5-sulfo-OSu]-streptavidin-[biotin-AC5-sulfo- OSu], miRNA probe, target miRNA, 535nm QDs, chromatophore, bacteriorhodopsins (BRs), the linking system of lipid-biotin-streptavidin-[biotin-AC5-sulfo-OSu]-Polylysine, and the glass surface, respectively. (b)Results of different concentration of miRNA. RNA was extracted from MCF-7 cells. **a** without RNA; from **b** to **e** the amounts of miRNA was summed from $10, 10^2, 10^4$ and 10^6 cells respectively. Base-pair reaction was hold at 37°C(Liao et al., 2009).

The chromatophores (100 μL) were resuspended in buffer A (50mM tricine-NaOH, 5mM MgCl$_2$, 10mM KCl, pH 6.5) and incubated for 3 h at room temperature with 100 μL CdTe QDs ($1\times10^{15}/\mu$L, dissolved in water)(Zhang et al., 2007). Free QDs were washed away by centrifuging at 13 000 rpm for 30 min at 4 °C in three times. The precipitate (QD-labeled chromatophores) was resuspended in 100 μL of 50mM tricine buffer (pH 6.5). Meanwhile, 2 μL of 2 μM biotin was added in 20 μL β subunit antibody at room temperature for 30 min, followed by adding 2 μL of 2 μM streptavidin at room temperature for 30 min. The streptavidin-biotinlabeled β-subunit antibody was incubated with 5 μL QDs labeled chromatophores fixed on the glass slips at 37°C for 1 h. Redundant free biotin-streptavidin-labeled β-subunit antibody was rinsed with 50mM TSM buffer (50mM Tricine-NaOH pH 7.0, 0.25M sucrose, and 4mM MgCl$_2$). Then 100 μL 10μM miRNA probe labeled with biotin was added and incubated at room temperature for 30 min. Free probes were washed out by 50mM TSM buffer. The δ-free F_0F_1-ATPase with chromatophore was immobilized on the glass surface through the biotin-streptavdin-biotin. miRNA probe system was hybridized with miRNA target in 100μL formamide hybridization solution at 37°C.

Before the detection, the sample was exposed under the 570 nm cool light for one hour to initiate the rotation of the F_0F_1-ATPase. During illumination, the buffer containing 2mM NaN_3 and 2 mM ATP was infused into the chamber to inhibit the hydrolysis activity of the F_0F_1-ATPase and prevent relative sliding between $\alpha_3\beta_3$ crown and γ subunit.

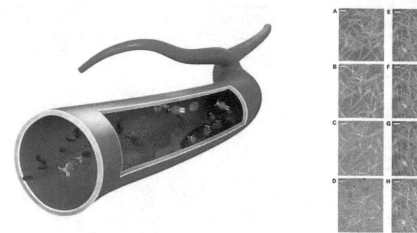

(a) Cartoon of submarine cruising in artery to promote thrombolysis.   (b)   Results   of
                                                                            experiment *in vitro*.

Fig. 8. (a) Cartoon of submarine cruising in artery to promote thrombolysis. (b) Results of experiments *in vitro*. Left row (A-D) represents the course of fibrinolysis in 30 min with lumbrokinase and δ-free F_0F_1 motor, while right row (E-H) does that of fibrinolysis in 30 min only with lumbrokinase(Tao et al., 2008).

7. A potential activator to promote thrombolysis

Cardiovascular disease such as ischemic stroke is a substantial cause of morbidity and mortality. The primary aim of thrombolysis in acute ischemic stroke is recanalization of an occluded intracranial artery. Recanalization is an important predictor of stroke outcome as timely restoration of regional cerebral perfusion helps salvage threatened ischemic tissue. At present, intravenously administered tissue plasminogen activator (IV-TPA) remains the only FDA-approved therapeutic agent for the treatment of ischemic stroke within 3 hours of symptom onset. Recent studies have demonstrated safety as well as efficacy of IV-TPA even in an extended therapeutic window. However, the short therapeutic window, low rates of recanalization, and only modest benefits with IV-TPA have prompted a quest for alternative approaches to restore blood flow in an occluded artery in acute ischemic stroke. Although intra-arterial delivery of the thrombolytic agent seems effective, various logistic constraints limit its routine use and as yet no lytic agent have not received full regulatory approval for intra-arterial therapy. Mechanical devices and approaches can achieve higher rates of recanalization but their safety and efficacy still need to be established in larger clinical trials(Sharma et al., 2010). The δ-free F_0F_1 motor has a potential to be designed a self-driven nanomachine, which serve as a submarine cruising in artery to promote thrombolysis. Our experiment *in vitro* has demonstrated that the motor may be one of alternative approaches to restore blood flow in an occluded artery in acute ischemic stroke. However, the mechanism of promoting thrombolysis has not been uncovered.

FITC Labeling on fibrinogen and fibrin formation: Fibrinogen (1 ml, 0.03 mM) was dissolved in PBS buffered saline containing 137 mM NaCl, 3 mM KCl, 8 mM Na$_2$HPO$_4$, 1 mM KH$_2$PO$_4$, pH 8.5. FITC was added to the fibrinogen solution under intensive stirring to a final concentration of 50 mg/ml(Sakharov et al., 1996). The fibrin fiber obtained from fibrinogen was polymerized with thrombin (0.5 U/μl) and fixed on the glass surface. After incubation at 37 °C for 30 min, a fibrin network with an approximate length of 200 μm was formed.

Fig.8(b) shows the morphological features of the fibrinolysis process observed directly under a fluorescence microscope. At the outset, two fibrin networks A and E, including fiber size, density, and branch point density, were similar. However, promotion of the fibrinolysis by δ-free F$_o$F$_1$ motor can be observed by comparing left and right rows. After 30 min, the fibrin almost disappear due to δ-free F$_o$F$_1$ motor (D), while the control one (H) still partly exist. It can be imaged that the many self-driven nanomachines will specially bind to fibrin and promote thrombolysis because of cooperative effect of collective propellers.

8. Self-assembly of ghost with the nanomachine

Nanotechnology aims to construct materials and operative systems at nanoscale dimensions. Several potential applications can be envisioned: targeted drug delivery systems, tissue engineering scaffolds, photonic crystals, and micro/nano fluidic and computational devices. The fundamental challenge in nanotechnology is to construct systems with varied functional features and predictably manipulate processes at the nanometer length scale. Conventional construction methods based on photolithography can successfully generate two-dimensional structures using a "top-down" approach, in which patterned surfaces are prepared by etching with light. Feature sizes on the order of 50 nm are easily achieved with commonly available technologies. Advances in specialized lithographic techniques (e.g. scanning probe lithography) have extended the resolution to below 20 nm. Molecular self-assembly serves as an alternative paradigm for preparing functional nanostructures, is perhaps one of the most intriguing phenomena in the fields of chemistry, materials, and bioscience, as well as is characterized by spontaneous diffusion and specific association of molecules dictated by non-covalent interactions. There are numerous recent examples involving different molecular entities: organic molecules, proteins, peptides, DNA and molecular motors(Kumar et al., 2011; Lo et al., 2010; Rajagopal & Schneider, 2004; Tao et al., 2009; Yin et al., 2008; Zhao et al., 2010).

A current challenge in molecular self-assembly is to achieve controlled organization in three-dimensions, to provide tools for biophysics, molecular sensors, enzymatic cascades, drug delivery, tissue engineering, and device fabrication. Ghosts (Erythrocyte membranes) are promising bioactive materials and have a great potential of application in drug delivery. The ghost is a kind of flexile membrane, composed of a lipid bilayer and cytoskeleton. One of special shapes is concave disk with the diameter about 8 μm and the thickness about 1.7μm respectively. Ghosts loaded with drugs or other therapeutic agents have been exploited extensively, owing to their remarkable degree of bio-compatibility, biodegradability, and a series of other potential advantages. We have been motivated to design a novel self-organized material using ghosts with δ-free F$_o$F$_1$ motor. A lot of interesting phenomena appear: Most chromatophores combined with δ-free F$_o$F$_1$ motor arrayed in a filament-like fashion through biotin-streptavidin-biotin interaction. The filament-like nanomachines were able to stick around the surface of the ghost with the F_1 part against the ghost. Moreover, many ghosts, which were stuck around by filament-like nanomachines, assembled spontaneously to a larger scale complex with two or three layers. This sandwich structure may be useful for the self-driven delivery of drugs or other therapeutic agents.

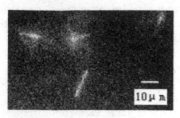
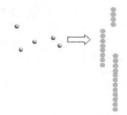
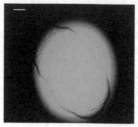

(a)   Micrograph   of
chromatophore-filaments.

(b) Possible mechanism
of   self-assembly   of
filament.

(c) Micrograph of larger
scale assembly structure.

Fig. 9. (a) Self-assembled filaments of δ-free F_0F_1 motors observed by fluorescence microscopy. (b) Possible mechanism of self-assembly of filament. Green ball represents individual δ-free F_0F_1 motor with chromatophore. Green lines represent chromatophores linked through biotin-streptavidin-biotin into filament structures. Scale bar represents 10 μm. (c) Micrograph of larger scale assembly structure. Ghosts with fluorescence-labeled δ-free F_0F_1 motors aggregate together and self-assemble into a large structure about 0.6 mm $\times$ 1.2 mm in size, which is stable for more than one week.(Tao et al., 2009).

Here, we present a novel type of self-assembled complex consisting of filaments of chromatophores with δ-free F_0F_1-ATPases and ghost, the detailed structure of which was observed by fluorescence microscopy and confocal microscopy. In the absence of light, biotin-labeled chromatophores embedded F_0F_1-ATPase are joined together by streptavidin to form filaments. These filaments can attach to ghost surface, such that the ghosts will aggregate into a larger scale self-assembled complexes with two or three layers, held together in head to head fashion between the rotary F_1's. However, if the complex is illuminated, it will disassemble due to rotation of F_1 caused by light energy. The diameter of these macroscopic complexes is more than 1 mm. δ-free F_0F_1-ATPase act as a switch to control the ghosts' self-assembly and self-disassembly, while the remote control signal (power) is light. This system, thus, has a great potential to be developed into a controllable micronmachine of drug delivery.

Ghost Preparation: Fresh blood of pig was washed three times with cold 0.15 M NaCl buffer, pH 8.0, and plasma and leukocytes were discarded. Ghosts were obtained by hypotonic lysis. Red blood cells were obtained from fresh blood and washed three times with PBS buffer (isotonic phosphate-buffered saline, pH 8.0). The washed cells were added to 40 volumes of ice-cold 5P8 buffer (5 mM sodium phosphate, pH 8.0) and left at room temperature for 20 min before centrifuging at 20 000g for 1 h at 4 °C. The pale ghost layer was collected and washed three more times with lysis solution(Steck et al., 1970).

Observation of Self-Assembly: Ghosts attached chromatophore-filaments were resuspended in 40 volumes of ice-cold buffer (0.5 mM sodium phosphate, pH 7.6) for 1 h. Addition of 5 mM NaN$_3$, 2 mM MgCl$_2$, 50 mM KCl, and 2 mM adenosine 50-diphosphate (ADP) to the buffer created conditions for light driven rotation of δ-free ATPase within the ghosts. The complexes were put into a cell, in which the chromatophores were illuminated by 570 nm light for 30 min at 4 °C. This illumination initiated proton transfer across the membrane of the chromatophores, and the rotation of δ-free F$_o$F$_1$-ATPase was then driven by the p.m.f. Once proton transfer was initiated, the cell was incubated at 37 °C throughout the whole experiment. The self-assembly and self-disassembly process was observed with an Olympus IX71 fluorescence microscope and recorded with a digital CCD camera (iXon CCD, ANDOR Technology). Confocal microscopy (Olympus FV500, optical scanning confocal microscope) was used during the scanning process of multiple layers of self-assembled complexes. FV1000 software was used to reconstruct the three-dimensional images.

9. Conclusion

In contrast to human-made machines, protein motors are self-assembled by natural biomaterial or elements, and operate in a world where Brownian motion and viscous forces dominate. The relevant energy scale is $k_B T$, which amounts to 4 pN·nm. This may be compared to the $\sim$ 80 pN·nm of energy derived from hydrolysis of a single ATP molecule at physiological conditions. Thermal, nondeterministic motion is thus an important aspect of the dynamics of molecular motors.

ATP hydrolysis does spontaneously occur in F$_1$, whereas the thermodynamically unfavorable reaction, ATP synthesis, has to be driven by harnessing the transmembrane proton flow in F$_o$. The mechanism of ATP formation in the F$_1$ part is well described by the "binding change mechanism". This has been developed in great detail by many techniques, and understanding of the mechanism has been claimed to be "almost complete". However, if the motor functions as a synthase, the two substrates, ADP and P$_i$, are recombined into one product, ATP. The binding order of the two substrates is still unclear(Watanabe et al., 2010). Another challenging question is whether the main kinetic enhancement occurs upon filling the second or the third site(Boyer, 2000; Milgrom & Cross, 2005; Senior et al., 2002). For F$_o$, the torque generation between a and c$_n$ in F$_o$ is still covered(Pogoryelov et al., 2010). In addition, it has remained unsettled whether the entropic (chemical) component of $\Delta\tilde{\mu}_{H^+}$ relates to the difference in the proton activity between two bulk water phases (ΔpH^B) or between two membrane surfaces (ΔpH^S)(Cherepanov et al., 2003).

It is of interest to ponder whether we can employ F$_o$F$_1$-ATPase nanomachine in artificial environments outside the cell to perform tasks that we design to our benefit(Martin et al, 2007)? One striking demonstration is the construction of a nickel nanopropeller that rotates through the action of an engineered F$_1$-ATPase motor(Soong et al., 2000). A metal-binding site was engineered into the motor and acted as a reversible on-off switch by obstructing the rotation upon binding of a zinc ion(Liu et al., 2002), similar to the action of putting a stick between two cogwheels. The other high light examples are the sol-gel packaging of vesicles containing bacteriorhodopsin, a light driven proton pump, and F$_o$F$_1$-ATP synthase(Choi & Montemagno, 2005; Luo et al., 2005), or F$_o$F$_1$-ATPase embedded chromatophore(Cui et al., 2005). Upon illumination, protons are pumped into the vesicles and ATP is created outside the vesicle by the ATP synthase. Besides the excellent stability of these gels (bacteriorhodopsin continued functioning for a few months), this technology provides a convenient packaging method and a way to use light energy for fueling devices. Therefore, these nanodevices with a battery can be employed to design a rapid, no labeled, sensitive and selective biosensor(Cheng et al., 2010; Deng et al., 2007; Liu et al., 2006b; Zhang et al., 2007), or construct a self-propelled nano-machine which can serves for nano-submarine in artery to promote thrombolysis(Tao et al., 2008). With ghost, the motor also has a great potential for drug delivery(Tao et al., 2009). Of course, all of these application tries are very coarse, and little more than proof-of-principle examples. Thus, there are many questions to be investigated for application.

10. Acknowledgements

This work was supported by the National Basic Research Program of China (973 Program) under the grant No. 2007CB935903 and No. 2007CB935901, the National Natural Science Foundation of China (90923009 and 20873176), Knowledge Innovation Program of the Chinese Academy of Sciences (YYYJ-0907), Instrument Program of Chinese Academy of Sciences (07CZ203100), and Starting Mérieux Research Grants 2011-Institute of Biophysics-Prof. JiachangYue.

11. References

Abrahams, J. P.; Leslie, A. G. W.; Lutter, R.; Walker, J. E. (1994). Structure at 2.8 Å resolution of F_1-ATPase from bovine heart mitochondria. *Nature*. 370., 621-628

Adachi, K.; Oiwa, K.; Nishizaka, T.; Furuike, S.; Noji, H.; Itoh, H.; Yoshida, M. & Kinosita, K. Jr. (2007). Coupling of rotation and catalysis in F_1-ATPase revealed by single-molecule imaging and manipulation. *Cell*. 130., 309-321

Aksimentiev, A.; Balabin, I. A.; Fillingame, R. H. & Schulten, K. (2004).Insights into the molecular mechanism of rotation in the F_0 sector of ATP synthase. *Biophys. J.* 86., 1332-1344

Ballmoos, C. von; Wiedenmann, A. & Dimroth, P. (2009). Essentials for ATP synthesis by F_1F_0 ATP synthase. *Annu. Rev. Biochem.* 78., 649-672

Boyer, P. D.; Cross, R. L. & Momsen, W. (1973). A new concept for energy coupling in oxidative phosphorylation based on a molecular explanation of the oxygen exchange reactions . *Proc. Natl. Acad. Sci. USA*. 70., 2837-2839

Boyer, P. D. (1997). The ATP synthase-A splendid molecular machine. *Annu. Rev. Biochem.* 66.,717-749

Boyer, P. D. (2000). Catalytic site forms and controls in ATP synthase catalysis. *Biochim. Biophys. Acta*. 1458., 252-262

Cheng, J.; Zhang, X. A.; Shu, Y. G. & Yue, J. C. (2010). F_0F_1-ATPase activity regulated by external links on β subunits. *Biochem. Biophys. Res. Commun.* 391., 182-186

Cherepanov, D. A.; Feniouk, B. A.; Junge, W. & Mulkidjanian, A. Y. (2003). Low dielectric permittivity of water at the membrane interface: effect on the energy coupling mechanism in biological membranes. *Biophys. J.* 85., 1307-1316

Choi, H. J. & Montemagno, C. D. (2005). Artificial Organelle: ATP Synthesis from cellular mimetic polymersomes. *Nano. Lett.* 5., 1538-1542

Cui, Y. B.; Fan, Z. & Yue, J. C. (2005). Detecting proton flux across chromatophores driven by F_0F_1-ATPase using N-(fluorescein-5-thiocarbamoyl)-1,2-dihexadecanoyl-sn-glycero-3-phosphoethanolamine, triethylammonium salt. *Anal. Biochem.* 344., 102-107

Deng, Z. T.; Zhang, Y.; Yue, J. C.; Tang, F. Q. & Weil, Q. (2007). Green and Orange CdTe Quantum Dots as Effective pH-Sensitive Fluorescent Probes for Dual Simultaneous and Independent Detection of Viruses. *J. Phys. Chem. B*. 111., 12024-12031

Diez, M.; Zimmermann, B.; Börsch, M.; König, M.; Schweinberger, E.; Steigmiller, S.; Reuter, R.; Felekyan, S.; Kudryavtsev, V.; Seidel, C. A. M. & Gräber, P. (2004). Proton-powered subunit rotation in single membrane-bound F$_1$F$_o$-ATP synthase. *Nat. Struct. Mol. Biol.* 11., 135-141

Düser, M. G.; Zarrabi, N.; Cipriano, D. J.; Ernst, S.; Glick, G. D.; Dunn, S. D. & Börsch, M. (2009). 36° step size of proton-driven *c*-ring rotation in F$_1$F$_o$-ATP synthase. *EMBO J.* 28., 2689-2696

Elston, T.; Wang, H. & Oster, G. (1998). Energy transduction in ATP synthase. *Nature.* 391., 510-513

Feniouk, B. A. & Yoshida, M. (2008). Regulatory mechanisms of proton-translocating F$_1$F$_o$-ATP synthase. *Results Probl. Cell Differ.* 45.,279-308

Ishmukhametov, R.; Hornung, T.; Spetzler, D. & Frasch, W. D. (2010). Direct observation of stepped proteolipid ring rotation in *E. coli* F$_o$F$_1$-ATP synthase. *EMBO J.* 29.,3911-3923

Itoh, H.; Takahashi, A.; Adachi, K.; Noji, H.; Yasuda, R.; Yoshida, M. & Kinosita, K. (2004). Mechanically driven ATP synthesis by F$_1$-ATPase. *Nature.* 427., 465-468

Jiang, W. P.; Hermolin, J. & Fillingame, R. H. (2001). The preferred stoichiometry of c subunits in the rotary motor sector of *E. coli* ATP synthase is 10. *Proc. Natl. Acad. Sci. USA.* 98., 4966-4971

Junesch, U. & Gräber, P. (1987). Influence of the redox state and the activation of the chloroplast ATP synthase on proton-transport-coupled ATP synthesis/hydrolysis. *Biochim. Biophys. Acta.* 893., 275-288

Junesch, U. & Gräber, P. (1991). The rate of ATP-synthesis as a function of ΔpH and Δψ catalyzed by the active, reduced H$^+$-ATPase from chloroplasts. *FEBS. Lett.* 294., 275-278

Junge, W. (2004). Protons, Proteins and ATP. *Photosynthesis Res.* 80.,197-221

Kaim, G.; Prummer, M.; Sick, B.; Zumofen, G.; Renn, A.; Wild, U. P. & Dimroth, P. (2002). Coupled rotation within single F$_1$F$_o$ enzyme complexes during ATP synthesis or hydrolysis. *FEBS Lett.* 525., 156-163

Kothen, G.; Schwarz, O. & Strotmann, H. (1995). The kinetics of photophosphorylation at clamped ΔpH indicate a random order of substrate binding. *Biochim. Biophys. Acta.* 1229., 208-214

Kumar, P.; Pillay, V.; Modi, G.; Choonara, Y. E.; du Toit, L. C.& Naidoo, D. (2011). Self-assembling peptides: implications for patenting in drug delivery and tissue engineering. *Recent Pat Drug Deliv. Formul.* 5., 24-51

Li, M.; Shu, Y. G. & Ou-Yang, Z. C. (2009). Mechanochemical Coupling of Kinesin Studied with a Neck-Linker Swing Model. *Commun. Theor. Phys.* 51., 1143-1148

Liao, J. Y.; Yin, J. Q. & Yue, J. C. (2009). A novel biosensor to detect microRNAs rapidly. *Journal of Sensors.* 2009., 671896

Liu, H. Q.; Schmidt, J. J.; Bachand, G. D.; Rizk, S. S.; Looger, L. L.; Hellinga, H. W. & Montemagno, C. D. (2002). Control of a biomolecular motorpowered nanodevice with an engineered chemical switch. *Nat. Mater.* 1., 173-177

Liu, X. L.; Zhang, X. A.; Cui, Y. B.; Yue, J. C.; Luo, Z. Y. & Jiang, P. D. (2006a). Mechanically driven proton conduction in single δ-free F$_o$F$_1$-ATPase. *Biochem. Biophys. Res. Commun.* 347., 752-757

Liu, X. L; Zhang, Y.; Yue, J. C.; Jiang, P. D. & Zhang, Z. X. (2006b). F$_o$F$_1$-ATPase as biosensor to detect single virus. *Biochem. Biophys. Res. Commun.* 342., 1319-1322

Lo, P. K.; Metera, K. L. & Sleiman, H. F. (2010). Self-assembly of three-dimensional DNA nanostructures and potential biological applications. *Curr Opin Chem Biol.* 14., 597-607

Luo, T. J. M.; Soong, R.; Lan, E.; Dunn, B. & Montemagno, C. D. (2005). Photo-induced proton gradients and ATP biosynthesis produced by vesicles encapsulated in a silica matrix. *Nat. Mater.* 4., 220-224

Martin, G. L.; Heuvel, V. D. & Dekker, C. (2007). Motor proteins at work for nanotechnology. *Science.* 317., 333-336

Matsui, T. & Yoshida, M. (1995). Expression of the wild-type and the Cys-/Trp-less $\alpha_3\beta_3\gamma$ complex of thermophilic F_1-ATPase in *E. coli. Biochim. Biophys. Acta.* 1231., 139-146

Meier, T.; Morgner, N.; Matthies, D.; Pogoryelov, D.; Keis, S.; Cook, G. M.; Dimroth, P. & Brutschy, B. (2007). A tridecameric c ring of the adenosine triphosphate (ATP) synthase from the thermoalkaliphilic *Bacillus* sp. strain TA2.A1 facilitates ATP synthesis at low electrochemical proton potential. *Mol. Microbiol.* 65., 1181-1192

Milgrom, Y. M. & Cross, R. L. (2005). Rapid hydrolysis of ATP by mitochondrial F_1-ATPase correlates with the filling of the second of three catalytic sites. *Proc. Natl. Acad. Sci. USA.* 102., 13831-13836

Mitome, N.; Suzuki, T.; Hayashi, S. & Yoshida, M. (2004). Thermophilic ATP synthase has a decamer c-ring: Indication of noninteger 10:3 H^+/ATP ratio and permissive elastic coupling. *Proc. Natl. Acad. Sci. USA.* 101., 12159-12164

Montemagno, C. & Bachand, G. (1999). Constructing nanomechanical devices powered by biomolecular motors. *Nanotechnology.* 10., 225-231

Moriyama, Y.; Iwamoto, A.; Hanada, H.; Maeda, M. & Futai, M. (1991). One-step purification of *E. coli* H^+-ATPase (F_1F_0) and its reconstitution into liposomes with neurotransmitter transporters. *J. Biol. Chem.* 266., 22141-22146

Muneyuki, E.; Makino, M.; Kamata, H.; Kagawa, Y.; Yoshida, M. & Hirata, H. (1993). Inhibitory effect of NaN_3 on the F_0F_1 ATPase of submitochondrial particles as related to nucleotide binding. *Biochim. Biophys. Acta.* 1144., 62-68

Nishizaka, T.; Oiwa,K.; Noji, H.; Kimura, S.; Muneyuki, E.; Yoshida, M. & Kinosita, K. (2004). Chemomechanical coupling in F_1-ATPase revealed by simultaneous observation of nucleotide kinetics and rotation. *Nat. Struct. Mol. Biol.* 11., 142-148

Noji, H.; Yasuda, R.; Yoshida, M.; Kinosita, K. Jr. (1997). Direct observation of the rotation of F_1-ATPase.*Nature.* 386., 299-302

Oster, G.; Wang, H. & Grabe, M. (2000). How F_0-ATPase generates rotary torque. *Phil. Trans. R. Soc. Lond. B.* 355., 523-528

Pänke, O. & Rumberg, B. (1996). Kinetic modelling of the proton translocating CF_0CF_1-ATP synthase from spinach. *FEBS Lett.* 383., 196-200

Pänke, O. & Rumberg, B. Kinetic modeling of rotary CF_0F_1-ATP synthase: storage of elastic energy during energy transduction. *Biochim. Biophys. Acta.* 1412., 118-128

Pogoryelov, D.; Yu, J. S.; Meier, T.; Vonck, J.; Dimroth, P. & Müller, D. J. (2005). The c_{15} ring of the Spirulina platensis F-ATP synthase: F_1/F_0 symmetry mismatch is not obligatory. *EMBO rep.* 6., 1040-1044

Pogoryelov, D.; Krah, A.; Langer, J. D.;, Yildiz, Ö.; Faraldo-Góez, J. D. & Meier, T. (2010). Microscopic rotary mechanism of ion translocation in the F_0 complex of ATP synthases. *Nat. Chem. Biol.* 6., 891-899

Rajagopal, K. & Schneider, J. P. (2004). Self assembling peptides and proteins for nanotechnological applications. *Curr Opin Struct Biol.* 14., 480-486

Ravshan, Z. S. & Yasunobu, O. (2004). Wide Nanoscopic Pore of Maxi-Anion Channel Suits its Function as an ATP-Conductive Pathway. *Biophys. J.* 87., 1672-1685

Rondelez, Y.; Tresset, G.; Nakashima, T.; Kato-Yamada, Y.; Fujita, H.; Takeuchi, S. & Noji, H. (2005). Highly coupled ATP synthesis by F$_1$-ATPase single molecules. *Nature.* 433., 773-777

Sakharov, D. V.; Nagelkerke, J. F. & Rijken, D. C. (1996). Rearrangements of the fibrin network and spatial distribution of fibrinolytic components during plasma clot lysis. *J. Biol. Chem.* 271., 2133-2138.

Saraste, M. (1999). Oxidative phosphorylation at the *fin desiécle. Science.* 283., 1488-1493

Seelert, H.; Poetsch, A.; Dencher, N. A.; Engel, A.; Stahlberg, H. & Müller, D. J. (2000). Structural biology: Proton-powered turbine of a plant motor. *Nature.* 405., 418-419

Senior, A. E.; Nadanaciva, S.; Weber, J. (2002). The molecular mechanism of ATP synthesis by F$_1$F$_o$-ATP synthase. *Biochim. Biophys. Acta.* 1553., 188-211

Sharma, V. K.; Teoh, H. T.; Wong, L. Y. H.; Su, J.; Ong, B. K. C. & Chan, B. P. L. (2010). Recanalization Therapies in Acute Ischemic Stroke: Pharmacological Agents, Devices, and Combinations. *Stroke Research and Treatment.* 2010., 672064

Shu, Y. G. & Shi, H. L. (2004). Cooperative effects on the kinetics of ATP hydrolysis in collective molecular motors. *Phys. Rev. E.* 69., 021912

Shu, Y. G. & Lai, P. Y. (2008). Systematic kinetics study of F$_1$F$_o$-ATPase: Analytic results and comparison with experiments. *J. Phys. Chem. B.* 112., 13453-13459

Shu, Y. G.; Yue, J. C. & Ou-Yang, Z. C. (2010). F$_1$F$_o$-ATPase, rotary motor and biosensor. *Nanoscale.* 2., 1284-1293

Soong, R. K.; Bachand, G. D.; Neves, H. P.; Olkhovets, A. G.; Craighead, H. G. & Montemagno, C. D. (2000).Powering an inorganic nanodevice with a biomolecular motor. *Science.* 290., 1555-1558

Steck, T. L.; Weinstein, R. S.; Straus, J. H.& Wallach, D. F. (1970). Inside-Out Red Cell Membrane Vesicles: Preparation and Puirification. *Science* 168.; 255-257

Steigmiller, S.; Turina, P. & Gräber, P. (2008). The thermodynamic H$^+$/ATP ratios of the H$^+$-ATP synthases from chloroplasts and *E. coli. Proc. Natl. Acad. Sci. USA.* 105., 3745-3750

Stock, D.; Leslie, A. G. W. & Walker, J. E. (1999). Molecular Architecture of the Rotary Motor in ATP Synthase. *Science.* 286., 1700-1705

Su, T.; Cui, Y. B.; Zhang, X. A.; Liu, X. L.; Yue, J. C.; Liu, N. & Jiang, P. D. (2006). Constructing a novel Nanodevice powered by δ-free F$_1$F$_o$-ATPase. *Biochem. Biophys. Res. Commun.* 350., 1013-1018

Sun, S. X.; Wang, H. & Oster, G. (2004). Asymmetry in the F$_1$-ATPase and its implications for the rotational cycle. *Biophys. J.* 86., 1373-1384

Tao, N.; Cheng, J. & Yue, J. C. (2008). Using F$_1$F$_o$-ATPase motors as micro-mixers accelerates thrombolysis. *Biochem. Biophys. Res. Commun.* 377., 191-194

Tao, N.; Cheng, J.; Wei, L. & Yue, J. C. (2009). Self-Assembly of F0F1-ATPase Motors and Ghost. *Langmuir.* 25., 5747-5752

Toei, M.; Gerle, C,; Nakano, M.; Tani, K,; Gyobu, N.; Tamakoshi, M.; Sone, N.; Yoshida, M.; Fujiyoshi, Y.; Mitsuoka, K. & Yokoyama, K. (2007). Dodecamer rotor ring defines H$^+$/ATP ratio for ATP synthesis of prokaryotic V-ATPase from *Thermus thermophilus. Proc. Natl. Acad. Sci. USA.* 104., 20256-20261

Turina, P.; Samoray, D. & Gräber, P. (2003). H$^+$/ATP ratio of proton transport-coupled ATP synthesis and hydrolysis catalysed by CF$_o$F$_1$-liposomes. *EMBO J.* 22., 418-426

Ueno, H.; Suzuki, T.; Kinosita, K. Jr. & Yoshida, M. (2005). ATP-driven stepwise rotation of F$_o$F$_1$-ATP synthase. *Proc. Natl. Acad. Sci. USA.* 102., 1333-1338

Wang, H. & Oster, G. (1998). Energy transduction in the F_1 motor of ATP synthase. *Nature*. 396., 279-282

Watanabe, R.; Iino, R. & Noji, H. (2010). Phosphate release in F_1-ATPase catalytic cycle follows ADP release. *Nat. Chem. Biol.* 6., 814-820

Weber, J. & Senior, A. E. (2003). ATP synthesis driven by proton transport in F_1F_0-ATP synthase. *FEBS Lett.* 545., 61-70

Weber, J. (2006). ATP synthase: Subunit-subunit interactions in the stator stalk. *Biochim. Biophys. Acta*. 1757., 1162-1170

Xing, J.; J. C. Liao, J. C. & Oster, G. (2005). Making ATP. *Proc. Natl. Acad. Sci. USA*. 102., 16539-16546

Yang, Q.; Liu, X. Y.; Miyake, J. & Toyotama, H. (1998). Self-assembly and immobilization of liposomes in fused-silica capillary by avidin-biotin binding. *Supramol. Sci.* 5., 769-772.

Yasuda, Y.; Noji, H.; Kinosita, K. Jr.; Yoshida, M. (1998). F_1-ATPase is a highly efficient molecular motor that rotates with discrete 120° steps. *Cell*. 93., 1117-1124

Yin, P.; Choi, H. M. T.; Calvert, C. R. & Pierce, N. A. (2008). Programming biomolecular self-assembly pathways. *Nature*. 451., 318-322

Zhang, Y. H.; Wang, J.; Cui, Y. B.; Yue, J. C. & Fang, X. H. (2005). Rotary torque produced by proton motive force in F_1F_0 motor. *Biochem. Biophys. Res. Commun.* 331., 370-374

Zhang, Y.; Deng, Z. T.; Yue, J. C.; Tang, F. Q. & Wei, Q. (2007). Using cadmium telluride quantum dots as a proton flux sensor and applying to detect H9 avian influenza virus. *Anal. Biochem.* 364., 122-127

Zhao, X.; Pan, F.; Xu, H. Yaseen, M.; Shan, H.; Hauser, C. A.; Zhang, S.; Lu, J. R. (2010). Molecular self-assembly and applications of designer peptide amphiphiles. *Chem. Soc. Rev.* 39., 3480-98

9

Complete Healing of Severe Experimental Osseous Infections Using a Calcium-Deficient Apatite as a Drug-Delivery System

G. Amador Del Valle, H. Gautier et al.*
University of Nantes, Teaching Hospital of Nantes
France

1. Introduction

1.1 Classifications

Osteomyelitis represents the majority of severe bone infections. The localization of osteomyelitis originating in the bloodstream is most often the metaphysis of long bones [femur (36%), tibia (33%), and humerus (10%)] in children and vertebral bodies in adults (Lazzarini et al., 2004; Calhoun & Manring, 2005) (Figure 1).

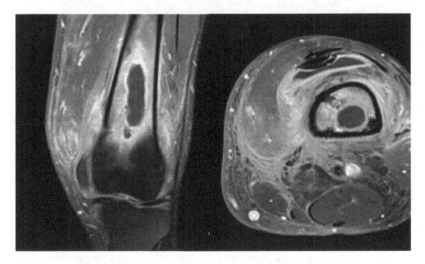

Fig. 1. Magnetic resonance tomography showing an osteolysis of the distal epiphysis of the left femur in an osteomyelitis case in a 40-year-old male patient.

Contiguous-focus bone infections from infected prosthetic devices are more frequently observed in adult males, who are more exposed to trauma (Jorge et al., 2009). Three

*A. Gaudin, V. Le Mabecque, A.F. Miegeville, J.M. Bouler, J. Caillon, P. Weiss, G. Potel and C. Jacqueline
University of Nantes, Teaching Hospital of Nantes, France

classifications are widely used in clinical practice. Waldvogel et al. (1970) described osteomyelitis according to duration, either acute or chronic. The disease is also classified according to the source of infection (i.e., hematogenous or contiguous focus). A third category defines osteomyelitis in terms of vascular insufficiency (Table 1).

Duration	Origin	Sub-divisions
Acute	Hematogenous	
	Contiguous focus	No generalized vascular disease
		Generalized vascular disease
Chronic	Necrotic bone	

Table 1. Osteomyelitis staging system (adapted from Waldvogel et al., 1970)

Nosocomial or traumatic transmissions are not considered in this classification system. Cunha (2002) suggested a simple classification based on acuteness (acute, subacute, or chronic) and microorganisms present for the elderly. The most recent classification system, based on anatomical, clinical, and radiologic features, was described by Cierny et al. (1985) (Table 2). Osteomyelitis is first defined by four stages, depending on the degree of extension: confined (medullary bone), superficial (cortical bone), localized (both), and diffuse. Second, the status of the patient (host) is considered, from A (healthy) to C (severely compromised).

Stages	Anatomical type	Description
1	Medullar	Endosteal focus
2	Superficial	Limited to the surface of the bone
3	Localized	Full thickness of the cortical bone
4	Diffused	Entire cortical bone is involved
Host	Description	Equivalent ASA status
A	Normal	ASA 1
B	Bs: systemic compromise	ASA 2 - 4
	Bl: local compromise	
	Bsl: local and systemic compromise	
C	Major comorbidities	ASA 5 -6

Table 2. Adult osteomyelitis staging system (adapted from Cierny et al., 1985)

1.2 Microbiology

In the case of acute osteomyelitis (AHO), the infection is caused by a hematogenous pathogen and is often located at a metaphysis (Table 3). *Staphylococcus aureus* is isolated in 60-80% of cases (Gafur et al., 2008) with an increasing minimal inhibitory concentration (MIC) to methicillin, followed by other Gram-positive cocci (i.e., coagulase-negative staphylococci, *Streptococcus* spp.), *Pseudomonas aeruginosa*, and *Escherichia coli* (Lew & Waldvogel, 1997; Gutierrez, 2005; Saavedra-Lozano et al., 2008) (Table 4). Bacteria are isolated from blood cultures or tissue biopsy in only 45% in children. Incidence of osteomyelitis was found to reach one in 808 to more than 2,000 admissions (Georgens et al., 2004; Weichert et al., 2008). Methicillin-resistant *S. aureus* (MRSA) represents approximately 10% of the causative bacteria, except in the USA (40-50%) (Weichert et al., 2008). The

presence of Panton-Valentine leukocidin could explain the persistence and rapid local
extension of AHO in humans (Crémieux et al., 2009; Labbé et al., 2010).

< 1 year	1 to 16 years	More than 16 years
Group B streptococci	*Staphylococcus aureus*	*Staphylococcus epidermidis*
Staphylococcus aureus	*Streptococcus pyogenes*	*Staphylococcus aureus*
Escherichia coli	*Haemophilus influenzae*	*Pseudomonas aeruginosa*
		Serratia marcescens
		Escherichia coli

Table 3. Organisms commonly isolated in osteomyelitis based on patient age (adapted from
Dirschl et al., 1993)

Bacteria	Circumstances
Staphylococcus aureus	All types of osteomyelitis
Coagulase-negative staphylococci or *Propionibacterium* species	Foreign-body–associated infection
Enterobacteriaceae sp or *Pseudomonas aeruginosa*	Nosocomial infections
Streptococci or anaerobic bacteria	Wounds infected by saliva, diabetic foot lesions, decubitus ulcers
Salmonella species or *Streptococcus pneumoniae*	Sickle cell disease
Bartonella henselae, *Aspergillus* sp, *Mycobacterium avium*-intracellulare or *Candida albicans*	Immunocompromised patients
Pasteurella multocida or *Eikenella corrodens*	Bites

Table 4. Main bacteria isolated in bacterial osteomyelitis (adapted from Lew et al., 1997)

1.3 Diagnosis and treatment

The clinical picture of AHO is often classic: it is commonly a child from 6 to 12 years of age
who suddenly presents with a disability absolved from the affected limb and associated
with a 39-40°C fever. After clinical investigation, the pain is extremely intense, and the
preferential location is the lower extremity of the thighbone or the superior extremity of the
shin. Emergency treatment must be initiated, associated with fixed immobilization in plaster
and intravenous antibiotic therapy. If the treatment is administrated early, cure is most often
achieved within 3 weeks. If a delay in diagnosis is made or the treatment is inadequate,
chronic osteomyelitis associated with a 38°C fever can develop and the affected limb aches,
is red and warm, and sometimes abscesses. Radiography shows osteolysis at the
metaphysis, with thickening or detachment of the periostium with ossification and
appearance of a sequestrum. The treatment of these forms, which can become subacute or
chronic, is complex and is often associated with 6 months to 1 year of medical treatment and
repeated surgical procedures to remove intra-osseous or under-periostium abscesses and
sequestra. The after-effects are important: osseous fragility with risk of fracture and
disorders of healing and growth in length or with deviation. The osteitis is usually subacute
with *S. aureus* and more or less painful. When osteitis affects a lower limb, patients have a

limp, and clinical examination shows amyotrophy regarding the skeletal area of interest. The biology shows all the signs of infection (leucocytosis, erythrocyte sedimentation rate, C-reactive protein); radiology reveals evidence of uni- or polycyclic osteolysis that is finely encircled by dense bone (Brodie's abscess). Surgical treatment is necessary, and osseous trepanning is performed to decompress this internal infection, administering antibiotics intravenously first and then orally. The duration of treatment is at least 3 weeks. If everything does not quickly normalize, oral antibiotics are necessary for several months. Osteomyelitis is an infective process that may also require numerous surgical interventions and leads to bone sclerosis and deformity, and even to a loss of limb.

2. Animal experimental models

Clinical trials for antibiotic treatment of osteomyelitis are rare and difficult to perform for many reasons. First, the anatomical localization of the lesions varies. Moreover, the treatment of patients suffering from severe bacterial infection with new drugs raises complicated ethical concerns that must be addressed. In vitro alternatives to replace animal tests, specifically to study osteomyelitis due to MRSA, are unrealistic and do not allow for surgical procedures. For these reasons, animal studies are the most appropriate and feasible way to assess the impact of antibiotic therapy on the outcome of osteomyelitis. Several different models exist and were developed to study hematogenous (or post-traumatic) osteomyelitis or osteomyelitis related to orthopedic implants and prosthetic joint infections. The features and history of these osteomyelitis models have been summarized by several authors (Mader, 1985; Norden, 1988; Rissing, 1990; Patel et al. 2009). Further, osteomyelitis studies have been conducted using various species, including rats (Power et al. 1990), rabbits (Andriole et al., 1973; Norden 1988), dogs (Deysine et al., 1976; Fitzgerald, 1983), and guinea pigs (Passl et al., 1984)., each with advantages and limitations.

2.1 Limitations and failures
The osteomyelitis experimental model is demanding but critical for testing new antibiotics because eradication of bacteria from bone represents a very difficult challenge (Yin et al., 2005). In experimental studies, viable bacteria can be retrieved from the bone despite prolonged antibiotic treatment (i.e., up to 4 weeks). The development and maturation of bacterial biofilms could explain the failure of antibiotic treatments and subsequent relapses (Brady et al. 2008). However, current animal models of osteomyelitis have a number of limitations, including low success rates for the induction of osteomyelitis, the elimination of causative bacteria by the host immune system, and the need for administration of sclerosing agents (SAs) in most cases (Patel et al., 2009). These SAs, as morrhuate sodium or its derivative arachidonic acid, are thought to induce varying degrees of aseptic bone necrosis, providing ideal conditions for bacterial proliferation and likely facilitating bone infection by occluding the microvasculature. In most animal models of osteomyelitis, SAs are usually injected prior to bacterial injection (Yoshii et al., 2001, Fukushima et al., 2005)

2.2 The acute rabbit model
In the acute model developed by Gaudin et al. (2011), devascularized bone made from a surgically induced bone defect provided a site in which to establish a productive infection.

Femoral trepanation using a biopsy needle was followed by injection of 1 mL of 10^9 colony-forming units (CFU)/mL *S. aureus* suspension directly into the knee cavity. Using this protocol, bacterial densities approached 9-$\log_{10}$ CFU/g infected tissue 3 days post-infection that persisted at least 14 days without treatment. Unlike chronic models of osteomyelitis, no spontaneous recovery of the bacterial infection was observed. Moreover, the rabbit long bone model is appropriate for the study of osteomyelitis because rabbits are more prone to infection than other animals, such as rats. The size of New Zealand white rabbits makes it possible to more closely mimic human surgical procedures such as bone debridement and computer-controlled pharmacokinetic .

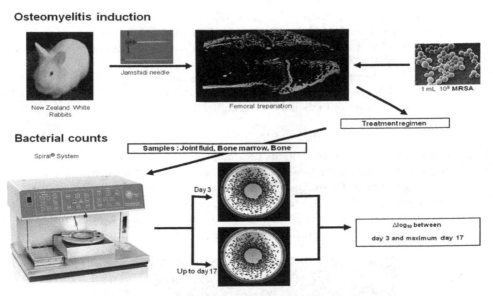

Fig. 2. The acute experimental osteomyelitis rabbit model (Gaudin et al., 2011)

3. Calcium phosphate as a matrix of antibiotic release

The term "biomaterial" has recently been defined as "a substance that has been engineered to take a form that, alone or as part of a complex system, is used to direct...the course of any therapeutic or diagnostic procedure" (Williams, 2009). Implantable biomaterials are inert or can promote biological activities, such as bone regeneration, or minimize undesirable activities, such as infection or blood clotting (Williams, 2008, 2009).

In the osseous and dental fields, biomaterials are often necessary to fill or treat different pathological situations, such as bone trauma, infections, irradiations, or various diseases such as osteoporosis and tumor resection (Campoccia et al., 2010). As alternatives to bone grafts, different biomaterials have been developed.

3.1 Biomaterials

Inorganic materials are frequently used as bone matrixes and are divided into three chemical families that represent current alternatives to biological bone grafts: calcium phosphate (CaP), calcium sulphate, and calcium carbonate. These materials can be shaped into different forms such as powders, granules, ceramics, cements, and coating, depending on the site, and the size and shape of the bone defect. Granules are more convenient than blocks, allowing the replacement of a large bone volume. As blocks are difficult to fit into cavities, vacant areas are often observed between blocks and bone. Vertebrate bone tissue is primarily composed of CaP, which explains why CaP materials are excellent candidates for bone reconstruction (Rush, 2005; Vallet-Regi, 2006: LeGeros, 1991). CaP materials are also interesting because of their cell resorption and osteoconductive properties. Calcium sulphate and calcium carbonate are less frequently used because they promote poor osseous formation because of their higher solubilities.

Based on composition, currently used synthetic CaP matrixes are classified as hydroxyapatite [HA: $Ca_{10}(PO_4)_6(OH)_2$], alpha- or beta-tricalcium phosphate [α or β-TCP : $Ca_3(PO_4)_2$], mixtures of these compounds, biphasic CaP (BCP), or unsintered apatites called calcium-deficient apatite (CDA).

HA and ß-TCP ceramics can be prepared by grinding CaO and P_2O_5 powders with Ca/P equal to 1.67 and 1.5, respectively. These mixtures must be sintered at more than 1100°C. These CaP biomaterials differ in their extent of dissolution (Chow, 2009):

$$\text{α-TCP} \gg \text{CDA} > \text{β-TCP} \gg \text{HA}$$

CDAs can be prepared either by aqueous precipitation from calcium and phosphate salts or alkaline hydrolysis of acidic CaP (Jarcho, 1981; Gauthier et al., 1998; Venesmaa et al., 2001; Nehme et al., 2003). For BCPs, the dissolution rate depends on the HA/TCP ratio: the higher the ratio, the higher the dissolution (LeGeros, 1991; Daculsi et al., 1997). HA, TCP, BCPs, and CDA are frequently described in the literature as excellent candidates for bone substitution because of their similarity to bone structures (Figures 3 and 4).

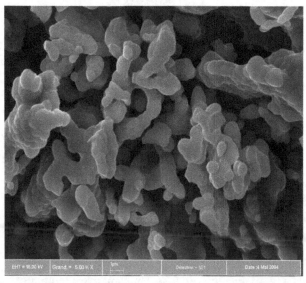

Fig. 3. Scanning electron micrograph picture of BCP at a magnification of 5000.

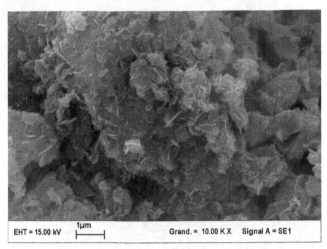

Fig. 4. Scanning electron microscopy picture of CDA at a magnification of x10 000.

These materials have all the necessary properties required for a graft: biocompatibility, bioactivity, biofunctionality, and osteoconductivity. Because of CDA's better solubility than BCP, bone colonization with CDA will be quicker and more significant and will thus provide a better reconstitution of the bone.

Others matrix properties are also very important. Macroporosity, which corresponds to pores larger than 100 µm, defines its capacity to be colonized by cells. Different agents can be associated with the matrix during the preparation process (naphthalene or sucrose particles and granules) and then calcinated or sublimated at high temperature (Lecomte et al., 2008; Le Ray et al.; 2010). Microporosity, corresponding to pores smaller than 10 µm, defines the matrix capacity to be impregnated by biological fluids. These micropores depend on the sintering process, and the microporosity depends mainly on the material composition and the used thermal cycle. Solubility and biological properties of these CaP materials depend on crystal size, ionic impurities, specific surface area, and porosity. The control of the macro- and micropore size and distribution of CaP bone substitutes represent the most important parameters to promote or induce bone formation. All these parameters have a specific influence on the final mechanical properties of the bioceramics (Bouler et al., 1996).

CaP biomaterials possess three fundamental properties that govern potential bone substitution:

- Biocompatibility: CaP ceramics are perfectly tolerated by the host organism, as described by numerous studies (Deligianni et al., 2001; Ooms et al., 2003; Julien et al., 2007; Williams, 2008),
- Bioactivity: After implantation, the biological fluids interact with the CaP ceramics and initiate the dissolution of the material. Depending on the chemical composition of the CaP ceramics, a precipitation of a layer of biological apatite can be obtained on their surfaces. The continuity thus obtained between the host bone tissue and the biomaterial promotes cellular colonization and the formation of bone tissue. The cellular resorption and degradation of the bone substitute results from the concomitant action of osteoclasts and macrophages, respectively (Anderson & Miller, 1984; Minkin & Marinho, 1999; Detsch et al., 2008). The resorption rate of the material and the *de novo*

bone tissue rate ideally must be similar to ensure stability of the interface (Zerbo et al., 2005). The biological, chemical, and mechanical properties at the bone/material interface are therefore essential to ensure good osteointegration of the implant (Ducheyne & Cuckler, 1992).

- Biofunctionality (Daculsi et al., 1999; Parikh, 2002; LeGeros, 2002): The material mechanical properties of CaP ceramics are limited by low initial mechanical properties compared to host bone mechanical properties. However if osteoconduction and resorption are favored (e.g., by a convenient porous structure), the fragility of the CaP ceramic implant is going to decrease, and an optimal final biofunctionality will be achieved with the total resorption/substitution process. Therefore, intrinsic material parameters [e.g., rate of porosity and solubility (Ca/P ratio)] and extrinsic parameters (e.g., primary stability, instrumentation) must be adapted to promote both complete implant resorption and tissue regeneration. Then, the three functions (mechanic, metabolic, and hematopoietic) of bone can be fully restored.

3.2 Biomaterials as drug delivery systems

The "fill-in" properties are interesting but rapidly it became necessary to not only fill in osseous or dental defects (Navarro et al., 2008) but to treat locally different pathologies. Thus, several combinations of biomaterial matrices and therapeutic agents were prepared. Such biomaterials are called drug delivery systems (DDS). First, polymethylmethacrylate cements were tried as innovative drug delivery systems, but these materials were progressively replaced by resorbable materials whose major advantage is to be left *in situ* in the bone defect and do not require surgical removal. These materials are numerous, ranging from inorganic to organic and from natural to semi-synthetic or synthetic.

Therapeutic agent-CaP biomaterial combinations prepared to produce an *in situ* DDS with a sustained release profile were numerous; a large panel of therapeutic agents loaded onto biomaterials was used, including growth factors (Verron et al. 2010) such as bone morphogenetic proteins (Ripamonti et al., 1992; Deckers et al., 2002), human growth hormone (Goodwin et al., 1995; Downes et al., 1995; Guicheux et al., 1998), transforming growth factor-beta (Kim et al., 2005), insulin-like growth factor (Matsuda et al., 1992); antiosteoporotics (Denissen et al., 1994, 1997; Golomb et al.,1992); anticancer drugs (Otsuka et al., 1995; Itokazu et al., 1998); insulin (Otsuka et al., 1994); steroid hormones (Bajpai & Benghuzzi, 1988); analgesic drugs (morphine and lidocaine (Gautier et al., 2010), and antibiotics (Penner et al., 1996; Suzuki et al., 1998).

Concerning antibiotics, the incorporation of antibacterial therapeutic agents in biomaterials dates back to the 1950s with the association of dental cements and resins with antibiotic drugs. The idea was to release locally therapeutic agent at the infection site. As cements and resins are not bioresorbable, other biomaterials that are resorbable and soluble were developed. Therapeutic agent release must be controlled to ensure adequate tissue concentrations several times higher than the MIC and maintained sufficiently to entirely cover the difficult post-surgery period, avoiding the systemic administration of intravenous or oral antibiotics and their subsequent side effects. Among the antibiotics (Sudo et al., 2008), gentamicin sulphate (Specht & Kühn, 1998) and crobefat (Joschek et al., 1998), cephalexin (Yu et al., 1992), tobramycin (Nijhof et al., 1997; Anaja et al., 2008), arbekacin (Itokazu et al., 1997), ciprofloxacin ((Wu et al., 1997), isepamicin sulphate (Itokazu et al., 1998; Kawanabe et al., 1998), gentamicin (Randelli et al., 2010), and vancomycin (Hamanishi et al., 1996) are commonly used for these associations. Recently, a new DDS using linezolid was developed (Gautier et al., 2010). Tetracyclines cannot be used with CaPs because their fixation to the matrix is irreversible (Misra, 1991). Tetracycline is moreover used as a tracer for forehead mineralization in histology studies but is not used for the treatment of children.

3.3 Associating therapeutic agents with biomaterials

Various techniques associating a therapeutic agent with a CaP biomaterial have been reported in the literature: powder-powder mixing (Yu et al., 1992; Dacquet et al., 1992; Hamanishi et al., 1996; Trécant et al., 1997); soaking of beads (Thomazeau & Langlais, 1996; Brouard et al., 1997), granules (Joschek et al., 1998), or blocks (Prat-Poiret et al., 1996) in a therapeutic agent solution; packing the therapeutic agent in a central, cylindrical cavity in porous blocks (Shinto et al., 1992) or in the central cavity of TCP capsules to maintain high-level, long-term release of the therapeutic agent (Wu et al., 1997); adsorption of the therapeutic agent in solution on the biomaterial (Guicheux et al., 1997; Trécant et al., 1997; Gautier et al., 1998); centrifugation (Itokazu et al., 1995; Nijhof et al., 1997; Itokazu et al., 1994a, 1998d, 1998e, 1998f); or immersion of a biomaterial block in a therapeutic agent solution followed by vacuum (Itokazu et al., 1998f; Kawanabe et al., 1998). Adsorption and soaking both allow the therapeutic agent to be incorporated at the surface of the biomaterial, whereas centrifugation and vacuum enable the therapeutic agent to enter the pores of the biomaterial. These different processes of therapeutic agent–matrix association are chosen to either facilitate contacts between the biomaterial and the therapeutic agent or achieve compaction. At the same time, our laboratory has dismissed the use of wet granulation and developed two compaction techniques: dynamic compaction and isostatic compression for the successful preparation of sustained-release forms.

The technique of wet granulation, a densification technique widely used in the pharmaceutical industry for the manufacture of granules and pellets, is commonly used for the association of CaP (CDA or BCP) with the therapeutic agent, making it possible to acquire a homogeneous distribution of the constituents of the granules and create close links between CDA and the therapeutic agent (Ormos, 1994). In addition, the acquired granules have a spherical form that is suitable for filling bone defects. This technique has already been used for bone substitute formulations with vancomycin and linezolid (Gautier H et al., 2000). A particle size analysis by laser light diffraction can be performed on acquired granules after sieving of the fraction (40- to 80-µm fraction, 80- to 200-µm fraction, 200- to 500-µm fraction, depending on the defect size). The results show that a large majority of the granules belong to the required fraction. If necessary, and to select more precisely the fraction desired, aspiration with an air jet sieving machine can be performed.

Dynamic compaction is a powder compaction technique developed in 1995 to consolidate CaP powders (Trécant et al., 1997). During this process, particle surfaces are highly deformed, producing interparticulate bonding in a one-step procedure. This process occurs during the passage of a shock wave through the powder. As this technique requires no external heat and allows the compaction to be formed without a sintering step, a heat-sensitive therapeutic agent can be associated with a CaP powder without denaturing the active element. The agent and powder can be melted and associated before compaction, and the pressure can vary between 0.5 and 2 MPa. Different studies showed the advantage of dynamic compaction to obtain compact CaP biomaterials (Trécant et al., 1995) and to associate therapeutic agents with those materials (Guicheux et al., 1997; Trécant et al., 1997). These studies investigated the association of growth factors (e.g., human growth hormone) and antibiotics, such as vancomycin and polymyxin B, with the CaP matrix (CDA and BCP).

The physicochemical characterization of CaP granules by X-ray diffraction, infrared spectroscopy, and nuclear magnetic resonance showed that the structures of BCP and vancomycin were unchanged by dynamic compaction at 1.9 MPa. This finding was concordant with another study (Trécant et al., 1995), showing that the structures of powders such as hydroxyapatite, β-CaP, BCP, and octacalcium phosphate were conserved after a 2-MPa dynamic compaction. Scanning electron microscopy showed that granule porosity depends on the manufacturing process, ranging between 37.7 ± 6.8 and 9.9 ± 4.7%. Granule porosity with dynamic compaction was 3-to 4-fold lower than with wet granulation. In fact, the wet granulation process is performed during a single step in which densification occurs, whereas granule preparation is done in two steps with the dynamic compaction process: densification by powder volume reduction (which gives a compact with lower density) followed by crushing. This volume reduction is correlated with the pressure applied (porosity is reduced when compaction pressure is high). As bone ingrowth correlates with material porosity (Lu et al., 1999), the choice of preparation process allows various granules to be obtained.

Polymyxin B, a polypeptidic antibiotic that undergoes thermodamage above 60°C, was also studied and associated with CaP by dynamic compaction (Kimakhe et al., 1999). The biological activity of polymyxin B-loaded CaP was determined by the effect of the antibiotic and monocyte/macrophage degradation on compact surfaces. The biological activities (i.e., antibacterial activity and inhibited lipopolysaccharide effects on monocyte/macrophage CaP degradation) of polymyxin B released from compacted calcium-deficient apatite were unaltered. Thus, dynamic compaction allows polymyxin B to be used with CaP ceramics without any loss in integrity or biological effects.

Isostatic compression is a technique based on the transmission of an isostatic omni-directionnal hydraulic pressure to powder, thus making the materials denser within a few minutes at room temperature. This cold technique allows the association of drugs without any degradation and allows the direct preparation of a correctly and directly molded implant. Compression pressure is applied uniformly and from all directions to consolidate the material (Gautier et al., 2000a, 2000b).

Physicochemical characterization of BCP granules by X-ray diffraction, infrared spectroscopy, and nuclear magnetic resonance showed that BCP, linezolid, and vancomycin structures remained the same. After association, release profiles must be determined to characterize the biomaterials. To establish the granule release profiles of the therapeutic agents, different tests can be used: culture chamber dissolution tests (Guicheux et al., 1997) or paddle apparatus dissolution tests (European Pharmacopoeia 7.1). Proportions of therapeutic agents released daily from a CaP matrix must be measured by an UV–visible spectrophotometric or high-pressure liquid chromatography (HPLC) assay.

Generally, using the culture chamber dissolution test, independent of the therapeutic agent (e.g., vancomycin or linezolid), after a waiting time of approximately 6 hours, the kinetics were observed to be order 0 up to a complete release in 3 to 26 days, depending on the amount of therapeutic agent loaded, its solubility, and the process of association. The waiting time of 6 hours, noticed before the beginning of the release of the antibiotic, corresponds to the time of the anchoring of grains, necessary at the beginning of the dissolution of the antibiotic in the medium.

For example, in wet granulation, the process allows a faster delivery, releasing the associated vancomycin in a maximum of 3 days. Dynamic compaction increases the period of vancomycin release to 4 to 6 days. Granules obtained by this process form a matrix that releases the therapeutic agent slowly, depending on the binding force (not yet determined) of vancomycin to CaP. The pressure of dynamic compaction has no significant influence on release time, and there was no significant difference in the vancomycin adsorbed on granules prepared by dynamic compaction or compacted with BCP granules. In the first case, the water of the dissolution medium penetrates into the pores to release the therapeutic agent; in the second case, a vancomycin dissolution-diffusion process operates from the periphery toward the center of the granule.

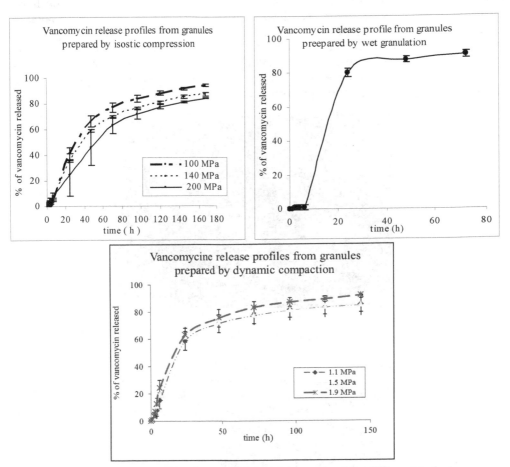

Fig. 5. Vancomycin release profiles from BCP granules prepared by different techniques.

Another study compared wet granulation and isostatic compression (Gautier et al., 2000b). Release was faster for granules prepared by wet granulation than for those prepared by isostatic compression. Moreover, vancomycin release time was prolonged as compression increased: an increase in isostatic compression from 100 to 200 MPa allowed a doubling of 75% vancomycin release. The use of isostatic compression allowed a 3- to 5-fold increase in the period of vancomycin release compared to granules prepared by wet granulation. These differences in the rate of vancomycin release may have been due to the nature of BCP-vancomycin binding strength. Vancomycin is always released faster when associated by adsorption at the surface of the granule compared to direct incorporation into the granule mass, regardless of the manufacturing process used. Release is also faster for wet granulation than for isostatic compression. Moreover, therapeutic agent release slows as isostatic pressure increases. Figure 5 shows different vancomycin release profiles from 200- to 500-μm BCP granules prepared by isostatic compression, wet granulation, and dynamic compaction.

Scanning electron micrographs show that granules prepared by wet granulation have a greater number of macropores and those prepared by isostatic compression possess a greater number of micropores (Figure 6). Image analysis also indicates that porosity is greater for granules prepared by isostatic compression. Pores of granules prepared by wet granulation appear to be more accessible to the release medium, thereby increasing the rate of vancomycin release. Moreover, the porosity percentage for granules prepared by isostatic compression is greater as isostatic pressure increases.

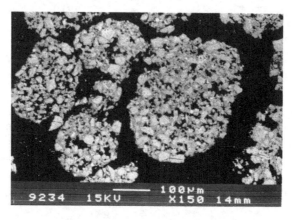

6a: porosity = 33.93 ± 4.29 %

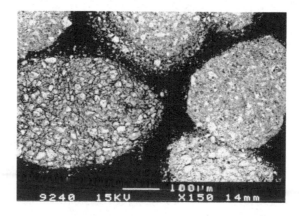

6c: porosity = 47.92 ± 5.94 %

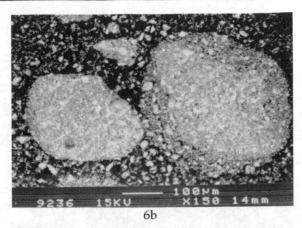

6b

porosity = 63.4 ± 14.30 %

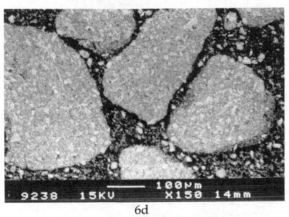

6d

porosity = 42.71 ± 7.48 %

Fig. 6. Scanning electron micrographs of BCP granules. BCP granules (200- to 500-μm) were prepared by wet granulation (a) and isostatic compression at 100 MPa (b), 140 MPa (c), and 200 MPa (d). Porosity percentages are expressed as the mean ± SD (Gautier et al., 2000b)

Another study was performed on CDA granules containing linezolid associated by a wet granulation process (Gautier H, Biomaterials 2010). Figure 5 shows images of CDA containing 10% linezolid (a) and 50% linezolid (b) acquired by scanning electronic microscopy. A comparison of the slope of the linear regression was made. For 10% linezolid-loaded granules, the slope (p) was equal to 17.068 with correlation coefficient r^2 = 0.994; for 50% linezolid-loaded granules, p = 5.11 and r^2 = 0.9969. For granules containing 10% linezolid, the release was rather quick (3.3 times more important for 10%-loaded granules than for 50%-loaded granules). After a waiting time of approximately 6 hours, the kinetics observed were order 0 up to a complete release in 9 days. The results of the release kinetics for CDA loaded with 10% linezolid were similar to those observed for vancomycin integrated into BCP, although with a slightly longer release time. For the release kinetics of CDA containing 50% linezolid, the release kinetics were similar, with a waiting time from approximately 6 hours, and kinetics of order 0. The release was complete after 26 days, which is three times greater than for grains loaded with 10% linezolid.

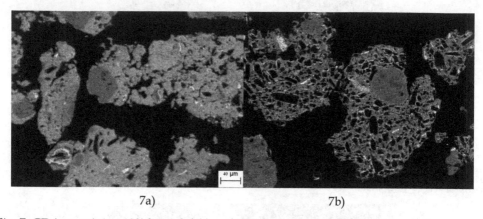

7a)   7b)

Fig. 7. CDA containing 10% linezolid (a) and 50% linezolid (b) acquired by scanning electronic microscopy at a magnification of ×250 (Gautier et al., 2010a)

Another laboratory (Kundu et al., 2010) developed HA-based porous scaffolds loaded with ceftriaxone-sulbactam (i.e., a drug combination consisting of an irreversible β-lactamase inhibitor and a β-lactam antibiotic) and presented that results of in vitro and in vivo drug elution after 41 days showed release rates higher than minimum inhibitory concentration of ceftriaxone-sulbactam against *S. aureus* in a chronic osteomyelitis model.

Additionally, there is no correlation between these in vitro release results, the release test used, and the in vivo therapeutic agent released. It appears to be important to choose the fabrication process in terms of the needed release time: a flash release of just a few days to avoid infections after surgical intervention or long-term release at high concentrations after bone infection.

It is important to demonstrate the effectiveness of the antibiotic released from the granules. This can be performed by nuclear magnetic resonance-mediated structural identification as well as by antibacterial assay. The analysis by 1H- nuclear magnetic resonance (1H-NMR) must be performed on samples of CaP granules to verify that the association process does not modify the CaP structure. 1H-NMR analysis must also be performed on samples of CaP granules loaded with therapeutic agent to identify the structure of the therapeutic agent molecule in the different samples regardless of the percentage of therapeutic agent associated. Analysis performed on BCP and CDA showed that wet granulation, isostatic compression, and dynamic compaction processes did not affect the structure of the CaP matrices. Analysis performed either on vancomycin or linezolid showed that the incorporation of pharmacological agents into CDA and BCP by wet granulation and isostatic compression did not affect the structure of the antibiotic. The chemical structure of the vancomycin and linezolid remained identical in granules even during release. In fact, no significant spectral differences were noticed during the NMR analyses of the therapeutic agent molecule released and extracted from the release profiles from 24 hours to 7 days.

The bacteriological test consists of measuring the amount of therapeutic agent still active in samples after its release. Bacterial strains must be shown to be sensitive to the therapeutic agent, and the matrices (i.e., CDA and BCP) do not inhibit the bacterial growth of the bacterial strain. The ratio of the therapeutic agent (i.e., vancomycin or linezolid) quantities calculated by bacteriological and assay measurements, derived from release kinetics of the granules after 24 hours, 5 days, or 7 days of release are determined and correlated to the NMR analyses, showing that the chemical structures of the released vancomycin and linezolid were maintained. It can be concluded that the manufacture of granules by wet granulation and isostatic compression, as well as the tests of release, changes neither the structure nor the activity of the vancomycin or linezolid, and thus, the antibiotics might be able to treat bone infection. However, a comparison of the amounts of activity detected by spectrophotometry and microbiological assay shows that only 28% of the vancomycin released from biomaterials prepared by dynamic compaction was active. This compaction technique is known to cause large but brief local temperature increases in compact materials, which are not quantifiable but high enough to induce grain joint formation. This process could denature vancomycin activity, which remains stable for 6 h at 80°C. As dynamic compaction reduces the microbiological activity of vancomycin, wet granulation and isostatic compression processes are preferred.

As a result, according to the nature of the implant and the release profiles of the different therapeutic agents, surgeons will be able to choose the most appropriate biomaterial (blocks, grains, or powders) for their patients.

4. CDA as a vancomycin delivery system: results

4.1 Rationale
In this study, we evaluated whether CDA could be used as a local DDS for vancomycin. The antibacterial activities of CDA loaded with 10% vancomycin over 14 days, in the presence or absence of a standard systemic treatment of vancomycin, were assessed using an in vivo model of acute MRSA osteomyelitis (Amador et al., 2010; Gaudin et al., 2011).

4.2 Materials and methods
4.2.1 Animals
Female New Zealand rabbits (2.0 to 2.5 kg) used in this study were individually caged and had free access to water and food. Experiments were performed according to the Committee of Animal Ethics of the University of Nantes, France. Animals soon to be moribund (i.e., having difficulty accessing water and food associated with 10% weight loss per day for 2 days) were euthanatized by lethal injection of thiopental under general anesthesia. A fentanyl patch (Durogesic®, Janssen-Cilag Lab.) was used for pain management. Due to the delay of action (approximately 12 hours), the patch was placed on the animals the night before beginning the experiment (induction) and changed every 72 hours.

4.2.2 Bacterial strain
The MRSA strain used in this study was isolated from a blood culture and exhibited heterogeneous, low-level methicillin resistance (methicillin MIC=16 µg/mL). Molecular characterization showed this strain has a cassette chromosome *SCCmec* type IVa and agr-1 and was Panton-Valentine leukocidin toxin- and toxic shock syndrome toxin-negative. The MRSA vancomycin MIC was 2 µg/mL. Inocula (CFU per mL) were adjusted to 10^9 CFU/mL.

4.2.3 Bacterial counts

Bacterial counts were determined after 48 hours of incubation at 37°C on tryptic soy agar plates. To evaluate whether vancomycin treatment induced the selection of in vivo-resistant variants, undiluted sample homogenates were spread on agar plates containing 8 µg/mL vancomycin, 4-fold greater than the MIC.

4.2.4 DDS synthesis

The most efficient concentrations of antibiotics were previously determined by in vitro and in vivo analyses (Amador et al., 2010). Granules containing 10% vancomycin were prepared by wet granulation. The size of the granules was determined to be 200-500 µm, compatible with common handling human practice.

4.2.5 Vancomycin tissue measurements

Dosages of vancomycin in joint fluid, bone marrow, and spongy bone were realized at λ=214 nm by HPLC (ThermoFisher Spectra System SCM1000/P1000XR, with automatic syringe AS3000 and UV6000LP detectors and FL3000). The column was a C18RP (Hypersil GOLD, 150-mm length, 5 µm × 4.6 mm, ThermoFisher). The isocratic mobile phase was 12% acetonitrile in an ammonium acetate buffer adjusted to pH 6 by phosphoric acid. Experiments with every range and dosage were performed in triplicate.

4.2.6 Experimental design

Animals were randomly assigned to six groups: (1) vancomycin group $V_{(IV)}$ [vancomycin constant intravenous infusion to reach a 20× MIC serum steady-state concentration (CIV)] for 4 days; (2) $V_{(CDA10\%)}$ (CDA loaded with 100 µg/mg vancomycin) for 4 days or (3) for 14 days; (4) $V_{(IV)}$ for 4 days + $V_{(CDA10\%)}$ (CDA loaded with 100 µg/mg) for 4 days (5) or 14 days (6) for vancomycin tissue measurement.

We used a percutaneous, transarticular route to perform femoral trepanation using a Jamshidi bone marrow biopsy needle under general anesthesia. The Jamshidi needle was inserted between the two femoral condyles and through the epiphysis, physis, and metaphysis to reach the medullar canal. After the needle was removed, the skin incision was closed. Subsequently a 1-mL suspension containing 10^9 CFU MRSA was injected parapatellarly into the knee cavity. At day 3, osteomyelitis was induced, causing unbridling, and the infected site was washed as recommended in human practice. Samples of joint fluid, bone marrow, and spongy bone were removed for bacterial counts. At day 7 or 17 post-inoculation, animals were euthanized to measure the bacterial load in the joint fluid, bone marrow, and bone. Results were expressed as the bacterial counts ($\log_{10}$/g of tissue) at day 3 (reference level) and either day 7 or 17. The lower limit of detection for this method was 1 CFU/50 µl undiluted tissue homogenate. Infusions of antibiotics began at day 3 and continued for only 4 days due to ethical reasons.

4.2.7 Statistical analysis

Statistical analyses were performed using Graphpad Prism® 4 for Windows (Graphpad Software, San Diego, CA, USA). Results were expressed as the means ± standard deviation. Regimens were compared using one-way analysis of variance. This analysis was performed using a post-hoc Student-Newman-Keuls test. Time-dependant efficacy was tested by a nonparametric t test associated with a Wilcoxon post-test. P less than 0.05 was considered statistically significant.

4.3 Results and discussion
4.3.1 Vancomycin tissue measurements

Wysocki et al. (2001) demonstrate that CIV patients (targeted plateau drug serum concentrations of 20 to 25 mg/L) reached the targeted concentrations faster, and fewer samples were required for treatment monitoring than with intermittent infusion patients (IIV). For comparable efficacy and tolerance, CIV may be a cost-effective alternative to IIV. Samples of plasma, spongy bone, and bone marrow were analyzed for vancomycin by HPLC in healthy and infected femurs. Vancomycin concentrations were 7.50 ± 2.48 µg/g in bone marrow and 6.11 ± 3.18 µg/g in spongy bone in healthy tissues, associated with a vancomycin plasma level of 19.09 ± 3.79 µg/mL. For infected bone tissues, vancomycin concentrations were 6.70 ± 2.23 µg/g, 12.63 ± 5.16, and 22.63 ± 8.53 for bone marrow, spongy bone, and plasma, respectively, related to the vancomycin MCIs of the causative MRSA (2 µg/mL). The constant infusion of vancomycin exhibits more than three times the MICs of the studied strain in any compartment.

For the CDA loaded with 10% vancomycin group (without a systemic approach), samples were taken at the maximum local delivering time (24 hours): plasma for vancomycin dosage and bone marrow and spongy bone, near the CDA implants, to assess local tissue delivery. Vancomycin plasma levels were 3.36 ± 0.81 µg/mL, corresponding to a very weak elevation. Local bone tissue concentrations were more than 100 times and 150 times the vancomycin MICs for the MRSA strain for bone marrow and spongy bone, respectively. Surprisingly, the introduction of CDA loaded with 10% vancomycin did not significantly increase the plasma concentration obtained at steady-state by continuous infusion of vancomycin, reducing the risk of general toxicity. In contrast, the contribution of local antibiotic-loaded material appeared to be considerable.

4.3.2 Bacterial counts

No vancomycin-resistant mutants were detected after either 4 or 14 days of treatment in any group and in any compartment.

Data from the in vivo experiments are summarized in Table 5. Because infusion caused major venous time-dependent impairment, the efficacy of $V_{(IV)}$ could not be assessed over the full 14-day treatment period. Moreover, $V_{(IV)}$ did not demonstrate significant antibacterial activity in any of the three tissues (joint fluid, bone marrow, and spongy bone) after the 4-day treatment. Of the different treatments [$V_{(CDA10\%)}$ and $V_{(CDA10\%)}$ + $V_{(IV)}$], only treatment with CDA-vancomycin plus constant infusion of vancomycin [$V_{(CDA10\%)}$ + $V_{(IV)}$] showed a significant inhibitory effect in joint fluid, with $P<0.05$ after 14 days of treatment.

Treatment with 10% vancomycin-loaded CDA alone exhibited a greater activity than $V_{(IV)}$ alone ($P<0.01$), but combining these treatments significantly enhanced treatment efficacy ($P<0.001$). $V_{(CDA10\%)}$ did not exhibit greater efficacy after 14 days compared with 4 days. In spongy bone and bone marrow, most samples were sterile after 14 days of treatment with CDA-vancomycin plus intravenous vancomycin [$V_{(CDA10\%)}$ + $V_{(IV)}$], but none after $V_{(CDA10\%)}$.

Furthermore, the combined $V_{(CDA10\%)} + V_{(IV)}$ treatment seemed to be the most effective. These data indicate the addition of a local delivery system enhanced the antibacterial effects of these drugs in a tissue-specific manner. One possible mechanism for the enhanced efficacy of the combined treatment is that the release of vancomycin loaded onto CDA is limited to the site of infection, with cortical bone acting as a semi-permeable membrane and preventing the elimination of vancomycin through the bloodstream.

Treatment regimens	n	Means ±SD log10 CFU/g tissue								
		day 3			day 7			day 17		
		JF	BM	Bo	JF	BM	Bo	JF	BM	Bo
$V_{(IV)}$	10	7.88 0.62	6.97 1.15	7.86 0.44	7.78 ± 0.75	6.38 ± 1.89	7.29 ± 0.80	ND	ND	ND
$V_{(CDA10\%)}$	21	7.86 0.55	8.47 0.80	8.11 0.05	7.81± 1.03	5.06 ± 1.43	5.76 ± 1.45	6.27 ± 2	4.80 ± 1.56 [a]	6.16 ± 1.36 [a]
$V_{(CDA10\%)}$ + $V_{(IV)}$	15	7.53 0.69	8.58 1.32	8.41 1.36	6.63 ± 0.39	4.55 ± 1.33 [a]	3.78 ± 1.28 [a]	2.52 ± 0.97* [a,b]	2.33 ± 0.34* [a,b]	2.30 ± 0.09* [a,b]

ND: not done n: number of animals [a] $P<0.05$ vs day 3 [b] $P<0.05$ vs $V_{(CDA10\%)}$ and $V_{(IV)}$
*under the lower limit of detection

Table 5. Bacterial counts in joint fluid (JF), bone marrow (BM), and spongy bone (Bo) at day 3 (post-inoculation) and 4 and 14 days after the beginning of the treatment.

5. Conclusion

Biomaterials as local DDS could reduce or eliminate the toxic side effects and complications of systemic antibiotic treatments, enhancing patient safety. From this perspective, the reference antibiotic against MRSA, vancomycin, was selected, and optimized concentrations were loaded into a CaP matrix (CDA) by wet granulation. The in vitro antibacterial activity of eluents from the DDS showed that the nature of the antibiotics was not altered either as a result of CDA loading or after sustained release from the granules. After a 14-day in vitro release, the CDA matrix was still able to deliver antibiotics at a concentration 50 times greater than the MIC of the MRSA strain used, providing local effective bactericidal concentrations of antibiotic and not inducing the development of antibiotic resistance from a slow residual release at suboptimal antibiotic concentrations. While more traditional antibiotic carrier systems are available, CDA has both desirable antibiotic release kinetics and a high osteogenic-promoting activity, including degradation of the apatite, obviating the need for a second surgery to remove the implanted material.

6. References

Amador, G., Gautier, H., Le Mabecque, V., Miegeville, A.F., Potel, G., Bouler, J.M., Weiss, P., Caillon, J. & Jacqueline, C. (2010). In vivo assessment of the antimicrobial activity of a calcium-deficient apatite vancomycin drug delivery system in a methicillin-resistant Staphylococcus aureus rabbit osteomyelitis experimental model. *Antimicrob Agents Chemother*, 54(2), pp. 950-952.

Anderson, J.M. & Miller K.M. (1984). Biomaterial biocompatibility and the macrophage. *Biomaterials*, 26, pp.1445-1451.

Andriole, V.T., Nagel, D.A. & Southwick, W.O. (1973). A paradigm for human chronic osteomyelitis. *J Bone Joint Surg Am*, 55, pp.1511-1515.

Aneja, A., Woodall, J., Wingerter, S., Tucci, M. &, Benghuzzi, H. (2008). Analysis of tobramycin release from beta tricalcium phosphate drug delivery system. *Biomed Sci Instrum*, 44, pp.88-93.

Bajpai, P.K. & Benghuzzi, H.A. (1988). Ceramic systems for long delivery of chemicals and biologicals. *J Biomed Mater Res*, 22, pp.1245-1266.

Bouler, J.M., Trecant, M., Delecrin, J., Royer, J., Passuti N. & Daculsi, G. (1996). Macroporous biphasic calcium phosphate ceramics: influence of five synthesis parameters on compressive strength. *J Biomed Mater Res*, 32, pp.603-609.

Brady, R.A., Leid, J.G., Calhoun, J.H., Costerton, J.W. & Shirtliff, M.E. (2008). Osteomyelitis and the role of biofilms in chronic infection. *FEMS Immunol Med Microbiol*, 52, pp.13-22.

Brouard, S., Lelan, J., Lancien, G., Bonnaure, M., Cormier, M. & Langlais, F. (1997). Phosphate tricalcique, vecteur d'antibiotiques : gentamicine et vancomycine. Caractérisation physicochimique *in vitro*, étude de la porosité du matériau et du relargage de la gentamicine et de la vancomycine. *Chirurgie*, 122, pp.397-403.

Calhoun, J.H. & Manring, M.M. (2005). Adult osteomyelitis. *Infect Dis Clin North Am*. 19(4), pp.765-786.

Calhoun, J.H., Manring, M.M. & Shirtliff, M. (2009). Osteomyelitis of the long bones. *Semin Plast Surg*,23(2), pp.59-72.

Campoccia, D., Montanaro, L., Speziale, P. & Arciola, C.R. (2010). Antibiotic-loaded biomaterials and the risks for the spread of antibiotic resistance following their prophylactic and therapeutic clinical use. *Biomaterials*, 25, pp.6363-6377.

Chow, L.C. (2009). Next generation calcium phosphate-based biomaterials. *Dent Mater J*, 1, pp. 1–10.

Cierny, G., Mader, J.T. & Pennick J.J. (1985). A clinical staging system for adult osteomyelitis. *Contemp Orthop*, 10, pp.17–37.

Crémieux, A.C., Dumitrescu, O., Lina, G., Vallee, C., Côté, J.F., Muffat-Joly, M., Lilin, T., Etienne, J., Vandenesch, F. & Saleh-Mghir, A. (2009). Panton-valentine leukocidin enhances the severity of community-associated methicillin-resistant *Staphylococcus aureus* rabbit osteomyelitis. *PLoS One*, 25, 4(9):e7204.

Cunha, B.A. (2002) Osteomyelitis in elderly patients. *Clin Infect Dis*, 35(3), pp.287-293.

Dacquet, V., Varlet, A., Tandogan, R.N., Tahon, M.M., Fournier, L., Jehl, F., Monteil, H. &, Bascoulergue, G. (1992). Antibiotic impregnated plaster of Paris beads - Trials with teicoplanin. *Clin Orthop*, 282, pp.241-249.

Daculsi, G., Bouler, J.M., LeGeros, R.Z. (1997). Adaptive crystal formation in normal and pathological calcifications in synthetic calcium phosphate and related biomaterials. *Int Rev Cytol*, 172, pp.129-191.

Daculsi, G., Weiss, P., Bouler, J.M., Gauthier, O., Millot, F. & Aguado E. (1999). Biphasic calcium phosphate/hydrosoluble polymer composites: a new concept for bone and dental substitution biomaterials. *Bone*, 25(2 Suppl), pp.59S-61S.

Deckers, M., van Bezooijen, R.L., van der Horst, G., Hoogendam, J., van Der Bent, C., Papapoulos, S.E. & Löwik, C.W. (2002). Bone morphogenetic proteins stimulate angiogenesis through osteoblast-derived vascular endothelial growth factor A. *Endocrinology*, 143(4), pp.1545-1553.

Deligianni, D.D., Katsala, N.D., Koutsoukos, P.G. & Missirlis, Y.F. (2001). Effect of surface roughness of hydroxyapatite on human bone marrow cell adhesion, proliferation, differentiation and detachment strength. *Biomaterials*, 22, pp.87-96.

Denissen, H., Van Beek, E., Löwik, C., Papapoulos, S. & van den Hooff, A. (1994). Ceramic hydroxyapatite implants for the release of bisphosphonate. *Bone Miner*, 25, pp.123-134.

Denissen, H., Van Beek, E., Martinetti, R., Klein, C., van der Zee, E. & Ravaglioli, A. (1997). Net-shaped hydroxyapatite implants for release of agents modulating periodontal-like tissues. *J Periodontal Res*, 32, pp.40-46.

Detsch, R., Mayr, H. & Ziegler, G. (2008). Formation of osteoclast-like cells on HA and TCP ceramics. Acta Biomater, 4, pp.139-148.

Deysine, M., Rosario, E. & Isenberg, H.D. (1976). Acute hematogenous osteomyelitis: an experimental model. *Surgery*, 79, pp.97-99.

Dirschl, D.R. & Almekinders, L.C. (1993). Osteomyelitis. Common causes and treatment recommendations. *Drugs*, 45, pp.29-43.

Downes, S., Clifford, C.J., Scotchford, C. & Klein C.P. (1995). Comparison of the release of growth hormone from hydroxyapatite, heat-treated hydroxyapatite, and fluorapatite coatings on titanium. *J Biomed Mater Res*, 29, pp.1053-1060.

Ducheyne, P. & Cuckler, J.M. (1992). Bioactive ceramic prosthetic coatings. *Clin Orthop Relat Res*, 276, pp.102-114.

European Pharmacopoea 7.1, Consil of Europe 2011.

Fitzgerald, R.H. (1983). Experimental osteomyelitis: description of a canine model and the role of depot administration of antibiotics in the prevention and treatment of sepsis. *J Bone Joint Surg Am*, 65, pp.371-380.

Fukushima, N., Yokoyama, K., Sasahara, T., Dobashi, Y. & Itoman, M. (2005). Establishment of rat model of acute staphylococcal osteomyelitis: relationship between inoculation dose and development of osteomyelitis. *Arch Orthop Trauma Surg*, 125, pp.169-176.

Gafur, O.A., Copley, L.A., Hollmig, S.T., Browne, R.H., Thornton, L.A. & Crawford, S.E. (2008). The impact of the current epidemiology of pediatric musculoskeletal infection on evaluation and treatment guidelines. *J Pediatr Orthop*, 28(7), pp.777-785.

Gaudin, A., Amador Del Valle, G., Hamel, A., Le Mabecque, V., Miegeville, A.F., Potel, G., Caillon, J. & Jacqueline, C. (2011). A new experimental model of acute osteomyelitis due to methicillin-resistant *Staphylococcus aureus* in rabbit. *Lett Appl Microbiol*, 52(3), pp.253-257.

Gautier, H., Guicheux, J., Grimandi, G., Faivre, A., Daculsi, G. & Merle, C. (1998). *In vitro* influence of apatite-granule-specific area on human growth hormone loading and release. *J Biomed Mater Res*, 40, pp.606-613.

Gautier, H., Caillon, J., Le Ray, A.M., Daculsi, G. & Merle, C. (2000a). Influence of isostatic compression on the stability of vancomycin loaded with a calcium-phosphate implantable drug-delivery device. *J Biomed Mater Res*, 52(2), pp.308-314.

Gautier, H., Merle, C., Auget, J.L. & Daculsi, G. (2000b). Isostatic compression, a new process for incorporating vancomycin into biphasic calcium phosphate: comparison with a classical method. *Biomaterials*, 21, pp.243-249.

Gautier, H., Plumecocq, A., Amador, G., Weiss, P., Merle, C. & Bouler J.M. (2010a). In vitro characterization of calcium phosphate biomaterial loaded with linezolid for osseous bone defect implantation. *J Biomater Appl*. Sep 28.

Gautier, H., Chamblain, V., Weiss, P., Merle, C. & Bouler, J.M. (2010b). In vitro characterisation of calcium phosphate biomaterials loaded with lidocaine hydrochloride and morphine hydrochloride. *J Mater Sci: Mater Med*, 21(12), pp. 3141-3150.

Gauthier, O., Bouler, J.M., Aguado, E., Pilet P. & Daculsi G. (1998). Macroporous biphasic calcium phosphate ceramics: influence of macropore diameter and macroporosity percentage on bone ingrowth. *Biomaterials*, 19: pp.133-139.

Goergens, E.D., McEvoy, A., Watson, M. &, Barrett, I.R. (2005). Acute osteomyelitis and septic arthritis in children. *J Paediatr Child Health*,41(1-2), pp.59-62.

Golomb, G., Levi, M., van Gelder, J.M. (1992). Controlled release of bisphosphonate from a biodegradable implant: evaluation of release kinetics and anticalcification effect. *J Appl Biomater*, 3, pp.23-28.

Goodwin, C.J., Braden, M., Downes, .S & Marshall, N.J. (1995). A comparison between two methacrylate cements as delivery system for bioactive human growth hormone. *J Mater Sci: Mater Med*, 6, pp.590-596.

Guicheux, J., Grimandi, G., Trécant, M., Faivre, A., Takahashi, S. & Daculsi, G. (1997). Apatite as carrier for growth hormone: in vitro characterization of loading and release. *J Biomed Mater Res*, 34, pp.165-170.

Guicheux, J., Heymann, D., Rousselle, A.V.,, Gouin, F., Pilet, P., Yamada, S. & Daculsi, G. (1998). Growth hormone stimulatory effects on osteoclastic resorption are partly mediated by insulin-like growth factor I: an in vitro study. *Bone*, 22(1), pp.25-31.

Gutierrez, K. (2005). Bone and joint infections in children. *Pediatr Clin North Am*,52(3), pp.779-794.

Hamanishi, C., Kitamoto, K., Tanaka, S., Otsuka, M., Doi, Y. & Kitahashi, T. (1996). A self-setting TTCP-DCPD apatite cement for release of vancomycin. *J Biomed Mater Res A*, 33, pp.139-143.

Itokazu, M., Matsunaga, T., Kumazawa, S. & Oka, M. (1994a). Treatment of osteomyelitis by antibiotic impregnated porous hydroxyapatite block. *Clin Mater*, 17, pp.173-179.

Itokazu, M., Matsunaga, T., Kumazawa, S. & Wenyi, Y. (1995b). A novel drug delivery system for osteomyelitis using porous hydroxyapatite blocks loaded by centrifugation. *J Appl Biomater*, 6, pp.167-169.

Itokazu, M., Ohno, T., Tanemori, T., Wada, E., Kato, N. & Watanabe, K. (1997c). Antibiotic-loaded hydroxyapatite blocks in the treatment of experimental osteomyelitis in rats. *J Med Microbiol*, 46, pp.779-783.

Itokazu, M., Aoki, T., Nonomura, H., Nishimoto, Y. & Itoh, Y. (1998d). Antibiotic-loaded porous hydroxyapatite blocks for the treatment of osteomyelitis and postoperative infection. A preliminary report. *Bull Hosp Joint Dis*, 57(3), pp.125-129.

Itokazu, M., Sugiyama, T., Ohno, T., Wada, E. & Katagiri, Y. (1998e). Development of porous apatite ceramic for local delivery of chemotherapeutic agents. *J Biomed Mater Res*, 39, pp.536-538.

Itokazu, M., Yang, W., Aoki, T., Ohara, A. & Kato, N. (1998f). Synthesis of antiobiotic-loaded interporous hydroxyapatite blocks by vacuum method and *in vitro* drug release testing. *Biomaterials*, 19, pp.817-819.

Jarcho, M. (1981). Calcium phosphate ceramics as hard tissue prosthetics. *Clin Orthop Relat Res*. 157, pp.259-278.

Jorge, L.S., Chueire, A.G. & Rossit, A.R. (2010). Osteomyelitis: a current challenge. *Braz J Infect Dis*, 14(3), pp.310-315.

Joschek. S., Krote, R., Nies, B. & Göpferich, A. (1998). Porous ceramics for local drug delivery. *Proc 2nd World Meeting APGI/APV*, Paris:353-354.

Julien, M., Khairoun, I., LeGeros, R.Z., Delplace, S., Pilet, P., Weiss, P., Daculsi, G., Bouler, J.M. & Guicheux, J. (2007). Physico-chemical-mechanical and in vitro biological properties of calcium phosphate cements with doped amorphous calcium phosphates. *Biomaterials*, 28, pp.956-965.

Kaplan, S.L. (2009). Challenges in the evaluation and management of bone and joint infections and the role of new antibiotics for gram positive infections. *Adv Exp Med Biol*, 634, pp.111-120.

Kawanabe, K., Okada, Y., Matsusue, Y., Ida, H. & Nakamura, T. (1998). Treatment of osteomyelitis with antibiotic-soaked porous glass ceramic. *J Bone Joint Surg*, 80-B, pp.527-530.

Kim, I.Y., Kim, M.M. & Kim, S.J. (2005). Transforming growth factor-beta : biology and clinical relevance. *J Biochem Mol Biol*, 38(1), pp.1-8.

Kimakhe, S., Bohic, S., Larrose, C., Reynaud, A., Pilet, P., Giumelli, B., Heymann, D. & Daculsi, G. (1999). Biological activities of sustained polymyxin B release from calcium phosphate biomaterial prepared by dynamic compaction: An *in vitro* study. *J Biomed Mater Res*, 47, pp.18-27.

Kundu, B., Soundrapandian, C., Nandi, S.K., Mukherjee, P., Dandapat, N., Roy, S., Datta, B.K., Mandal, T.K., Basu, D. & Bhattacharya, R.N. (2010). Development of new localized drug delivery system based on ceftriaxone-sulbactam composite drug impregnated porous hydroxyapatite: a systematic approach for in vitro and in vivo animal trial. *Pharm Res*, 27(8), pp.1659-1676.

Labbé, J.L., Peres, O., Leclair, O., Goulon, R., Scemama, P., Jourdel, F., Menager, C., Duparc, B. & Lacassin, F. (2010). Acute osteomyelitis in children: the pathogenesis revisited? *Orthop Traumatol Surg Res*, 96(3), pp.268-275.

Lazzarini, L., De Lalla, F. & Mader, J.T. (2002). Long bone osteomyelitis. *Curr Infect Dis Rep*, 4(5), pp.439–445.

Le Ray, A.M., Gautier, H., Bouler, J.M., Weiss, P. & Merle, C. (2010). A new technological procedure using sucrose as porogen compound to manufacture porous biphasic calcium phosphate ceramics of appropriate micro- and macrostructure. *Ceramics International*. 36(1), pp.93-101.

Lecomte, A., Gautier, H., Bouler, J.M., Gouyette, A., Pegon, Y., Daculsi, G. & Merle, C. (2008). Biphasic calcium phosphate: a comparative study of interconnected porosity in two ceramics. *J Biomed Mater Res B Appl Biomater*. 84(1), pp.1-6.

LeGeros, R.Z. (1991). Calcium phosphate in oral biology and medicine. *Monogr Oral Sci*, 15 pp.1-201.

LeGeros, R.Z.. (2002). Properties of osteoconductive biomaterials: calcium phosphates. *Clin Orthop*, 395, pp. 81-98.

Lew, D.P & Waldvogel, F.A. (1997). Osteomyelitis. *N Engl J Med*, 336, pp.999–1007.

Lu, J.X., Flautre, B., Anselme, K. & Hardouin, P. (1999). Role of interconnections in porous bioceramics on bone recolonization in vitro and in vivo. *J Mater Sci: Mater Med*, 10, pp.111-120.

Mader, J.T. (1985). Animal models of osteomyelitis. *Am J Med*, 78, pp.213-217.

Mader, J.T., Shirtliff, M. & Calhoun, J.H. (1997). Staging and staging application in osteomyelitis. *Clin Infect Dis*, 25(6), pp.1303-1309.

Matsuda, N., Lin, W.L., Kumar, N.M., Cho, M.I. & Genco, R.J. (1992). Mitogenic, chemotactic, and synthetic responses of rat periodontal ligament fibroblastic cells to polypeptide growth factors in vitro. *J Periodontol*, 63(6), pp.515-525.

Minkin, C. & Marinho, V.C. (1999). Role of the osteoclast at the bone-implant interface. *Adv Dent Res*,13, pp.49-56.

Misra, D.N. (1991). Adsorption and orientation of tetracycline on hydroxyapatite. *Calcif Tissue Int*, 48(5), pp.362-367.

Navarro, M., Michiardi, A., Castaño, O. & Planell, J.A. (2008). Biomaterials in orthopaedics. *J R Soc Interface*, 5(27), pp.1137-1158.

Nehme, A., Maalouf, G., Tricoire, J.L., Giordano, G., Chiron, P. & Puget, J. (2003). Effect of alendronate on periprosthetic bone loss after cemented primary total hip arthroplasty: a prospective randomized study. *Rev Chir Orthop Reparatrice Appar Mot*, 89(7), pp.593-8.

Nijhof, M.W., Dhert, W.J.A., Tilman, P.B.J., Verbaut, A.J. &, Fleer, A. (1997). Release of tobramycin from tobramycin-containing bone cement in bone and serum of rabbits. *J Mat Sci: Mater Med*, 8, pp.799-802.

Norden, C.W. (1988). Lessons learned from animal models of osteomyelitis. *Rev Infect Dis*,10, pp.103-110.

Ooms, E.M., Wolke, J.G., van de Heuvel, M.T., Jeschke, B. & Jansen J.A. (2003). Histological evaluation of the bone response to calcium phosphate cement implanted in cortical bone. *Biomaterials*, 24, pp.989-1000.

Ormos, Z.D. (1994). Granulation and coating. In: Williams JC, Allen T, advisory editors. Handbook of powder technology, volume 9, Powder technology and pharmaceutical processes. London, New York, Tokyo: Elsevier, pp.359-376.

Otsuka, M., Matsuda, Y., Suwa, Y., Fox, J.L. & Higuchi, W. (1994). A novel skeletal drug delivery system using self-setting calcium phosphate cement. 3: Physicochemical properties and drug release of bovin insulin and bovin albumin. *J Pharm Sci*, 83(2), pp.255-258.

Otsuka, M., Matsuda, Y., Fox, J.L. & Higuchi, W. (1995). A novel skeletal drug delivery system using self-setting calcium phosphate cement. 9: effects of the mixing solution volume on anticancer drug release from homogeneous drug-loaded cement. *J Pharm Sci*, 6, pp.733-736.

Parikh, S. (2002). Bone graft substitutes in modern orthopedics. *Orthopedics*, 2, pp. 1301-1310.

Passl, R., Muller, C., Zielinski, C.C. & Eibl, M.M. (1984). A model of experimental post-traumatic osteomyelitis in guinea pigs. *J Trauma*, 24, pp.323-326.

Patel, M., Rojavin, Y., Jamali, A.A., Wasielewski, S.J. & Salgado, C.J. (2009). Animal models for the study of osteomyelitis. *Semin Plast Surg,*23, pp.148-154.

Penner, M.J., Masri, B.A. & Ducan, C.P. (1996). Elution characteristics of vancomycin and tobramycin combined in acrylic bone cement. *J Arthroplasty*, 11(8), pp.939-944.

Prat-Poiret, N., Langlais, F., Bonnaure, M., Cormier, M. & Lancien, G. (1996). Phosphate tricalcique et gentamicine. Diffusion de l'antibiotique *in vitro* et *in vivo*, réhabitation en site osseux chez le mouton. *Chirurgie*, 121, pp.298-308.

Randelli, P., Evola, F.R., Cabitza, P., Polli, L., Denti, M. & Vlenti, L. (2010). Prophyllactic use of antibiotic-loaded bone cement in primary total knee replacement. *Knee Surg Sports Traumatol Arthrosc*, 18(2), pp. 181-186.

Ripamonti, U., Ma, S. & Reddi, A.H. (1992). The critical role of geometry of porous hydroxyapatite delivery system in induction of bone by osteogenin, a bone morphogenetic protein. *Matrix*, 12, pp.202-212.

Rissing, J.P. (1990). Animal models of osteomyelitis. Knowledge, hypothesis, and speculation. *Infect Dis Clin North Am*, 4, pp.377-390.

Rush SM. (2005). Bone graft substitute: osteologics. *Clin Podiatr Med Surg*, 22, pp.619-630.

Saavedra-Lozano, J., Mejías, A., Ahmad, N., Peromingo, E., Ardura, M.I., Guillen, S., Syed, A., Cavuoti, D. & Ramilo, O. (2008). Changing trends in acute osteomyelitis in children: impact of methicillin-resistant *Staphylococcus aureus* infections. *J Pediatr Orthop*, 28(5), pp.569-575.

Shinto, Y., Uchida, A., Korkusuz, F., Araki, N. & Ono, K. (1992). Calcium hydroxyapatite ceramic used as a delivery system for antibiotics. *J Bone Joint Surg*, 74-B, pp.600-604.

Specht, R. & Kühn, K. Palamed® and Palamed® G: new bone cements. *Proc 14th ESB Conference*, The Hague, The Netherlands 1998:169.

Sudo, A., Hasegawa, M., Fukuda, A. & Uchida, A. (2008). Treatment of infected hip arthroplasty with antibioticimpregnated calcium hydroxyapatite, *J Arthroplasty*, 23(1), pp.145-150.

Suzuki, Y., Tanihara, M., Nishimura, Y., Suzuki, K., Kakimaru, Y. & Shimizu, Y (1998). A new drug delivery system with controlled release of antibiotic only in the presence of infection. *J Biomed Mater Res*, 42, pp.112-116.

Thomazeau, H. & Langlais, F. (1996). Relargage d'antibiotiques par implantation osseuse de phosphate tricalcique. *Chirurgie*, 121, pp.663-666.

Trécant, M., Daculsi, G. & Leroy, M. (1995). Dynamic compaction of calcium phosphate biomaterials. *J Mater Sci*, 6, pp.545-551.

Trécant, M., Guicheux, J., Grimandi, G., Leroy, M. & Daculsi, G. (1997). Dynamic compaction: a new process to compact therapeutic agent-loaded calcium phosphate. *Biomaterials*, 18, pp.141-145.

Vallet-Regi, M. (2006). Revisting ceramics form medical appilications. *Dalton Trans*, 28, pp.5211-5220.

Venesmaa, P.K., Kroger, H.P., Miettinen, H.J., Jurvelin, J.S., Suomalainen O.T. & Alhav, E.M. (2001). Alendronate reduces periprosthetic bone loss after uncemented primary total hip arthroplasty: a prospective randomized study. *J Bone Miner Res*, 11, pp.2126-2131.

Verron, E., Khairoun, I., Guicheux, J. & Bouler J.M. (2010). Calcium phosphate biomaterials as bone drug delivery systems: a review. *Drug Discov Today.* 15(13-14, pp.547-52.

Waldvogel, F.A, Medoff, G. & Swartz, M.N. (1970). Osteomyelitis: a review of clinical features, therapeutic considerations and unusual aspects. 3. Osteomyelitis associated with vascular insufficiency. *N Engl J Med,* 282(6), pp.316-322.

Weichert, S., Sharland, M., Clarke, N.M. & Faust, S.N. (2008). Acute haematogenous osteomyelitis in children: is there any evidence for how long we should treat? *Curr Opin Infect Dis,* 21(3), pp.258-262.

Williams, D.F. (2008). On the mechanisms of biocompatibility. *Biomaterials*, 29(20), pp.2941-2953.

Williams, D.F. (2009). On the nature of biomaterials. *Biomaterials*, 30(30), pp. 5897-5909.

Wu, H., Zheng, O., Du, J., Yan, Y. & Liu, C. (1997). A new drug delivery system-ciprofloxacine/tricalcium phosphate delivery capsule (CTDC) and its in vitro drug release patern. *J Tongji Med Univ*, 17(3), pp.160-164.

Wysocki, M., Delatour, F., Faurisson, F., Rauss, A., Pean, Y., Misset, B., Thomas, F., Timsit, J.F., Similowski, T., Mentec, H., Mier, L. & Dreyfuss, D. (2001). Continuous versus intermittent infusion of vancomycin in severe Staphylococcal infections: prospective multicenter randomized study. *Antimicrob Agents Chemother*, 45(9), pp. 2460-2467.

Yin, L.Y., Lazzarini, L., Li, F., Stevens, C.M. & Calhoun, J.H. (2005). Comparative evaluation of tigecycline and vancomycin, with and without rifampicin, in the treatment of methicillin-resistant *Staphylococcus aureus* experimental osteomyelitis in a rabbit model. *J Antimicrob Chemother,* 55, pp.995-1002.

Yoshii, T., Nishimura, H., Yoshikawa, T., Furudoi, S., Yoshioka, A., Takenono, I., Ohtsuka, Y. & Komori, T. (2001). Therapeutic possibilities of long-term roxithromycin treatment for chronic diffuse sclerosing osteomyelitis of the mandible. *J Antimicrob Chemother*, 47, pp.631-637.

Yu, D., Wong, J., Matsuda, Y., Fox, J.L., Higuchi, W. & Otsuka, M. (1992). Self-setting hydroxyapatite cement: a novel skeletal drug delivery system for antibiotics. *J Pharm Sci*, 81(6), pp. 529-531.

Zerbo, R., Bronckers, A.L., de Lange G. & Burger, E.H. (2005). Localisation of osteogenic and osteoclastic cells in porous beta-tricalcium phosphate particles used for human maxillary sinus floor elevation. *Biomaterials*, 26, pp.1445-1451.

10

PLGA-Alendronate Conjugate as a New Biomaterial to Produce Osteotropic Drug Nanocarriers

Rosario Pignatello
Department of Pharmaceutical Sciences
Faculty of Pharmacy, University of Catania
Italy

1. Introduction

Targeting bone tissue to treat specific diseases, such as primary tumour or bone metastases from peripheral malignancies is a current and pressing research field for modern pharmaceutical technology, and nanomedicine in particular. Bone is the third most common site of metastasis and the incidence of bone metastases in patients died of cancer is reported to be around 70% [1,2]. Primary carcinomas of the lung, breast, prostate, kidney, and thyroid may develop skeletal metastases. In children affected by disseminated neuroblastoma bone metastases are also highly frequent.

Tumour osteolysis is responsible for pathologic fractures, intractable pain, nerve compression syndrome, and severe hypercalcemia. In addition, patients with bone metastases may have neurologic impairment from spinal lesions, anaemia, and complications exacerbated by immobilization. Bone matrix resorption is minimally due to direct cancer cell activity. In fact, bone-colonizing tumour cells also stimulate osteoclast-mediated bone resorption via the secretion of potent osteolytic agents [3]. The increased bone resorption that follows releases bone-derived growth factors into the extracellular milieu and systemic circulation, thereby further enhancing bone resorption, promoting tumour growth, and altering the tumour microenvironment. Vice versa, metastatic cancer cells are largely influenced by messages embedded within the bone matrix [4]. Under the influence of bone microenvironment, tumour cells proliferate and interact with osteoblasts and osteoclasts leading to lytic or sclerotic lesions.

Clinical management of metastatic bone disease is really hard. The probability of long-term survival decreases dramatically in patients with skeletal metastases. Current treatments are based both on systemic therapy (chemotherapy, immunotherapy, hormone therapy) [5,6] and local therapy (surgery and radiotherapy) [7,8].

The restoration of functionality and mobility, along with pain relief can improve patients' quality of life, but is unable to affect the negative progression of the disease. Because of the unique characteristics of tumours growth within bone tissues, conventional therapeutic strategies often lack efficiency in cure bone metastases. Moreover, most of the drugs used for the adjuvant therapy of osteolytic metastases interfere with signalling that induce osteoclast differentiation and osteoclast-mediated bone resorption, but they are not effective on tumour growth in the bone and their use is obviously associated with heavy side effects.

A number of drugs are effective for the treatment of bone tumours, but their systemic delivery is inevitably associated with significant side effects and lack of targeting. Thereby, targeting specific biochemical patterns inside bone cancer areas may theoretically provide a mean to improve the efficacy and reduce the required dose of anticancer drugs.

1.1 Bone targeting strategies

Development of osteotropic drug delivery systems (ODDS) is therefore an appealing issue in the wide field of innovative pharmaceutical technology. To realize an effective system, many obstacles must be overcome. Bones are covered with lining cells acting as a marrow-blood barrier; therefore, the contact of exogenous compounds to the bone surface is restricted. Furthermore, the expression of biomolecules having a specific targets, like enzymes or antigens is relatively low in mineralized tissues, thus restraining the chances for an active drug targeting.

The strategies proposed for targeting drugs to the bone can essentially be condensed in two fields: the passive targeting approach, realised by the encapsulation in or association of drugs to colloidal carriers, such as polymeric or lipid nanoparticles (NP), liposomes or dendrimers (strategy 1, **Figure 1**). Drug-loaded nanocarriers allow to achieve a selective release to some tissues, like tumours, by means of the well-known phenomenon called 'EPR effect' [9], due to the fact that all cancers are characterized by permeable (leaky) blood neovessels and an impaired lymphatic outflow. Because of their multifunctional properties, nanosized systems can carry both targeting molecules and drugs, and deliver the latter in very specific sites within the body. Another advantage of NPs is the possibility of carrying in the bloodstream poorly soluble or unstable compounds, such as peptides and proteins, preventing their premature inactivation by circulating enzymes.

However, active targeting should be in some case more useful to reach effective drug concentrations in specific tissues and organs. Thus, other approaches have also been explored in which a drug is covalently linked to a targetor moiety able to recognize the bone tissues, and selectively convey the whole compound (e.g., a prodrug or a polymeric conjugate) to the site of action (strategy 2, **Figure 1**) [10].

Since bones are made of a mineralized matrix, a logical solution to the problem of bone targeting would be the development of delivery systems that possess affinity for hydroxyapatite (HA) via osteotropic molecules, such as bisphosphonates (BP) [11,12]. BP are synthetic, non-hydrolysable compounds structurally related to pyrophosphate. The P-C-P structure of BP is responsible for the ability of binding divalent ions, such as Ca^{++}, and thereby for the high affinity to HA [13]. Upon administration, BP are hence rapidly cleared from the bloodstream and bind to bone mineral surfaces at sites of active bone remodelling, like the areas undergoing osteoclast resorption [13].

BP are the most effective antiresorptive agents for the treatment of bone diseases associated to an increase in the number or activity of osteoclasts, including tumour-related osteolysis and hypercalcemia [14]. Moreover, BP are also able to reduce the survival, proliferation, adhesion, migration, and invasion of tumour cells [15, 16] and to inhibit angiogenesis in experimental and animal tumour models [17]. Since HA crystals are only present in 'hard' tissues, like teeth and bones, conjugation to BP can represent a valid strategy for selectively deliver bioactives to the bones.

The scientific literature presents many papers and patents exploring such approach, sometimes carrying original ideas or integrating together different chemical and technological pathways. In particular, osteotropic drug delivery systems (ODDS) have been proposed some years ago as a possible mean to impart to drugs an affinity to bone tissues

[11, 12, 18, 19]. Bisphosphonates (BP) have been for instance conjugated to small drugs [20, 21], and proteins [22] with the aim at optimizing the treatment of osteoporosis, osteoarthritis, and bone cancer, and to radiopharmaceuticals to obtain novel agents for bone scintigraphy [23]. The conjugation of bisphosphonates to polymer backbones has been studied as a mean for bone targeting [24,25]. Recently, cholesteryl-trisoxyethylene-bisphosphonic acid (CHOL-TOE-BP), a new tailor-made BP derivative, has been used as a bone targeting moiety for liposomes [26]. In other works, the amino-bisphosphonate drug alendronate (ALE; Fosamax®) was co-conjugated to HPMA polymer backbones together with an anticancer agent. Thereby, passive targeting was achieved by extravasation of the nanoconjugates from the tumour vessels via the EPR effect, while active targeting to the calcified tissues was achieved by ALE affinity to HA [27].

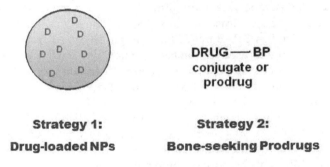

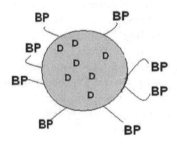

Fig. 1. The strategies described in the literature to achieve targeting to bone tumours: 1) an anticancer drug (D) is encapsulated/loaded into a nanocarrier (e.g., polymeric or lipid nanoparticles, liposomes, micelles, etc.) and passive targeting is expected (EPR effect); 2) a biologically active molecule is covalently linked to an osteotropic targetor moiety (e.g., a bisphosphonate, BP); 3) nanoparticles are made by an osteotropic polymer (e.g., a polymer-BP conjugate) and then loaded with a bioactive agent: in this way, both passive and active targeting possibilities can be achieved.

1.2 The scientific and technical rationale for a new targeting strategy

Targeted DDS should be preferable over drug-BP conjugates due to different factors, such as drug protection from biodegradation in the bloodstream, transport duration, and drug-payload. Thereby, in a recent and partially still on-going research, the two strategies depicted in **Figure 1** have been merged, leading to an innovative solution for active targeting of drugs to the bone. The working hypothesis was to realize a biocompatible nanocarrier showing high affinity to bone (i.e., an osteotropic nanocarrier), which can be loaded with different classes of drugs active against bone diseases, such as anticancer, anti-angiogenic, antibiotics, or anti-osteolytic agents.

To this aim, in a first step a new polymeric biomaterial showing osteotropic properties was produced through the conjugation of a poly(lactide-*co*-glycolide) (PLGA) to the BP agent alendronate (ALE). PLGA copolymers are diffusely used biocompatible and biodegradable materials for controlled drug release systems [28], including anticancer agents, and they have also been recognized as GRAS by US FDA. In this study, a copolymer made of 50:50 polylactic-*co*-glycolic acid was used (Resomer® RG 502 H; **Figure 2**) because of the presence of free carboxyl end groups susceptible to chemical derivatisation. The typical weight composition of this copolymer allows it to remain in the human body enough to let the bound BP moiety to recognize the bone proteins.

ALE (4-amino-1-hydroxybutyldiene-1,1-phosphoric acid, **Figure 2**) is an amino-BP, approved for the treatment and prevention of osteoporosis, treatment of glucocorticoid-induced osteoporosis in men and women, and therapy of Paget's disease of bone [29]. ALE was selected among BP agents because of some peculiar properties: a) the presence of a free amine group, able to create a stable covalent link with the carboxyl group present in the used PLGA; b) such amine group is not essential for the interaction of ALE with HA, and thus for its pharmacological effects, but exerts only a supportive role [30]; c) the possibility of easily converting the commercial sodium salt of ALE into its free acid form. The choice of an amide bond between the targeting BP and the polymer was also driven by the known relatively high resistance to enzymatic hydrolysis in plasma of this linkage, that should ensure the intact conjugate to reach the target (bone) tissues.

The haemo- and cytocompatibility of the PLGA-ALE conjugate was confirmed *in vitro*. Therefore, a nanoparticle system (NP) was produced starting from this new biomaterial. The NP were studied for their technological properties, as well as for their biocompatibility. Finally, PLGA-ALE NP were then loaded with a model cytotoxic drug, doxorubicin (DOX) and tested *in vitro* and *in vivo*.

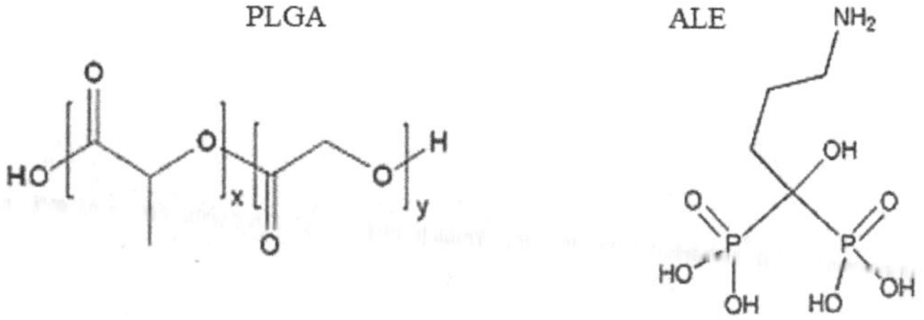

Fig. 2. Schematic structure of Resomer® RG 502 H (PLGA) and alendronic acid (ALE).

2. Synthesis and characterization of the PLGA-ALE conjugate

Polyl(D,L-lactic-co-glycolic acid) (50:50) containing a free carboxylic acid end group [Resomer® RG 502 H; inherent viscosity: 0.16-0.24 dl/g (0.1% in chloroform, 25°C)] was used (Boehringer Ingelheim, Ingelheim am Rhein, Germany). Sodium alendronate was converted into the acid form by treatment with aqueous acetic acid and lyophilisation. The conjugate was synthesized by two alternative methods, i.e., carbodiimide-assisted direct conjugation or preparation of an activated intermediate through N-hydroxysuccinimide [31]. In the first case, a solution of Resomer® RG 502 H in DMSO and dichloromethane (DCM) (1:1) was activated at 0°C for 2 h by N'-(3-dimethylaminopropyl)-N-ethyl carbodiimide hydrochloride (EDAC), in the presence of 1-hydroxy-benzotriazole (HOBt) and triethylamine. Alendronic acid was dissolved in DMSO and added to the reaction mixture, which was stirred for 2 h at 2°C and then at r.t. for 8 h. The solvent was partially removed under vacuum and the remaining solution was purified by dialysis water (CelluSep H1 MWCO 2000; M-Medical s.r.l., Cornaredo, Italy). In the alternative procedure, the PLGA was previously activated with N-hydroxysuccinimide (NHS) and dicyclohexylcarbodiimide in anhydrous dioxane at 15°C under stirring for 3 h [32]. The formed dicyclohexylurea was filtered off and the solution was poured in anhydrous diethyl ether. The solvent was decanted and the oily residue was purified by dissolution in anhydrous dioxane and precipitation with anhydrous diethyl ether (3 times), and finally dried in vacuo. A solution of NHS-PLGA in anhydrous DMSO was treated with triethylamine and sodium alendronate under stirring at r.t. for 12 h. At the end of the reaction the solvent was partially removed under vacuum and the remaining solution was purified by dialysis. The dialysed samples were frozen into using liquid nitrogen and lyophilised. Both methods resulted in similar production yields (70-75%) and purity of the final conjugate, therefore the first method could be better proposed as more direct and simple. The chemical structure of the PLGA-ALE conjugate was confirmed by MALDI-TOF MS and ^{1}H-NMR; analytical details are available [31].

In the view of using the PLGA-ALE copolymer to prepare bone-targeted NPs, the conjugate was evaluated for blood and cyto-compatibility, to individuate any negative effect which might have precluded any further biological investigation. Haemolysis was evaluated because erythrocytes are among the first cell lines that come into contact with injected materials. Experimental results did not show haemolytic effects of the conjugate; the plasmatic phase of coagulation was measured by the activated partial thromboplastin time (APTT) and prothrombin activity; they respectively evaluate the intrinsic and extrinsic phases of coagulation. In basal conditions, prothrombin activity was 140.2 ± 2.5 and APTT was 35.6 ± 0.3. In plasma incubated with PLGA-ALE at different dilutions, prothrombin activity and APTT were not significantly different from the plasma incubated with PBS (**Figure 3A** and **3B**). DMSO at the same dilutions did not affected either prothrombin activity or APTT.

In the bloodstream, nanoparticles come in contact with endothelium before passing through the vessel wall and reaching tissues. Therefore, the effect of PLGA-ALE on endothelial cells was tested to verify the lack of cytotoxicity. As expected, PLGA-ALE was not cytotoxic for human umbilical vein endothelial cells (HUVEC), as proven by the neutral red test (**Figure 3C**). Absence of cytotoxicity was also shown in cultures of human primary trabecular osteoblasts (BMSC) (**Figure 3D**).

In conclusion, PLGA-ALE conjugate did not cause either haemolysis on human erythrocytes, or alterations of the plasmatic phase of coagulation or cytotoxic effects on endothelial cells and trabecular osteoblasts [31].

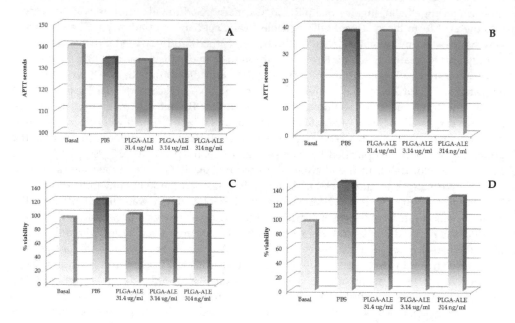

Fig. 3. Biocompatibility results of the PLGA-ALE conjugate: (A) mean prothrombin activity and (B) APTT of human plasma incubated with different concentrations of the conjugate; (C) viability of human umbilical vein endothelial cells (HUVEC) and (D) human primary osteoblasts from trabecular bone, respectively, after incubation with the conjugate. No haemolytic activity was given by the tested compound (not shown) (adapted from ref. [31]).

3. PLGA-ALE nanoparticles

NP were produced by the PLGA-ALE conjugate by a nanoprecipitation method, using an opportunely adapted emulsion/solvent evaporation technique [33]. The conjugate was dissolved in acetone, DMSO or their 1:1 mixture (v:v). The organic solution was added drop wise into phosphate buffered saline (PBS), pH=7.4, containing Pluronic F68. After stirring at r.t. for 10 min, the solvent was partially removed at 30 °C under reduced pressure and the concentrated suspension was purified by dialysis against water.

In **Figure 4** the size analysis of the formed systems, obtained by photon correlation spectroscopy is illustrated. DMSO was used in the NP production due to the low solubility of the conjugate in acetone (from which low production yields were achieved), but it did not appear to be an ideal solvent; in fact, NP obtained from pure DMSO solution showed a higher mean size with respect to those obtained using an acetone/DMSO mixture. These NP showed a homogeneous distribution, with an average size of 198.7 nm and a polidispersity index of about 0.3. However, in all cases mean sizes between 200-300 nm were obtained, an interesting feature for a further development of these systems as injectable drug carriers.

Also a dialysis method using a DMSO solution of the conjugate was attempted to prepare the NP [34], but it resulted in much larger particles (around 400 nm) (not shown).

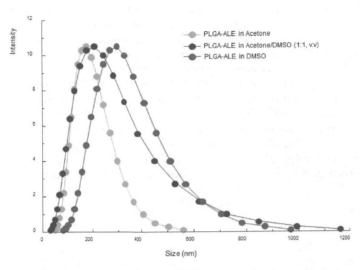

Fig. 4. Size distribution patterns of PLGA-ALE NP prepared using different organic phases (adapted from [31].

The PLGA-ALE NPs showed a net negative surface charge (ζ-potential of –38 mV), close to the value given by the NPs obtained from pure PLGA (-41.8 mV). SEM analysis revealed spherical particles with a smooth surface (**Figure 5**). The system was also shown to be sterilisable by gamma irradiation at 10 kGy, showing only minimal particle size changes [33]. This finding prospects the possibility of using sterilized NPs for further *in vivo* studies of the system.

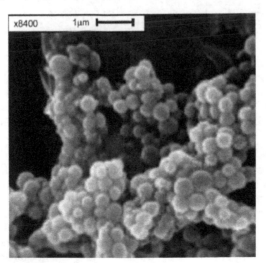

Fig. 5. SEM picture of PLGA-ALE NPs produced in 1:1 acetone/DMSO.

To assess the affinity for HA, PLGA-ALE and PLGA NPs were loaded with a lipophilic probe (Red Oil O) and incubated with two different HA concentrations (1 and 5 mg/ml) for 15 or 30 min. PLGA-ALE NPs showed a relative increase of affinity towards the phosphate salt compared to pure PLGA NPs (**Figure 6**). The affinity increased with the incubation time and was proportional to the concentration of HA in the suspension. This latter observation would suggest that some form of chemical interaction occurred between PLGA-ALE and HA, reinforcing the mere physical absorption of the phosphate on NP surface, which justifies the affinity already measured for pure PLGA NPs.

The biocompatibility profile of PLGA-ALE NPs was assessed by means of several *in vitro* assays, able to demonstrate their effects on biological systems which use to come in contact with a material injected into the body [33, 35, 36]. The use of NPs for drug delivery necessitates an accurate assessment of their biocompatibility [37, 38]. For their nanoscale size, NPs may have a reduced blood compatibility in comparison with the starting material: even if the biocompatibility of a macromolecule is well-established, the enormous increase of its surface when in the form of NPs may bring on negative effects that are not given by the bulk material.

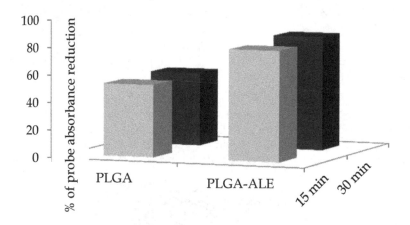

Fig. 6. Affinity of PLGA-ALE and PLGA NPs for hydroxyapatite (HA). Oil Red O-loaded NP suspensions were incubated at r.t. for either 15 or 30 min with an aqueous suspension containing 5 mg/ml of the phosphate salt. Results are expressed as the percentage decrease of light absorbance at 523 nm with respect to the corresponding NPs incubated without HA [*cf.* ref. 33].

3.1 Biocompatibility studies

Blood-biomaterial interactions are complex events that involve erythrocyte and leukocyte damage, and activation of platelet, coagulation, and complement. Damage of red blood cells, as well as complement activation may favour haemolysis and other forms of general toxicity. Analogously, NPs should not activate platelets and the plasmatic phase of coagulation, nor damage endothelial cells to avoid thrombogenesis [39, 40]. In the meantime, they should not reduce the levels of the plasmatic factors of coagulation, to prevent haemorrhagic accidents. Finally, with the aim of bone targeting, when NP will reach bone tissues they should inhibit osteoclast activity without altering osteoblasts. Therefore, a preliminary evaluation of NP biocompatibility has been necessary before their loading with actives.

The PLGA-ALE NP at different concentrations did not show any haemolytic effects towards a suspension of human erythrocytes. The percentage of haemolysis was in fact similar to the erythrocytes incubated with PBS (Table 1).

Sample	NP concentration	% of haemolysis
PLGA-ALE NP	56 µg/ml	0.001±0.165
	5.6 µg/ml	0.289±0.320
	560 ng/ml	0±0.272
	56 ng/ml	0.356±0.309
	5.6 ng/ml	0.167±0.191
	0.56 ng/ml	0±0.155
PBS	-	0
Saponin	-	132.72±2.74
Distilled water	-	100

Table 1. Hemolytic activity (arithmetic mean ± S.E. of 6 experiments) of PLGA-ALE NPs. Their concentration was expressed as the amount of ALE in each sample.

As a further proof of their compatibility with blood components, at all the tested concentrations PLGA-ALE NPs did not induce any significant effect either on the total leukocyte number or on their subpopulations percentage. Analogously, the NPs did not cause platelet adhesion or activation (release reaction), as assessed by the platelet factor 4 measurement (**Figure** 7), all process that may induce thrombotic phenomena after NP injection [33].

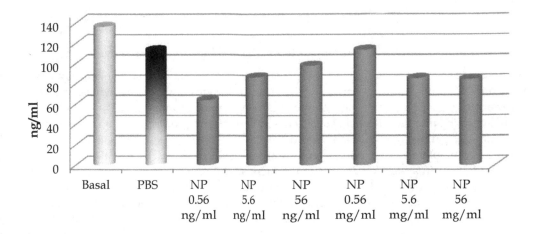

Fig. 7. Platelet factor 4 concentration after incubation with PLGA-ALE NP.

To assess the lack of alterations of blood proteins, we evaluated the effects of PLGA-ALE NPs on the plasmatic phase of coagulation and on complement. A decrease of the coagulation factors levels favours haemorrhage, while an increase of their activity may induce thrombotic phenomena. In our experiments, only the highest tested concentration of NPs caused a decrease of the prothrombin activity, while all the lower concentrations increased it, with changes however always ranging within normal physiological values (**Figure 8**). Since APTT (i.e., the intrinsic and the common phase of coagulation) was also not significantly affected by the NPs (not shown), the observed changes could be due to an alteration of Factor VII of the extrinsic pathway of coagulation. Probably, Factor VII was adsorbed on the NPs surface at high concentration and was less available for coagulation; conversely, lower concentrations of PLGA-ALE NPs could activate factor VII, in a way similar to the effect of tissue factor. Another hypothesis could involve the activation of Factors XII and XI by the NPs, similarly to silica gel or glass (*cf.* [33] for more details).

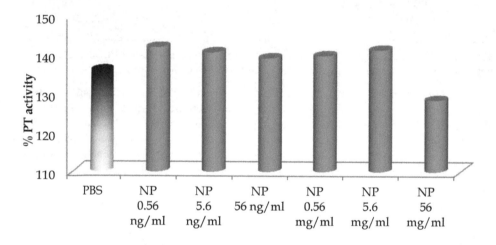

Fig. 8. Protrombin activity induced by different PLGA-ALE NP concentrations.

Activation of complement induces the production and release of small biologically active peptides. C3a and C5a are chemo-attractive for leukocytes and favour their aggregation. Furthermore, C5a induces the adhesion of granulocytes and monocytes to the endothelium, their migration into the external tissues, enzyme release and production of pro-coagulant or platelet aggregating compounds. C3a and the C5b-9 complex can directly activate platelets. Therefore, complement activation should not be considered as a strictly local phenomenon, but results also in systemic effects. Complement activation may occur by the classical and the alternative pathways. In the classical pathway, the protein C1q recognises activators (usually immune complexes) and binds to them. The activation via the alternative pathway starts by the binding of C3b to the activator surface (such as microbial polysaccharides or lipids or surface antigens present on some viruses, parasites and cancer cells) and then follow the same events of the classical pathway. NPs predominantly activate the complement through the alternative pathway.

In our experiments PLGA-ALE NPs did not activate complement by none of the two pathways, as shown by a non-significant different complement consumption from PBS (**Figures 9A** and **9B**). Conversely, the positive control zymosan induced a 70% complement consumption, twice the amount consumed by PBS. Also the Bb fragment, which is produced during the complement activation by the alternative pathway, was not significantly affected by the PLGA-ALE NPs (not shown).

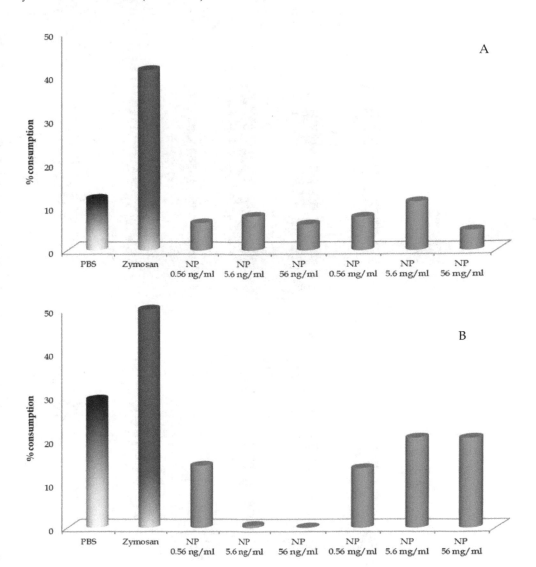

Fig. 9. Percentage consumption of human serum complement activity via the classical pathway (A) or the alternative pathway (B), after incubation with the PLGA-ALE NPs (adapted from ref. [33]).

In the bloodstream, NP come rapidly in contact with vessel endothelium before passing to the outer tissues; therefore, absence of damage to endothelial cells must be ensured. Moreover, bone oriented NPs should not affect the vitality and function of normal osteoblasts. The cytotoxicity of the prepared PLGA-ALE NPs was excluded on both endothelial (HUVEC) cells and osteoblasts derived by bone marrow stromal cells (BMSC). Cell viability was always higher than 80% upon 24 h-exposure to the various concentrations of NPs or to PBS. Phenol, used as a positive control, reduced the cell viability to 19.0% (HUVEC) and to 27.5% (BMSC) (**Figure 10**).

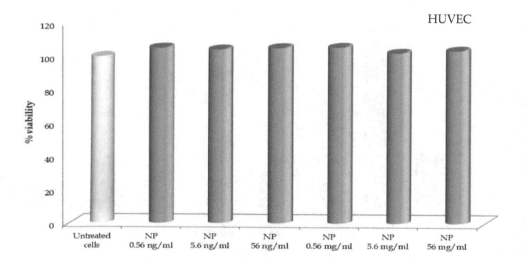

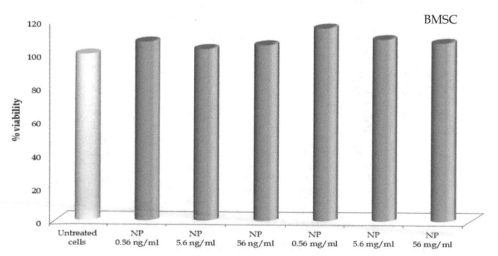

Fig. 10. Viability of endothelial (HUVEC) cells and osteoblasts (BMSC) exposed to various concentrations of PLGA-ALE NPs (adapted from ref. [33]).

In conclusion, PLGA-ALE NPs did not affect platelets, leukocytes and complement, did not induce haemolysis and did not exert cytotoxic effects on endothelial cells and osteoblasts [33]. To assess if the PLGA-ALE NPs are able to retain the antiosteoclastic properties of the bisphosphonate, osteoclast cultures obtained from human peripheral blood mononuclear cells (PBMC) were incubated with either PLGA-ALE or pure PLGA NPs, at an equivalent concentration of 0.64 µM or 6.4 µM of ALE; free ALE was tested as a positive control. Experiments showed that ALE retained the ability of inhibiting the osteoclast-mediated degradation of type I human bone collagen, determined a dose-dependent reduction of osteoclast number, and induced apoptosis in osteoclast cultures, also when conjugated with the copolymer PLGA and in the form of NPs [41]. Interestingly, pure PLGA NPs also showed similar effects, and this can be considered an useful phenomenon in the view of the overall aim of this study: since the conjugation of ALE to PLGA, and the resulting NP formation was aimed at targeting antitumor drugs to osteolytic bone metastases, the additional antiosteoclastic effect observed for polymer-bound ALE and also of PLGA could even contribute to the inhibition of the associated osteolysis.

4. Drug-loaded nanoparticles

Doxorubicin (DOX) is an anticancer agent of wide clinical use, from leukaemia and Hodgkin's lymphoma to symptomatic metastatic breast cancer, from neuroblastoma to many other cancers (prostate, thyroid, bladder, stomach, lung, ovary). Its therapeutic applications are nevertheless limited by the strong cardiac and bone marrow toxicity. DOX effectiveness has been greatly improved when specific targeting at the tumour sites has been achieved, for instance by loading the drug into liposomes (e.g., Caelyx®/Doxil®) [42, 43].
DOX was loaded in the previously described PLGA-ALE NPs and the anti-tumour effect of the carrier was assessed *in vitro* and *in vivo* [44]. In a first instance, the intracellular accumulation and distribution of DOX-loaded NPs was assessed by fluorescence and confocal microscopy, in comparison with free DOX. A panel of potential target cells was used in these experiments: MDA-MB-231 and MCF7 breast adenocarcinoma cell lines, Saos-2 and U-2 OS osteosarcoma cell lines, SH-SY5Y neuroblastoma cell line, and ACIIN renal adenocarcinoma cell line. The above tumour histotypes were chosen because all originate from or can metastasize to the bone.
The final localization of DOX in cell nucleus is important because of it mechanism of action [45]. We observed that the incubation of free DOX with cells resulted in its accumulation in the nuclei, while it was absent in the cytoplasm (**Figure 11**). Conversely, cells treated with DOX-loaded NPs showed also fluorescent spots localized in the cytoplasmic vacuoles. Polymeric NPs typically accumulate in lysosomal vesicles, from which the drug is released into the cytoplasm [46, 47]. Therefore, it is likely that the observed cytoplasmic fluorescence was due to the same phenomenon, and that the DOX-loaded NPs were trafficked through the endo-lysosomal compartment.
The incubation of the above cell lines with DOX-loaded PLGA-ALE NPs (48 and 72 h) gave a cell growth inhibition profile very similar to that one of the free drug [44]. To evaluate the *in vivo* activity, DOX-loaded NPs were injected into a mouse model of breast cancer bone metastases: osteolytic lesions were induced by intratibial inoculation of the human breast carcinoma cells MDA-MB-231 that can induce prominent bone metastases. Histological analysis confirmed that the NP did not cause any organ abnormality, hence they should not exert any systemic cytotoxic effect. Control mice treated with PBS developed pronounced

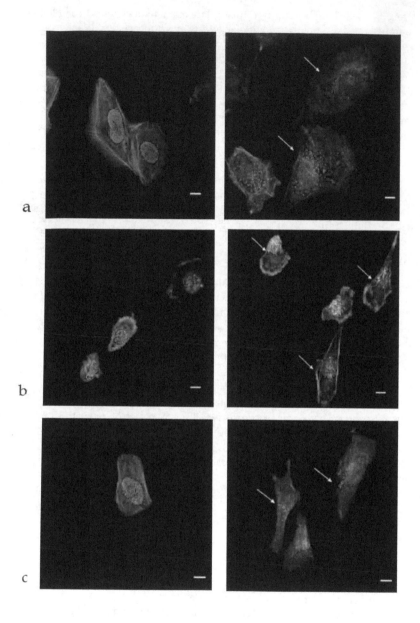

Fig. 11. Confocal analysis of cellular uptake of DOX-loaded PLGA-ALE NPs. Free DOX (left) or NP samples (right) were incubated for 24 h with U-2 OS (a), MDA-MB-231 (b), or SH-SY5Y cells (c). Cytoplasm fluorescence (red spots) was evidenced by arrows. Bars, 10 μm; magnification, 60X (adapted from ref. [44]).

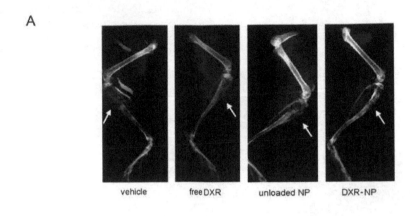

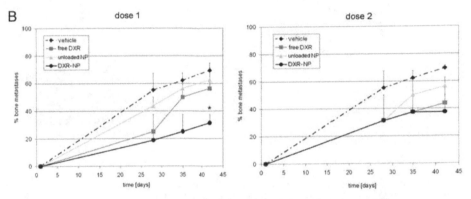

Fig. 12. Effect of DOX-loaded NPs on the incidence of osteolytic bone metastases *in vivo*.
BALB/c-nu/nu mice were injected intratibially with a suspension of MDA-MB-231 cells.
Mice were weekly treated for six weeks with PBS, free DOX, unloaded NPs, or drug-loaded
NPs (DOX-NP) at the dose of 0.2 or 1 mg/kg. *A*, X-ray of hind limbs at day 42 of MDA-MB-
231-injected mice and treated with PBS, free DOX, unloaded NPs or DOX-NP at an
equivalent drug dose of 0.2 mg/kg (arrows: osteolytic areas). *B*, incidence of osteolytic bone
metastases after the same treatments at the lower (left panel) and higher dose (right panel).
Means ± SE, n = 8 (modified from ref. [44]).

osteolytic lesions detectable by X-ray analysis starting from the 28th day after the tumour
cell inoculation (**Figure 12A**). The free drug was effective in retarding the onset of
metastases and reducing their incidence compared to the animals treated with PBS or blank
NPs (**Figure 12B**). However, a significant effect was observed only in the DOX-loaded NP-
treated group at the dose of 0.2 mg/kg (**Figure 12B**, left panel; *P*= 0.028 vs. vehicle).
The extension of tumour size was significantly smaller in animal groups which received
both the free drug and DOX-loaded NPs at a drug concentration of 0.2 mg/kg or 1 mg/kd
(**Figure 13A**), whereas unloaded NPs were ineffective. A trend of reduction of the osteolytic
areas was measured in mice treated with either free DOX, DOX-loaded NPs or unloaded
NPs. However, DOX-loaded NPs induced a higher inhibition of osteolysis than unloaded

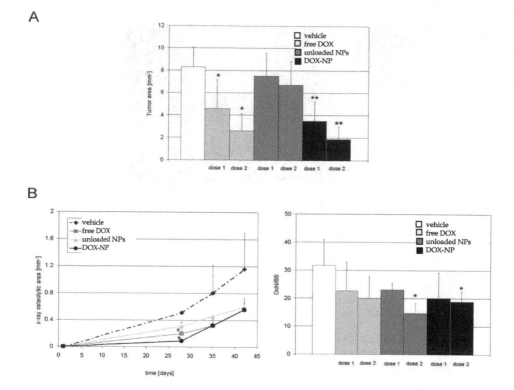

Fig. 13. Effects of DOX-loaded NPs on tumour area and osteolysis. Mice were treated with either PBS, free DOX, unloaded NPs, or DOX-loaded NPs (DOX-NP) at 0.2 mg/kg (dose 1) or 1 mg/kg (dose 2). At the end point, the extension of the osteolytic area was determined by X-ray analysis; sections of the tibiae were histologically examined to evaluate tumour area and the number of osteoclasts on the bone surface. A, tumour area (mean ± SD); B, osteolytic areas quantified on X-ray images of mice treated with dose 1 (mean± SD); C, number of osteoclasts found on the bone surface (OcN/BS) in TRAP stained sections of the tibiae (mean ± SD). * $P < 0.05$, ** $P < 0.005$ (modified from ref. [44]).

NPs (0.090±0.009 vs. 0.310±0.040 mm2, P = 0.033); both free and NP-loaded DOX reached a similar effect at the end of the experiment (day 42) (Figure 13B). Similarly, the histomorphometric analysis of sections stained for TRAP activity showed a trend of reduction for the number of osteoclasts found at the bone surface by either free DOX, unloaded NPs, and DOX-loaded NPs (Figure 13C). However there was a significant inhibition only for unloaded NPs and DOX-loaded NPs at the highest dose (P= 0.04 and P = 0.014 vs. vehicle, respectively).

In conclusion, loading of DOX in the osteotropic PLGA-ALE did not affect the drug efficacy on bone metastases formation; the reduction of the incidence of metastases induced by DOX-loaded NPs was significantly higher than that allowed by the free drug. The enhanced efficacy of the drug when loaded in these NPs can be used as an indirect demonstration of the successful delivery of DOX to the bones. The modest activity registered with unloaded PLGA-ALE NPs could be related to the inhibitory effect of ALE conjugated to PLGA on osteoclast activity, that indirectly reduced tumour expansion, and of a direct effect exerted by ALE on tumour cells [48]. Treatment of mice with both free or NP-loaded DOX significantly reduced also the tumour area.

All the above experimental findings provide *in vitro* and *in vivo* evidences of the effectiveness of a new osteotropic delivery system for DOX, and possibly other antitumour agents, in which a synergism between the antineoplastic activity of the drugs and the antiosteolytic activity of ALE can afford a better inhibition of tumour development and progression. In the meantime, loading of DOX in biodegradable and biocompatible NPs, made from a conjugate between PLGA and ALE, can allow a site-specific delivery of the drug to osteolytic areas, possibly reducing its systemic side effects. A potential tool for the development of innovative regimens for metastatic bone diseases can thus be exploited by this novel nanocarrier.

5. Acknowledgments

The wide research project described in this chapter was originally supported by a grant from the Associazione Italiana per la Ricerca sul Cancro (AIRC): "Targeting skeletal metastases by nanoscale multifunctional bone-seeking agents". Thanks are due to all the researchers from the Istituto Ortopedico Rizzoli of Bologna (N. Baldini, E. Cenni and co-workers), the University of L'Aquila (A. Teti and co-workers), and the University of Catania (Italy) (F. Castelli and co-workers), who have actively contributed to the project.

6. References

[1] Hanahan D, Weinberg RA. The hallmark of cancer. Cell. 2000;100:57.

[2] Mundy GR, Yoneda T. Facilitation and suppression of bone metastasis. Clin. Orthop. 1995;312:34.

[3] Guise TA, Mohammad KS, Clines G, Stebbins EG, Wong DH, Higgins LS, et al. Basic mechanisms responsible for osteolytic and osteoblastic bone metastases. Clin. Cancer. Res. 2006;12:6213s.

[4] Couzin J. Tracing the steps of metastases, cancer's menacing ballet. Science. 2003;299:1002.

[5] Houston SJ, Rubens RD. The systemic treatment of bone metastases. Clin. Orthop. 1995;312:95.

[6] Pritchard KI. The best use of adjuvant endocrine treatments. Breast. 2003;12:497.

[7] Lin A, Ray ME. Targeted and systemic radiotherapy in the treatment of bone metastasis. Cancer Metastasis Rev. 2006;25:669.

[8] Sim FH, et al. Orthopaedic management using new devices and prostheses. Clin. Orthop. 1995;312:160.

[9] Torchilin VP. Passive and active drug targeting: drug delivery to tumours as an example. Handb. Exp. Pharmacol. 2010;(197):3-53.

[10] Hirsjärvi S, Passirani C, Benoit JP. Passive and active tumour targeting with nanocarriers. Curr. Drug Discov. Technol. 2011 (in press)

[11] Hirabayashi H, Fujisaki J. Bone-specific drug delivery systems: approaches via chemical modification of bone-seeking agents. Clin. Pharmacokinet. 2003;42:1319.

[12] Wang D, Miller SC, Kopeckova P, Kopecek J. Bone-targeting macromolecular therapeutics. Adv. Drug Del. Rev. 2005;57:1049-1076.

[13] Masarachia P, et al. Comparison of the distribution of 3H-alendronate and 3H-etidronate in rat and mouse bones. Bone. 1996;19:281.

[14] Coleman RE. Metastatic bone disease: clinical features, pathophysiology, and treatment strategies. Cancer Treat. Rev. 2001;27:165.

[15] Clezardin P, Ebetino FH, Fournier PGJ. Bisphosphonates and cancer-induced bone disease: beyond their antiresorptive activity. Cancer Res. 2005;65:4971.

[16] Hashimoto K, Morishige K, Sawada K, Tahara M, Kawagishi R, Ikebuchi Y. et al. Alendronate inhibits intraperitoneal dissemination in in vivo ovarian cancer model. Cancer Res. 2005;65:540.

[17] Giraudo E, Inoue M, HanahanD. An amino-bisphosphonate targets MMP-9-expressing macrophages and angiogenesis to impair cervical carcinogenesis. J. Clin. Invest. 2004;114:623.

[18] Fujisaki J, Tokunaga Y, Takahashi T, Hirose T, Shimojo F, Kagayama A, et al. Osteotropic drug delivery system (ODDS) based on bisphosphonic prodrug. I: synthesis and in vivo characterization of osteotropic carboxyfluorescein.. J. Drug Target. 1995;3:273-282.

[19] Hirabayashi H, Sawamoto T, Fujisaki J, Tokunaga Y, Kimura S, Hata T. Relationship between physicochemical and osteotropic properties of bisphosphonic derivatives: rational design for osteotropic drug delivery system (ODDS). Pharm. Res. 2001;18:646-651.

[20] Niemi R, Vepsalainen J, Taipale H, Jairvinen T. Bisphosphonate prodrugs: synthesis and in vitro evaluation of novel acyloxyalkyl esters of clodronic acid. J. Med. Chem. 1999;2:5053-5058

[21] Ezra A, Hoffman A, Breuer E, Alferiev S, Monkkonen, El Hanany- Rozen N, et al. A peptide prodrug approach for improving bisphosphonate oral absorption. J. Med. Chem. 2000;43:3641-3652

[22] Wright JE, Gittens SA, Bansal G, Kitov PI, Sindrey D, Kucharski C, et al. A comparison of mineral affinity of bisphosphonate-protein conjugates constructed with disulfide and thioether linkages. Biomaterials. 2006; 27(5):769-784.

[23] Ogawa K, Mukai T, Inoue Y, Ono M, Saji H. Development of a novel 99mTc-chelate conjugated bisphosphonate with high affinity for bone as a bone scintigraphic agent. J. Nucl. Med. 2006;47:2042-2047.

[24] Uludag H, Yang J, Targeting systemically administered proteins to bone by bisphosphonate conjugation. Biotechnol. Prog. 2002;18:604-611.

[25] Wang D, Miller S, Sima M, Kopeckova P, Kopecek J. Synthesis and evaluation of water-soluble polymeric bone-targeted drug delivery systems. Bioconj. Chem. 2003;14:853-859.

[26] Hengst V, Oussoren C, Kissel T, Storm G. Bone targeting potential of bisphosphonate-targeted liposomes. Preparation, characterization and hydroxyapatite binding in vitro. Int. J. Pharm. 2007;331:224-227.

[27] Miller K, Erez R, Segal E, Shabat D, Satchi-Fainaro R. Targeting bone metastases with a bispecific anticancer and antiangiogenic polymer-alendronate-taxane conjugate. Angew Chem. Int. Ed. Engl. 2009;48:2949-2954.

[28] Bala I, Hariharan S, Kumar MN. PLGA nanoparticles in drug delivery: the state of the art. Crit. Rev. Ther. Drug Carrier Syst. 2004;21:387-422.

[29] http://www.drugs.com/pro/alendronate.html; revision May, 2011 (last visit: July 2011).

[30] De Ruiter J, Clark R. Bisphosphonates: calcium antiresorptive agents. http://www.duc.auburn.edu/~deruija/endo_bisphos.pdf; revision Spring 2002 (last visit: July 2011).

[31] Pignatello R, Cenni E, Miceli D, Fotia C, Salerno M, Granchi D, et al. A novel biomaterial for osteotropic drug nanocarriers. Synthesis and biocompatibility evaluation of a PLGA-alendronate conjugate. Nanomed. 2009;4:161-175.

[32] Tosi G, Rivasi F, Gandolfi F, Costantino L, Vandelli MA, Forni F. Conjugated poly(D,L-lactide-co-glycolide) for the preparation of in vivo detectable nanoparticles. Biomaterials 2005;26:4189-4195.

[33] Cenni E, Granchi D, Avnet S, Fotia C, Salerno M, Micieli D, et al. Biocompatibility of poly(D,L-lactide-co-glycolide) nanoparticles conjugated with alendronate. Biomaterials. 2008;29:1400-1411.

[34] Choi SW, Kim JH. Design of surface-modified poly(D,L-lactide-co-glycolide) nanoparticles for targeted drug delivery to bone. J. Control. Release. 2007;122:24-30.

[35] Salerno M, Fotia C, Avnet S, Cenni E, Granchi D, Castelli F, et al. Effects of bone-targeted nanoparticles on bone metastasis. Calcified Tissue Int. 2008;82(Suppl. 1):S91.

[36] Cenni E, Salerno M, Fotia C, Avnet S, Granchi D, Castelli F, et al. Osteotropic poly(D,L-lactide-co-glycolide)-alendronate nanoparticles for the treatment of bone cancer. Cancer Treat. Rev. 2008;34(Suppl. 1):S74.

[37] Oberdorster G, Maynard A, Donaldson K, Castranova V, Fitzpatrick J, Ausman K, et al. Principles for characterizing the potential human health effects from exposure to nanomaterials: elements for a screening strategy. Particle Fibre Toxicol. 2005;2:8.

[38] Borm PJA, Robbins D, Haubold S, Kuhlbusch T, Fissan H, Donaldson K, et al. The potential risk of nanomaterials: a review carried out for ECETOC. Particle Fibre Toxicol. 2006;3:11.

[39] Radomski A, Jurasz P, Alonso-Escolano D, Drews M, Morandi M, Malinski T, et al. Nanoparticle-induced platelet aggregation and vascular thrombosis. Br. J. Pharmacol. 2005;146:882.

[40] Salvador-Morales C, Flahaut E, Sim E, Sloan J, Green MLH, Sim RB. Complement activation and protein adsorption by carbon nanotubes. Mol. Immunol.2006;43:193.

[41] Cenni E, Avnet S, Granchi D, Fotia C, Salerno M, Micieli D, et al. The effect of poly(D,L-lactide-co-glycolide) nanoparticles conjugated with alendronate on human osteoclast precursors. J. Mat. Sci. Polym. Med. 2011 (in press)

[42] http://www.drugs.com/pro/doxil.html (last visit: July 2011).

[43] Andreopoulou E, Gaiotti D, Kim E, Downey A, Mirchandani D, Hamilton A, et al. Pegylated liposomal doxorubicin HCL (PLD; Caelyx/Doxil®): Experience with long-term maintenance in responding patients with recurrent epithelial ovarian cancer. Ann. Oncol. 2007;18:716-721.

[44] Salerno M, Cenni E, Fotia C, Avnet S, Granchi D, Castelli F, et al. Bone-targeted doxorubicin-loaded nanoparticles as a tool for the treatment of skeletal metastases. Curr. Cancer Drug Targets. 2010;10:649-659.

[45] Calabresi P, Chabner A. In Goodman and Gilman's the pharmacological basis of therapeutics. Goodman Gilman A, Rall TW, Nies AS, Taylor P., eds. Chemotherapy of neoplastic diseases. The McGraw-Hill Companies: New York, 1991, pp. 1202-1263.

[46] Panyam J, Zhou WZ, Prabha S, Sahoo SK, Labhasetwar V. Rapid endo-lysosomal escape of poly(D,L-lactide-co-glycolide) nanoparticles: implications for drug and gene delivery. FASEB J. 2002;16:1217-1226.

[47] Vasir JK, Labhasetwar V. Biodegradable nanoparticles for cytosolic delivery of therapeutics. Adv. Drug. Deliv. Rev. 2007;59: 718-728.

[48] Clézardin P, Ebetino FH, Fournier PGJ. Bisphosphonates and cancer-induced bone disease: beyond their antiresorptive activity. Cancer Res. 2005;65:4971-4974.

11

Transfection of Bone Cells *In Vivo* Using HA-Ceramic Particles - Histological Study

Patrick Frayssinet and Nicole Rouquet
Urodelia, Rte de St Thomas,
France

1. Introduction

The non-viral introduction of genes into mammalian cells (transfection) is of growing interest for tissue engineering and used as an alternative to viral transfer of recombinant genes. The introduction of a foreign gene into cells *in vivo* is often limited to the use of viral vectors such as adeno or retroviruses (Rochliz, C.F., 2001, Kahn, A., 2000). Viral vectors may present several disadvantages or side effects, which can be disastrous. Adenoviruses produce proteins, which can trigger immune reactions. Furthermore, the expression of a gene transduced with a viral vector is transient and can be shortened when an immune reaction occurs against the viral proteins. It must also be noted that the selection of cells, which are transduced by the virus is very poor and its efficiency is dependent on the stage the cell is in.

A number of non-viral vectors have been explored and used to date i.e. lipid-based carriers, hydrogel polymers, polycationic lipids, polylysine, polyornithine, histones and other chromosomal proteins, hydrogen polymers, precipitated calcium phosphate (Maurer, N., et al., 1999; Cullis, P.R., Chonn, A., 1998; Zauner, W., 1998; Ramsay, E., et al., 2000 ; Schwartz, B, 1999; Leong, W., 1998; Perez, C., et al., 2001; Graham, F.J. et al, 1973). Most of these vectors are usable *in vitro* but are difficult to apply *in vivo*, especially when a local transfection to a specific cell line must be achieved.

Transfection using polymer matrices i.e. gel, foams or bulk material have recently been developed to overcome these difficulties (Lauffenburger, D.A., and Schaffer, D.V., 1999). They are polycationic and are able to adsorb the negatively charged DNA molecules on their surfaces (Bonadio et al.). This concept is also extended to calcium phosphate ceramics which are widely used in human surgery as bone substitutes, cell carriers, or even thin layers at the surface of metal alloys to improve their integration by bones (Frayssinet, P., et al., 1998; Frayssinet, P., et al., 1992). The use of calcium phosphate ceramics for gene delivery presents several advantages. These matrices are biocompatible and are totally degradable by the cells of the monocyte lineage (Frayssinet, P., et al., 1994). Their behaviour in the organism is well known.

This matrix was tested in jaw bones in order to transfect bone and dental ligament cells to increase bone formation during parodontal disease. We adsorbed a plasmid DNA containing an *Escherichia coli* galactosidase gene (Lac-Z) at the surface of hydroxyapatite ceramic particles which were implanted at the junction between the incisor dental ligament and bone of rabbit jaws.

2. Materials and methods

2.1 Surgical implantation

Four white New Zealand rabbits were used for each implantation period (21 and 90 days). A pouch was created at the junction between the right incisors and the bone. 0.5 mg of HA-powder (Urodelia, St Lys, France) was introduced in the pouch using a curette. The powder was aggregated in the curette using PBS and the implanted particles were covered with a mucosal flap.

Control animals: in one animal the HA-particles were implanted without any contact with plasmid and in another one, the same amount of plasmid solution as used for particle adsorption was injected at the implantation location. The histological sections were done at 21 days and 90 days.

2.2 Particle characteristics

The hydroxylapatite particle characteristics are given in table 1.

Form :	irregularly shaped micro-particles
Colour :	White
Molecular formula :	$Ca_{10}(OH)_2(PO_4)_6$
Molecular weight :	1004.6
Solubility :	Stable at neutral and basic pH, soluble in acidic pH.
Granulometry range :	45 - 80 μm
Apparent density :	1.4 ± 0.2 g/ml
Composition	HA ≥ 97%
Ca/P :	$1.663 \le Ca/P \le 1.728$
Surface area :	0.7 m²/g
Surface potential :	- 35 mV
Surface pH :	7,8
BSA binding capacity :	> 22 mg/g
DNA binding capacity :	> 0.1 mg/ml (pCMV□ plasmid – Contech)
Dry weight/volume :	2 g/ml

Table 1. Characteristics of the implanted powder

2.3 Plasmid adsorption

10 mg of powder was soaked in 0.5 ml of a 0.1 M phosphate buffer pH 7 at 60°C for 4-8 hours. The buffer was removed and the powder was washed with new phosphate buffer. The excess buffer was removed and the powder was introduced in 1 ml of a phosphate buffer solution (0.1 M phosphate buffer pH 7) containing 25 μg of plasmid DNA (Clontech, Palo Alto, California) and incubated 2 hours at 37°C. The excess solution was then removed and the powder was dried at room temperature.

2.4 Bone histology

The jaw was fixed in a mixture ethanol/acetone (50/50 V/V) at room temperature and partially decalcified in a 4% solution of diNa-EDTA for 6 days. The jaw fragments were then embedded inside hydroxyl-ethylmethacrylate. 5 μm thick sections were then performed using a microtome for calcified tissues (Reicher-Jung type K). The galactosidase activity was evidenced using a X-gal solution at 37°C for two hours (100 mM sodium phosphate pH 7.3, 1.3 mM $MgCl_2$, 3 mM $K_3Fe(CN)_6$, 3mM $K_4Fe(CN)_6$ and 1mg/ml X-Gal). The sections were observed under a light microscope, and then counterstained by a Giemsa solution. The cells expressing the LacZ gene were stained in blue. The sections were done through the implanted particles and the same zone in the controlateral region.

3. Results

Macroscopically, the particles can be seen at the basis of the incisors at the first implantation time and they were stained in blue (fig. 1).

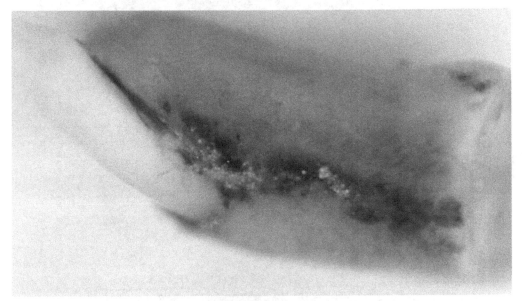

Fig. 1. Photograph of the implantation site at 21 days. The particles were visible at the junction between the incisor and the bone. The particles are stained in blue indicating that the cells having ingrown the material express the Lac-Z gene.

At 21 days, the particles were surrounded by a mild foreign body reaction constituted by mono and plurinucleated cells (fig. 2). These cells contained fragments of calcium phosphate ceramics.

The monocytes and multinucleated cells located around the particles were stained in blue (fig. 3). In the controlateral site, blue stained cells were dispersed in the stromal tissue evidenced in the bone pores. They were circulating cells such as monocytes and multinucleated cells (fig. 4). These late cells were often evidenced at the bone surface and sometimes in Howship's lacunae (fig. 4).

Some other cells expressing the galactosidase gene were found inside stromal tissue and showed a fibroblastic aspect (fig. 5). Some of these cells were identified as pericytes as they were evidenced in the immediate proximity to the capillaries.

Blue stained cells were also evidenced in the dental ligament (fig. 6). Some of them have the morphology of circulating cells as others are ligament fibroblasts.

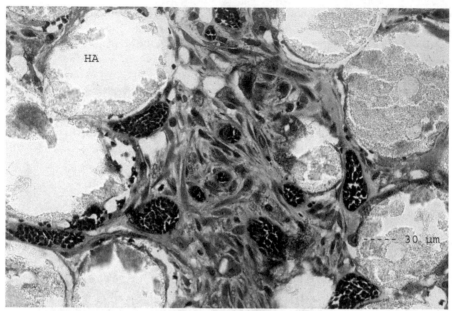

Fig. 2. Microphotograph of the implantation zone at 21 days showing that at an early implantation time, the microparticles (HA) were embedded in a mild foreign body reaction made of monocytes and multinucleated cells. Giemsa staining.

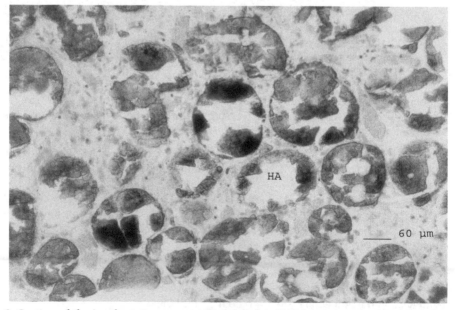

Fig. 3. Section of the implantation zone at 21 days after X-Gal staining showing that almost all the foreign body reaction cells were stained in blue. X-Gal and neutral red staining.

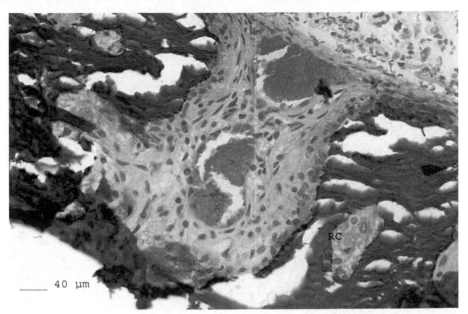

Fig. 4. Section of bone at remote distance from the implantation zone at 21 days. There were monocytes stained in blue in the pores of the bone tissue. Cells expressing the galactosidase gene were evidenced in Howship's lacunae or resorption cavities (RC). X-Gal and neutral red staining.

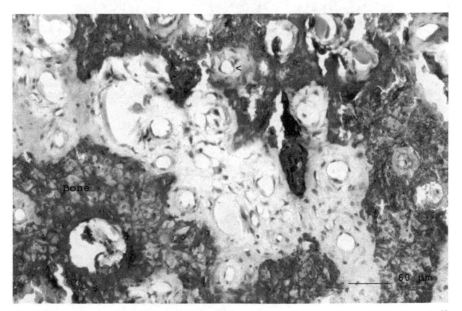

Fig. 5. At 21 days, the bone stromal tissue contained blue stained cells which were stellar shaped. Some of these cells were perivascular (<). X-Gal and neutral red staining.

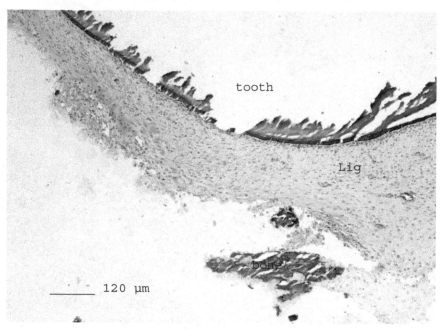

Fig. 6. At 21 days, section of the dental ligament (lig) of the implanted incisor. Some ligament cells were stained in blue. X-Gal and neutral red staining

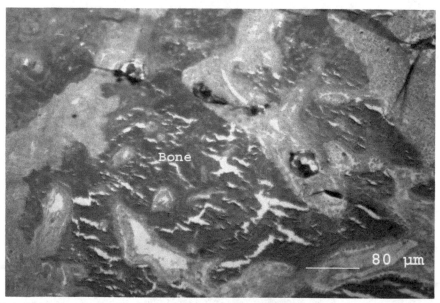

Fig. 7. At 3 months after implantation, the histological sections showed that the HA-particles (grey) were dispersed and integrated in the bone tissue without sign of foreign body reaction. Giemsa staining.

At 90 days (fig. 7), the particles were degrading and some of them were integrated inside bone trabeculae.

There were almost no circulating cells around the microparticles. The cells expressing the lac-Z gene were dispersed in the connective tissue. Some other cells showed a blue staining. Odontoblasts and fibroblasts were among these cells (fig. 8). The percentage of the labelled cells was low.

Sections of the control animals did not show any staining at any time.

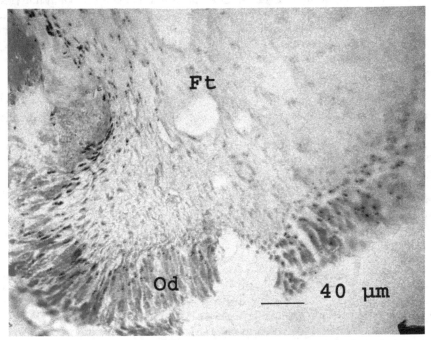

Fig. 8. Histological section of the incisor connective tissue of a three month implanted site. There were still some cells like odontoblasts showing a galactosidase gene expression. Numerous other cells mainly fibroblasts were also expressing the gene. X-Gal staining.

4. Discussion

This experiment showed that a transient transfection can be obtained using calcium phosphate ceramics with some level of specificity limited to the cells being in contact with the ceramic or located to its proximity. This "geo-specificity" allows to transfect the circulating cells i.e. monocytes, macrophages, multinucleated cells which are the first cells to come in contact with the material.

The transfection does not seem to interfere with the differentiation of the cells, as the monocytes transfected at the ceramic contact are found in Howship's lacunae and identified as osteoclasts. Furthermore, they are also found in various locations of bone indicating that the cells of the foreign body reaction are still able to circulate and differentiate from macrophages into osteoclasts. Thus, it indicates that contact with the ceramic and the phagocytosis of the ceramic particles would not impair the migration of cells toward the lymph node and their role of antigen presenting cells. It is also indicated that the degradation of the ceramic does not release toxic particles or products responsible for a cell death or apoptosis in the site of implantation.

The cell transfection with calcium phosphate/DNA coprecipitates has been used for decades *in vitro* (Schenborn, E.T., and Goiffon, V., 2000), it is almost impossible to obtain *in vivo* in an open medium. The use of nanoparticles which are already precipitated are also difficult to use *in vivo* because it is not possible to maintain them in a particular location.

It has been reported that a direct injection of a plasmid suspension in rodent muscles could trigger a significant transfection of the muscle cells (Danko, I., et al., 1997). However, it is not known what are the other cells transfected and what is the transfection kinetic and yield. It is also difficult to ensure any specificity of the transfected cells by this way. In this study, plasmid injection did not bring a significant transfection in the injection site, probably because the injected solution did not stay in the site.

Macrophages have the reputation of being difficult to transfect. This material can thus be of interest to target these cells. During the first time, only the circulating cells are labelled, while at three months, some other cells could be evidenced such as odontoblasts or fibroblasts of the connective tissue.

The mechanism of transfection is not clear and cannot totally be dissociated from that of the co-precipitate. Furthermore, the degradation of the ceramic takes place at the grain boundaries of the ceramic particles. A release of particle grains occurs in the proximity of the implantation zone explaining the localisation of the transfected cells (Frayssinet, P., and Guilhem, A., 2004; Frayssinet, P., et al., 2006).

The material degradation leads to the release of several particle sizes and shapes depending on the degradation stage. The ceramic grains after the dissolution of the grain boundaries, can be released alone or aggregated. At this stage, they are micronic in size. Then the particles are degraded inside the low pH compartments of the cells and their size decreases and they become nanosized (Frayssinet, P., et al., 1999; Jallot, E., et al., 1999). During this time, the shape becomes round with a disappearance of the particle angles. The dissolution/precipitation process occurring at the particle surface is very complex as there is a carbonated apatite epitaxial growth at neutral pH and finally a dissolution at low pH.

The physical interaction with between the HA and the hydroxylapatite chemically stabilizes the DNA molecules increasing the denaturation temperature (Martinoson, H.G., 1978). This stabilization can partly explain the transfection mechanism as the complex DNA/calcium phosphate could impair or slow the DNA destruction in the cytoplasm (Orrantia, E., Chang, P.L., 1990).

The adsorption mechanism at the HA surface is not clear. The DNA molecule is negatively charged as is the ceramic surface. Thus the adsorption is not driven by electrostatic forces. The surface modifications occurring during the culture or implantation make it difficult for the elucidation of the adsorption mechanism.

These results have to be compared to those obtained *in vitro* with isolated cells or tissue culture. It was shown that the percentage of transfected cells was time dependent and could be very high after a few days of contact. It was also shown that, regarding bone tissue, all the cell types could be transfected by this way.

5. Conclusions

Hydroxyapatite ceramics have numerous applications relating to the field of human and animal health. Their surface properties can explain the molecule adsorption and the ability of these materials for transient cell transfection both *in vitro* and *in vivo*. Applications for cell transfection could be numerous as the material is safe, degradable, and shows a good transfection yield. Furthermore, this material demonstrates interesting properties allowing to target antigen presenting cells. These cells can show some deficiencies in their role of antigen presentation which is essential in very different pathology such as cancers, infectiology or autoimmune diseases. It could be particularly appropriate as a DNA vaccine vector in order to bring the antigen presenting cells the properties they would need to overcome the immune evasion strategies of cancer cells.

6. References

Bonadio, J., Smiley, E., Patil, S., Goldstein. S., (1999) , Localized, direct plasmid gene delivery *in vivo*: prolonged therapy results in reproducible tissue regeneration. Nature Medicine 5 (7):753-759.

Cullis, P.R., Chonn, A. (1998) Recent advances in liposome technologies and their applications for systemic gene delivery. Adv Drug Deliv Rev, 30: 73-83

Danko,I., Williams, P., Herweijer, H., Zhang, G., Latendresse, J.S., Bock, I., Wolff, J.A., (1997) High expression of naked plasmid DNA in muscles of young rodents. Human Molecular Genetics 6 (9):1435-1443.

Frayssinet,P., Fages, J., Bonel,G., Rouquet,N., (1998) Biotechnology, material sciences and bone repair. European Journal of Orthopaedic Surgery & Traumatology 8: 17-25.

Frayssinet, P., Guilhem, A., (2004) Cell transfection using HA-ceramics. Bioprocessing Journal, 3, 4

Frayssinet, P., Hardy, D., Rouquet, N., Giammara, B., Guilhem, A., Hanker, J.S., (1992) New observations on middle term hydroxylapatite-coated titanium alloy hip prostheses. Biomaterials , 13, 10: 668-673.

Frayssinet, P., Rouquet, N., Mathon, D., (2006) Bone cell transfection in tissue culture using hydroxyapatite microparticles. Journal of Biomedical Material Research. 79: 225-8

Frayssinet, P., Rouquet, N., Tourenne, F., Fages, J., Bonel, G. (1994) *In vivo* degradation of calcium phosphate ceramics.Cells and materials 4: 383-394.

Frayssinet, P., Schwartz, C., Beya, B., Lecestre, P., (1999) Biology of the calcium phosphate integration in human long bones. European Journal of Orthopaedic Surgery & Traumatology 9: 167-170

Graham, F.L., van der Eb, A.J., A new technique for the assay of infectivity of human adenovirus 5 DNA. 1973, Virology 52, 456-467.

Jallot, E., Irigaray,J.L., Oudadesse, H., Brun,V., Weber,G., Frayssinet,P. (1999) Resorption kinetics of four hydroxyapatite-based ceramics by particle induced X-ray emission and neutron activation analysis. The European Physical Journal-Applied Physics 6, 205-215.

Kahn, A., (2000) Dix ans de thérapie génique: déceptions et espoirs. Biofutur 202:16-21

Lauffenburger, D.A., Schaffer, D.V., (1999). The matrix delivers. Nature Medicine 7 (5):733-734

Leong, W. (1998) DNA-polycation nanospheres as non-viral gene delivery vehicles. J Contr Rel 53: 183-193

Martinoson, H.G., (1973) The nucleic acid-hydroxyapatite interaction. I. Stabilization of native double-stranded deoxyribonucleic acid by hydroxylapatite. Biochemistry, 12, 139-143

Maurer, N., Mori, A., Palmer, L., Monck, M.A., Mok, K.W., Mui, B., Akhong, Q.F., Cullis, P.R., (1999) Lipid-based systems for the intracellular delivery of genetic drugs. Mol Membr Biol 16, 129-140

Orrantia, E., Chang, P.L., (1990). Intracellular distribution of DNA internalized through calcium phosphate precipitation. Experimental Cell Research 190 (2):170-174.

Perez, C., Sanchez, A., Putnam, D., Ting, D., Langer, R., Alonso, M.J. , (2001) Poly(lactic acid)-poly(ethylene glycol) nanoparticles as new carriers for the delivery of plasmid DNA. J Contr Rel 75: 211-224

Ramsay, E., Headgraft, J., Birchall, J., Gumbleton, M., (2000). Examination of the biophysical interaction between plasmid DNA and the polycations, polylysine, and polyornithine, as a basis for their differential gene transfection *in vitro*. Int J Pharm 210: 97-107

Rochliz C. F. (2001) Gene therapy of cancer. Swiss Med Wkly 131:4-9,.

Schenborn, E.T., Goiffon, V., (2000) Calcium phosphate transfection of mammalian cultured cells. Tymms, M.J.,Totowa NJ, (eds) Humana Press Inc, p. 135-144.

Schwartz, B., (1999) Synthetic DNA-compacting peptides derived from human sequence enhanced cationic lipid-mediated gene transfer *in vitro* and *in vivo*. Gene Ther 6, 282-292

Zauner, W., Ogris, M., Wagner, E., (1998). Polylysine-based transfection system using receptor-mediated delivery. Adv Drug Del Rev 30: 97-113

12

Magnetite Nanoparticles for Cell Lysis Implanted Into Bone - Histological and TEM Study

Patrick Frayssinet[1], Didier Mathon[2],
Marylène Combacau[1] and Nicole Rouquet[1]
[1]*Urodelia, Rte de St Thomas, St Lys,*
[2]*Ecole Nationale Vétérinaire, Toulouse,*
France

1. Introduction

Magnetite nanoparticles are frequently used to eliminate by heating in a high frequence oscillating magnetic field the tumor cells into which they are introduced in order to directly kill the cells or to make them more sensitive to radiotherapy (Ito, A., et al., 2005; Jordan, A., et al., 2001).

The appearance of bone metastases is a sign of a dissemination of primitive cancers. They rapidly become resistant to chemotherapy and radiotherapy and are often very painful necessitating local and/or alternative treatments in order to reduce the osteolysis triggered by the cancerous cells. The osteolysis is due to local activation of the osteoclasts and macrophages by factors synthesized by the tumor cells (Shimamura, T., et al., 2005). It is the osteolysis that is very often responsible for the pain.

We have developed a biomaterial containing magnetite nanoparticles which can be introduced into bone metastases in order to release naked nanoparticles in the contact with both the cancerous and the osteolytic cells. The material is made of a calcium sulphate paste containing a small percentage of nanoparticles which can be injected inside the metastasis (fig. 1). It sets within a few minutes *in situ*. The degradation of the calcium sulphate matrix within a few days releases the nanoparticles which are then available for cell internalisation. *In vitro*, these particles can be internalised in high amounts by metastatic cells from adenocarcinoma. The number of nanoparticles found inside the cells depends on the nanoparticle size, however the mass internalized seems to be almost independent of their size (Frayssinet, P., et al., 2005).

The nanoparticles did not show *in vitro* any signs of cell toxicity. This is consistent with previous reports which showed that cytotoxicity of magnetite nanoparticles could be due to several factors such as coating (Häfeli & Pauer, 1999). Furthermore, they are intented for use in very low doses (a few mgs). The degradation products of iron oxide are well known. They do not have a reported toxicity and are easily eliminated from the organism (Schoepf, U., et al. 1998, Okon, E.E., et al. 2000, Okon, F., et al. 1994).

Migration of the nanoparticles can however be a cause of concern due to the possible unwanted heating of other regions of the organism when submitted to a magnetic field.

When injected as a suspension in the blood, they were shown to be mostly taken up by the spleen and liver in the days following injection (Magin, R.L. et al., 1991). They can also migrate into the lymph nodes when directly injected into tissues.

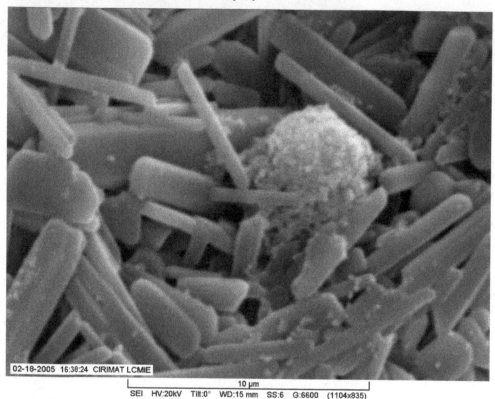

Fig. 1. SEM of calcium sulphate (flat crystals) matrix containing nanoparticles of magnetite. Isolated nanoparticles can be evidenced at the surface of the calcium sulphate crystals or as agregates between the crystals.

We have demonstrated that the nanoparticles used in this device penetrate adenocarcinoma cells by endocytosis *in vitro* (Frayssinet et al. 2004). The aim of this experiment was to check the uptake of these nanoparticles by the various types of bone tissue cells *in vivo*, their migration in the lymphatic tissue and the time *needed* for their *elimination*.

Thus, the nanoparticles were introduced through a bone defect drilled into the cancellous bone while the implantation zone and lymph nodes draining the region were examined by light and transmission electron microscopy.

2. Materials and methods

2.1 animal model

In order not to lose the nanoparticles, they were placed inside an open titanium alloy chamber implanted inside the cancellous bone of external condyles in the sheep. A titanium alloy was used because it was demonstrated that there was no or a very limited foreign body reaction against this kind of alloy and device implanted inside the bone (Aspenberg et al., 1996). The chamber in which the particles were inserted was tunnel shaped and open at the ends communicating with the bone allowing tissue at all stages of bone regeneration to cross the tunnel and come in contact with the nanoparticles . Using this device it is straight forward to locate the nanoparticles for histological and TEM sections.

The device containing the chamber can be screwed into the cancellous bone to avoid any micromovement between the bone and the chamber which would shear the regenerating tissue. It can also be opened to facilitate the collection of the tissue to analyse (fig. 2).

Two sheep were used for each sample implanted for a 3 weeks. 0.1 mg of sterile nanoparticles were placed inside the chambers which were then implanted in the external condyle by a lateral approach.

After the three-week exposure the animals were killed by a Nembutal injection and the chambers the inguinal and aortic lymph nodes draining the implantation zone retrieved. The operation and the care of the animals followed the European commission guidelines concerning animal experimentation.

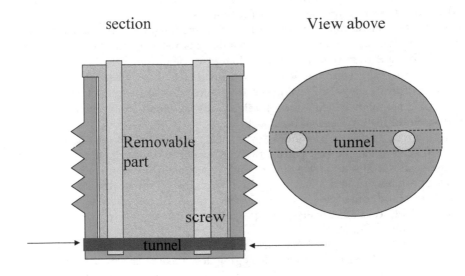

section   View above

Removable part

screw

tunnel

tunnel

Fig. 2. The titanium device containing the tunnel in which the nanoparticles were introduced was screwed in the cancellous bone of the condyles. The healing tissue ingrews the tunnel according to the arrows. After the implantation period, the removable part was extracted to open the tunnel and the tissue containing the nanoparticles was available for histology.

2.2 Magnetite powder characteristics

The powders were constituted by Fe_3O_4 (99%). Their shape was polyhedral. Three different particle size groups were used: 70 nm, 150 nm, 500nm.

2.3 Histological methods

The retrieved tissues were immediately immersed in isotonic phosphate buffer containing 2% glutaraldehyde for 2 days at 4°C. All the samples were then cut and either processed for light microscopy or TEM.

For light microscopy, the samples were dehydrated in increasingly concentrated ethanol solutions and embedded in hydroxyethyl methacrylate. 5 µm thick sections were cut and coloured with Perl's stain to reveal the nanoparticles in the sections. The tartrate resistant acid phosphatase activity (TRAP) of the cells was evidenced using a commercial leukocyte acid phosphatase kit (Sigma, St Louis, MO).

For TEM, the sections were dehydrated in increasingly concentrated ethanol solution and embedded in an epoxy polymer before ultrathin sections were performed and stained with uranyl acetate. Observations were made at 20 kV.

3. Results

3.1 Bone healing in the titanium tunnels

After the three-week experimental period, the tunnel was filled by loose connective tissue which did not show any signs of ossification.

Under light microscopy, the tissue in the tunnels showed that numerous cells contained nanoparticles. Some of the cells showed a black tattoo while in others the nanoparticles were not visible but were revealed by the blue-grey color of the cell after Perl's staining (fig. 3). The nanoparticles were either contained inside TRAP+ or TRAP- cells. These TRAP+ cells were uniformly dispersed inside the tunnel volume and were not aggregated around the foreign material as is usual for a foreign body reaction (fig. 4). The tissue appearance was the same for the three size of nanoparticles.

Under TEM, all tissues present in the tunnels contained cells loaded with the nanoparticles. It seemed that the smallest particles (70nm) penetrated the cells in larger numbers than the biggest ones (500 nm); at least their density was more uniform inside the cells. The 500 nm sized particles formed smaller aggregates in the cells than the 70 nm ones. These late particles could constitute large aggregates at the contact of which multinucleated cells were found. The cells dissociated or fragmented the aggregates before internalising the nanoparticules (fig. 5).

Inside the cells, the nanoparticles were found inside lysosomes, or phagolysosomes depending on the size of the particle aggregates. There were almost no particles alone inside cell vesicles (fig. 6). They occurred in groups of a few units to several dozen.

3.2 Lymph nodes

Using light microscopy, it appeared in most sections that nanoparticles had migrated to the lymph nodes after the three-week contact. Their number was very low, as only a few cells on each section were blue from Perl's stain. The nanoparticles were not found in the lymphoid follicles but in the capsule and subcapsular sinus. The migration was identical for the three types of nanoparticles.

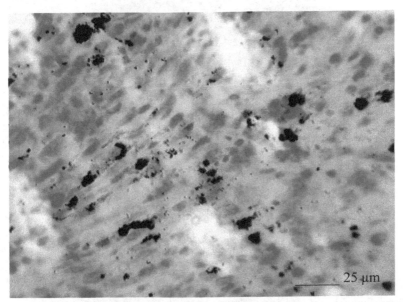

Fig. 3. The particles (70 nm) under light microscopy appear uniformly dispersed in the ingrown tissue in the titanium chambers. They can form aggregates inside the cells which are visible under the microscope or with Perl'staining a kind of blue grey tattoo

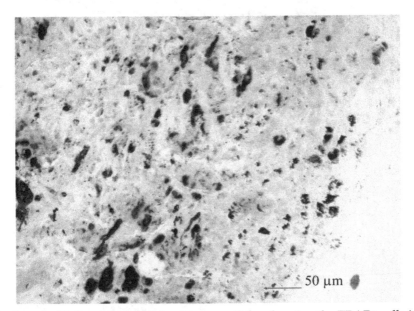

Fig. 4. Section of a Ti chamber containing 70 nm particles showing the TRAP+ cells in red. The particles are not necessarily internalised within the TRAP+ cells.

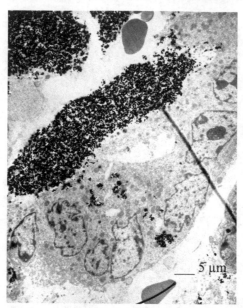

Fig. 5. When aggregates of 70 nm sized nanoparticles are formed, there can be multinucleated cells in contact with the material. The aggregate is dissociated by the cells which internalize the nanoparticles under the form of much smaller groups of particles.

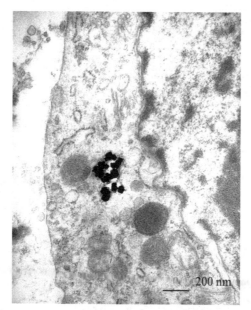

Fig. 6. Inside the cells the magnetite particles are found inside cell vesicles such as endosomes, lysosomes or phago- lysosomes.

By TEM, the nanoparticles were observed in the vesicles of macrophages and lymphocytes (fig. 7, 8,9, 10). All the particles seen in the lymph nodes showed one or several degradation signs. Nanoparticles of all three sizes were found in the lymph nodes, however in very low number.

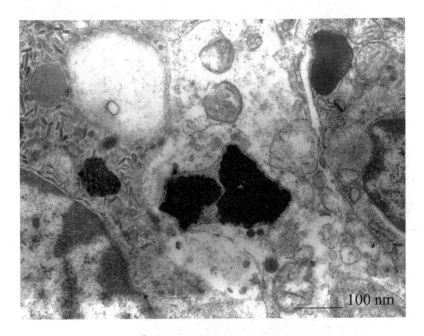

Fig. 7. TEM of 70 nm particles observed inside the lysosome of a lymph node macrophage. The particles show fuzzy edges, a modified shape and some have merged.

3.3 Degradation

Signs of nanoparticle degradation were evidenced both in the bone tissue and the lymph nodes (fig. 7, 8, 9, 10). The degradation took place in the cell vesicles. The big particles were sometimes fragmented. The small ones became fuzzy and lost their shape suggesting that material had dissolved. Very fine and needle like particles were sometimes observed in the periphery of the nanoparticles suggesting precipitation. Most of the particles, whatever their size, showed a modification of the shape and some particles fused together.

4. Discussion

Direct implantation of magnetite nanoparticles into the tumor instead of injection into bloodstream avoids their concentration inside liver, lung or spleen. It allows the use of lower doses of magnetite limiting its toxicity, if any, and side effects such as heating of the reticulo endothelial cells in these organs.

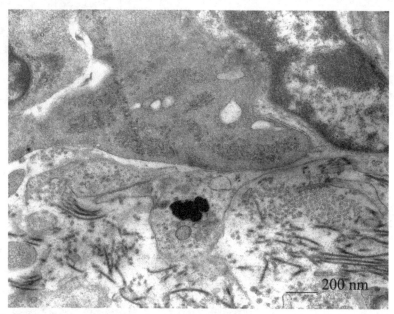

Fig. 8. TEM of 70 nm nanoparticles showing a precipitate formed in the lysosome around the nanoparticles.

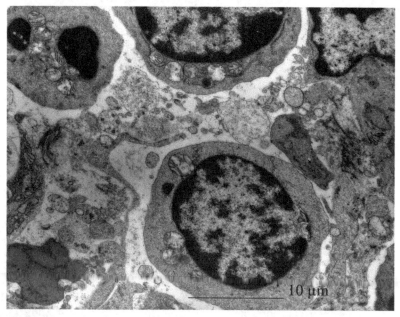

Fig. 9. 70 nm nanoparticles showing degradation signs in vesicles located inside a lymphocyte from a lymph node.

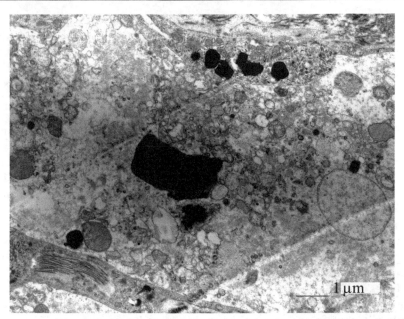

Fig. 10. 500 nm sized particles inside the vesicles of a cell going into apoptosis inside a lymph node. The nanoparticles have lost their shape and show a core surrounded by a fuzzy zone.

This experimentation shows that when implanted into bones the magnetite nanoparticles can migrate within the cells having internalised them. At this time however, the nanoparticles did not seem to be present in sufficient amounts to induce secondary heating as only a few particles appeared in each section of the lymph nodes.

The particles were found inside lysosomes or phagolysosomes. The physico-chemical environment in these vesicles is very aggressive with a low pH and many hydrolytic enzymes (Dell'Angelica et al., 2001). These conditions could explain the degradation of the material which was seen to occur in some of them. It must be noted that magnetite degradation at a low pH has already been demonstrated (Florindo et al., 2003, Gruendle et al., 2002). The rate depends on the pH and the type of acid present.

It is not clear how the endocytosis takes place. There is no indication of specific endocytosis. The amount of nanoparticles endocytosed by non- transformed cells is lower than the amount endocytosed by cancer cells. It is suggested that fast dividing cells show a large particle uptake (Jordan et al., 1999). This means that, in this case, the cells of the regenerating tissue would internalise fewer nanoparticles than bone metastasis cells.

From the TEM pictures it seemed that, when the nanoparticles formed aggregates in the implantation zone, isolated nanoparticles or small groups were able to penetrate inside the cells in contact with the aggregates. This suggests that the cells are able to separate the nanoparticles which are internalized from the aggregates.

There was no true foreign body reaction against this material even when large aggregates formed as TRAP+ cells were uniformly dispersed in the tunnel volume and not aggregated in contact with the material. Furthermore, the internalisation of the particles was not limited to the TRAP+ cells which are known to be among professional macrophages. This suggests that in bone metastasis these particles can potentially penetrate both the cancer cells and the cells of the monocyte lineage involved in osteolysis.

After three weeks of implantation, the healing tissue was similar to that occurring when there are no particles (Frayssinet, unpublished results). This result must be compared to *in vitro* experiments showing that when grown with a primary line of monocytes the small particles do not trigger the synthesis of cytokines or TGF and so do not activate these cells (Frayssinet, unpublished results) suggesting that the cells do not recognize the magnetite nanoparticle having this range of size as a foreign body.

Breakdown of iron oxides in the organism can form several kinds of degradation products: fragments of the material; salts such as iron chloride or hydroxide; complexes of the salts with organic molecules (Michel, A., Bénard, J., 1964). It was demonstrated that the iron released from magnetite can be incorporated into haemoglobin, erythrocytes or feritin (Weissleder et al., 1989). It is important to know the degradation rate of these nanoparticles and the location of the degradation because the degradation products show altered magnetic properties. Thus, knowing the migration and degradation rates of the material will help avoid heating unwanted zones.

All three types of particles tested migrated from the bone into the lymph nodes, however, the proportion of particles found in the lymph nodes was very low and the percentage of the lymph node cells containing nanoparticles was also very low.

It must also be pointed out that the nanoparticles were not found only in the macrophages of the lymph nodes but also in the lymphocytes.

This has direct consequences on the functionality of the biomaterials using iron oxide as seen to heat tissues under oscillating magnetic fields. The heating ability (SAR) of the nanoparticles decreases within weeks after implantation. Thus, the heating protocol must be performed in a window of time to be specified.

It is also probable that the material does not persist in the organism for a very long time. However, as long as a magnetic core persists in the particles it is possible to follow the migration of the cells containing the particles by MRI; It could be very useful to follow the migration of metastatic cells before they can form a visible tumor by MRI.

5. Conclusions

Magnetite nanoparticles can easily penetrate the cells with which they are in contact whether or not they are professional phagocytes. This property is particularly useful and is the essential rationale for injecting a medical device releasing iron oxide nanoparticles inside a bone metastasis. The aggregation of the magnetic nanoparticles outside the cells does not seem to impair their endo or phagocytosis inside the cells as isolated nanoparticles.

Magnetite nanoparticles able to be used for heating bone tumors can migrate with the cells in which they are internalised. They are degradable in the cell vesicles indicating that they will lose their magnetic properties in a few weeks to months depending on the structural modifications they undergo during their migration through the different cell compartments and the different cells of the site. During this time, their heating properties will decrease but as long as they have some magnetic properties they will be able to serve as a probe to follow the cells migrating from the tumor.

6. References

Aspenberg, P., Tägil, M., Kristensson, C., Lidin, S., (1996) Bone graft proteins influence osteoconduction : A titanium chamber study in rats, Acta orthopaedica Scandinavica, 67: 377-382

Dell'Angelica, E.C., Mullins, C., Caplan, S., Bonifacino, J.S., (2001) Lysosome-related organelles. FASEB J, 14: 1265-78

Florindo, F., Roberts, A.P., Palmer, M.R., Magnetite dissolution in siliceous sediments, (2003) Geochem Geophys Geosyst, 7: 1053

Frayssinet, P., Combacau, M., Gougeon, M., Mathon, D., RouquetN., (2005) Migration and degradation of magnetite nanoparticles in lymph nodes. Society for Thermal Medicine. Annual Meeting, Bethesda. Maryland.

Frayssinet, P., Goujeon, M., Lebugle, A., Boetto, S., Rousset, A., Rouquet, N., (2004) Magnetite nanoparticles for thermal therapy. Influence of the particle size for their uptake in cells of breast carcinoma metastasis. 9th International Congress on Hyperthermic Oncology. April 20-24, 2004, St Louis, Missouri, USA

Gruendle, K.V., Noll, M.R., Magnetite dissolution rates in acidic solutions, The Geological Society of America 2002 Annual Meeting, Denver Colorado, October 2002

Häfeli, U.O., Pauer, G.J., In vitro and in vivo toxicity of magnetic microspheres. Journal of Magnetism and Magnetic Materials, 1999, 194: 76-82.

Ito, A., Shinkai, M., Honda, H., Kobayashi, T., (2005) Medical application of functionalized magnetic nanoparticles, Journal of Bioscience and Bioengineering, 100: 1-11

Jordan, A., Scholz, R., Maier-Hauff, K., Johansen, M., Wust, P., Nadobny, J., Schirra, H., Schmidt, H., Deger, S., Loening, S., Lanksch, W., Felix, R.,(2001) Presentation of a new magnetic field therapy system for the treatment of human solid tumors with magnetic fluid hyperthermia. Journal of Magnetism and Magnetic Materials, 225: 118-126

Jordan, A., Scholz, R., Wust, P., Schirra, H., Schiestel, T., Schmidt, H., Felix, R., (1999) Endocytosis of dextran and silan-coated magnetite nanoparticles and the effect of intracellular hyperthermia on human mammary carcinoma cells in vitro. Journal of Magnetism and Magnetic Materials, 194: 185-196.

Magin, R.L., Bacic, G., Niesman, R.L., Alameda, J.C., Wright, S.M., Swartz, S.W., (1991). Dextran magnetite as a liver contrast agent. Magnetic Resonance in Medicine, 20: 1-16.

Michel, A., Bénard, J., in: Chimie Minérale. Généralités et Etude Particulière des Eléments. Masson et Cie eds. Paris 1964 : 646-49

Okon, F., Pouliquen, D., Okon, F., Kovaleva, Z.V., Stepanova, T.P., Lavit, S.G., Kudryavtsev, B.N., Jallet, P., Biodegradation of magnetite dextran nanoparticles in the rat. A histologic and biophysical study, Lab Invest, 1994, 71: 895-903.

Okon, E.E., Pulikan, D., Pereverzev, A.E., Kudriavtsev, B.N., Zhale, P., Toxicity of magnetite-dextran particles: morphological study. Tsitologia, 2000, 42: 358-366

Schoepf, U., Marecos, E.M., Melder, R.J., Jain, R.K., Weissleder, R., Intracellular magnetic labelling of lymphocytes for in vivo trafficking studies, Biotechniques, 1998, 24 : 642-646.

Shimamura, T., Amizuka, N., Li, M., Freitas, P.H.L., White, J.H., Henderson, J.E., Shingaki, S., Nakajima, T., (2005) histological observations on the microenvironment of osteolytic bone metastasis by breast carcinoma cell line. Biomedical Research, 26, 159-172

Weissleder, R., Stark, D.D., Engelstad, B.L., Bacon, B.R., Compton, C.C., White, D.L., Jacobs, P., Lewis, J., (1989) Superparamagnatic iron oxide: pharmacokinetics and toxicity. AJR, 152: 167-173

Permissions

The contributors of this book come from diverse backgrounds, making this book a truly international effort. This book will bring forth new frontiers with its revolutionizing research information and detailed analysis of the nascent developments around the world.

We would like to thank Prof. Rosario Pignatello, for lending his expertise to make the book truly unique. He has played a crucial role in the development of this book. Without his invaluable contribution this book wouldn't have been possible. He has made vital efforts to compile up to date information on the varied aspects of this subject to make this book a valuable addition to the collection of many professionals and students.

This book was conceptualized with the vision of imparting up-to-date information and advanced data in this field. To ensure the same, a matchless editorial board was set up. Every individual on the board went through rigorous rounds of assessment to prove their worth. After which they invested a large part of their time researching and compiling the most relevant data for our readers. Conferences and sessions were held from time to time between the editorial board and the contributing authors to present the data in the most comprehensible form. The editorial team has worked tirelessly to provide valuable and valid information to help people across the globe.

Every chapter published in this book has been scrutinized by our experts. Their significance has been extensively debated. The topics covered herein carry significant findings which will fuel the growth of the discipline. They may even be implemented as practical applications or may be referred to as a beginning point for another development. Chapters in this book were first published by InTech; hereby published with permission under the Creative Commons Attribution License or equivalent.

The editorial board has been involved in producing this book since its inception. They have spent rigorous hours researching and exploring the diverse topics which have resulted in the successful publishing of this book. They have passed on their knowledge of decades through this book. To expedite this challenging task, the publisher supported the team at every step. A small team of assistant editors was also appointed to further simplify the editing procedure and attain best results for the readers.

Our editorial team has been hand-picked from every corner of the world. Their multi-ethnicity adds dynamic inputs to the discussions which result in innovative outcomes. These outcomes are then further discussed with the researchers and contributors who give their valuable feedback and opinion regarding the same. The feedback is then collaborated with the researches and they are edited in a comprehensive manner to aid the understanding of the subject.

Apart from the editorial board, the designing team has also invested a significant amount of their time in understanding the subject and creating the most relevant covers. They scrutinized every image to scout for the most suitable representation of the subject and create an appropriate cover for the book.

The publishing team has been involved in this book since its early stages. They were actively engaged in every process, be it collecting the data, connecting with the contributors or procuring relevant information. The team has been an ardent support to the editorial, designing and production team. Their endless efforts to recruit the best for this project, has resulted in the accomplishment of this book. They are a veteran in the field of academics and their pool of knowledge is as vast as their experience in printing. Their expertise and guidance has proved useful at every step. Their uncompromising quality standards have made this book an exceptional effort. Their encouragement from time to time has been an inspiration for everyone.

The publisher and the editorial board hope that this book will prove to be a valuable piece of knowledge for researchers, students, practitioners and scholars across the globe.

List of Contributors

Selestina Gorgieva
University of Maribor, Institute for Engineering Materials and Design, Maribor, Slovenia

Vanja Kokol
University of Maribor, Institute for Engineering Materials and Design, Maribor, Center of Excellence NAMASTE, Ljubljana, Slovenia

Sayed Mahmood Rabiee
Babol University of Technology, Iran

Miroslav Petrtyl, Jaroslav Lisal and Jana Danesova
Laboratory of Biomechanics and Biomaterial Engineering, Department of Mechanics, Faculty of Civil Engineering, Czech Technical University in Prague, Czech Republic

Ladislav Senolt, Marketa Polanska and Hana Hulejova
Institute of Rheumatology, The First Faculty of Medicine, Charles University in Prague, Czech Republic

Zdenek Bastl
J. Heyrovsky Institute of Physical Chemistry, Academy of Sciences of the Czech Republic, Czech Republic

Zdenek Krulis
Institute of Macromolecular Chemistry, Academy of Sciences of the Czech Republic, Czech Republic

Pavel Cerny
ORTOTIKA, s.r.o., Prague, Czech Republic

Samit Kumar Nandi
Department of Veterinary Surgery and Radiology, West Bengal University of Animal and Fishery Sciences, Kolkata, India

Biswanath Kundu and Someswar Datta
Bioceramics and Coating Division, Central Glass and Ceramic Research Institute, Kolkata, India

Uwe Walschus, Jürgen Meichsner, Rainer Hippler and Michael Schlosser
University of Greifswald, Greifswald, Germany

Karsten Schröder and Birgit Finke
Leibniz Institute for Plasma Science and Technology, Greifswald, Germany

Barbara Nebe, Rainer Bader and Andreas Podbielski
University of Rostock, Rostock, Germany

Linying Cui
Department of Physics, Tsinghua University, Beijing, China

Fei Liu and Zhong-can Ou-Yang
Center for Advanced Study, Tsinghua University, Beijing, China

Ying-Chieh Chen
Institute of Cellular and System Medicine, National Health Research Institutes, Miaoli, Taiwan, Center for Biomedical Engineering, Department of Medicine, Brigham and Women's Hospital, Harvard Medical School, Boston, USA

Don-Ching Lee
Institute of Cellular and System Medicine, National Health Research Institutes, Miaoli, Taiwan

Ing-Ming Chiu
Institute of Cellular and System Medicine, National Health Research Institutes, Miaoli, Department of Life Sciences, National Chung Hsing University, Taichung, Taiwan, Department of Internal Medicine, The Ohio State University, Columbus, USA

Jia-Chang Yue, Pei-RongWang and Xu Zhang
Institute of Biophysics, Chinese Academy of Sciences, China

Yao-Gen Shu
Institute of Theoretical Physics, Chinese Academy of Sciences, China

G. Amador Del Valle, H. Gautier, A. Gaudin, V. Le Mabecque, A.F. Miegeville, J.M. Bouler, J. Caillon, P. Weiss, G. Potel and C. Jacqueline
University of Nantes, Teaching Hospital of Nantes, France

Rosario Pignatello
Department of Pharmaceutical Sciences Faculty of Pharmacy, University of Catania, Italy

Patrick Frayssinet and Nicole Rouquet
Urodelia, Rte de St Thomas, France

Patrick Frayssinet, Marylène Combacau and Nicole Rouquet
Urodelia, Rte de St Thomas, St Lys, France

Didier Mathon
Ecole Nationale Vétérinaire, Toulouse, France